Problems in Anaesthesia
Paediatric Anaesthesia

Dedication

We would like to dedicate this book to our spouses Helen and Simon
and to our children Michael, Sophie, Isabelle, Matthew, Shona, Roslyn and Johnny.

Problems in Anaesthesia
Paediatric Anaesthesia

Edited by

Peter A Stoddart MB BS BSc MRCP FRCA
Consultant Anaesthetist
Bristol Royal Infirmary for Children
Bristol
UK

Gillian R Lauder MB BCh FRCA
Consultant Paediatric Anaesthetist
Bristol Royal Infirmary for Children
Bristol
UK

CRC Press
Taylor & Francis Group
Boca Raton London New York

CRC Press is an imprint of the
Taylor & Francis Group, an **informa** business

CRC Press
Taylor & Francis Group
6000 Broken Sound Parkway NW, Suite 300
Boca Raton, FL 33487-2742

First issued in paperback 2019

ISBN-13: 978-1-84184-212-7 (hbk)
ISBN-13: 978-0-367-39445-5 (pbk)

A CIP record for this book is available from the British Library.

Library of Congress Cataloging-in-Publication Data available on application

Visit the Taylor & Francis Web site at
http://www.taylorandfrancis.com

and the CRC Press Web site at
http://www.crcpress.com

Contents

Contributors

Louise Aldridge MBChB FRCA DCH
Consultant in Paediatric Anaesthesia
Department of Anaesthesia
Royal Hospital for Sick Children
Edinburgh
UK

Lauren Barker MB BCh FRCA
Consultant Anaesthetist
Royal Devon and Exeter Hospital
Barrack Road
Exeter
UK

Robert Bingham MB BS FRCA
Consultant Paediatric Anaesthetist
Great Ormond Street Hospital for Children NHS Trust
Great Ormond Street
London
UK

Ann E Black MB BS FRCA
Consultant Paediatric Anaesthetist
Great Ormond Street Hospital for Children NHS Trust
Great Ormond Street
London
UK

Liam J Brennan BSc MB BS FRCA
Consultant in Paediatric Anaesthesia and Director of Paediatric Day Surgery
Addenbrooke's Hospital
Cambridge
UK

Alison S Carr MBBS FRCA
Consultant Paediatric Anaesthetist
Directorate of Anaesthesia, Critical Care Medicine and Pain Management
Plymouth Hospitals NHS Trust
Derriford Hospital
Plymouth
UK

Philip MD Cunnington MB BS FRCA
Consultant Paediatric Anaesthetist
Great Ormond Street Hospital for Children NHS Trust
Great Ormond Street
London
UK

Judith Dunnet MB ChB MRCP FRCA
Consultant Paediatric Anaesthetist
Frenchay Hospital
Bristol
UK

Julia Ely MB ChB FRCA
Clinical Research Fellow
Birmingham Children's Hospital NHS Trust
Birmingham
UK

John M Goddard MB BS MRCP FRCA
Consultant in Paediatric Anaesthesia and Pain Management
Sheffield Children's Hospital
Western Bank
Sheffield
UK

David William Green MB BS FRCA MBA
Consultant Anaesthetist
Kings College Hospital
Denmark Hill
London
UK

Deborah J Harris LMS FRCA
Consultant in Anaesthesia and Intensive Care
Frenchay Hospital
Frenchay Park Road
Bristol
UK

Anna Johnson BSc MBChB FRCA
Consultant paediatric anaesthetist
Derriford Hospital
Plymouth
UK

Gillian R Lauder MB BCh FRCA
Consultant Paediatric Anaesthetist
Bristol Royal Infirmary for Children
Bristol
UK

Stephen C Marriage MBBS BSc
Consultant in Paediatric Intensive Care
Bristol Royal Infirmary for Children
Bristol
UK

Stephen J Mather MBBS LRCP MRCS DRCOG FRCA
Consultant in Anaesthesia and Peri-operative Medicine
United Bristol Healthcare Trust
Bristol
UK

Alexander Mayor BSc MBBS MRCP FRCA
Directorate of Anaesthesia, Critical Care Medicine and Pain Management
Plymouth Hospitals NHS Trust
Derriford Hospital
Plymouth
UK

Angus McEwan MB ChB FRCA
Consultant Paediatric Anaesthetist
Great Ormond Street Hospital
London
UK

Anthony Moriarty MB BS FRCA
Consultant in Paediatric Anaesthesia and Pain Management
Birmingham Children's Hospital NHS Trust
Birmingham
UK

Hamish M Munro FRCA
Pediatric Cardiac Anesthesia
Congenital Heart Institute
Arnold Palmer Hospital
92 W Miller Street
Orlando
FL 32806
USA

Peter J Murphy MB ChB DA FRCA
Consultant in Paediatric Anaesthesia and Critical Care
Bristol Royal Infirmary for Children
Bristol
UK

J A Nolan BSc MB BS MRCP FRCA
Consultant Paediatric Anaesthetist
Bristol Royal Infirmary for Children
Bristol
UK

Jennifer E O'Flaherty MD MPH
Assistant Professor of Anesthesiology and Pediatrics
Department of Anesthesiology
PO Box 800710
University of Virginia Health System
Charlottesville
VA 22908-0710
USA

Jane M Peutrell MB BS FRCP (Edin) FRCA
Consultant Paediatric Anaesthetist
Royal Hospital for Sick Children
Yorkhill NHS Trust
Glasgow
UK

Anthony Pickering MB ChB PhD FRCA
Lecturer in Anaesthesia
Sir Humphrey Davy Department of Anaesthesia
Bristol Royal Infirmary
Bristol
UK

Miguel Plaza-Barrera LMS FRCA DA GP
Consultant Anaesthetist
Kings College hospital
London
UK

Dylan Parry Prosser MB BCh FRCA
Consultant Paediatric Anaesthetist
Department of Anaesthesia
Bristol Children's Hospital
Southwell Street
Bristol
UK

Paul Reynolds MD
Chief of Pediatric Anesthesiology
Clinical Associate Professor of Anesthesiology
University of Michigan Medical Center
Ann Arbor, MI
USA

Peter A Stoddart MB BS BSc MRCP FRCA
Consultant Anaesthetist
Bristol Royal Infirmary for Children
Bristol
UK

MRJ Sury MB BS FRCA
Consultant Paediatric Anaesthetist
Great Ormond Street Hospital for Children NHS Trust
Great Ormond Street
London
UK

Andy Tatman MBBS BSc MRCP FRCA
Consultant Paediatric Anaesthetist
Department of Anaesthesia
Birmingham Children's Hospital NHS Trust
Steelhouse Lane
Birmingham
UK

Isabeau Walker BSc BChir FRCA
Consultant Paediatric Anaesthetist
Great Ormond Street Hospital for Children NHS Trust
Great Ormond Street
London
UK

Robert Weatherly MD
Chief of Pediatric Anesthesiology
Clinical Associate Professor of Anesthesiology
University of Michigan Medical Center
Ann Arbor
MI
USA

Patricia M Weir MB ChB DRCOG DCH FRCA
Consultant in Paediatric Anaesthesia and Intensive Care
Paediatric Intensive Care Unit
Bristol Royal Infirmary for Children
Bristol
UK

Michelle White MB ChB DCH FRCA
Specialist Registrar
Bristol School of Anaesthesia
Bristol
UK

Kathy Wilkinson FRCA MRCP
Consultant Anaesthetist
Norfolk and Norwich University Hospital
Colney Lane
Norwich
UK

Andrew R Wolf MD FRCA
Consultant in Paediatric Anaesthesia and Intensive Care
Professor of Anaesthesia and Critical Care
University of Bristol
Bristol
UK

AER Young BSc MB BCh FRCA
Consultant Paediatric Anaesthetist
Frenchay Hospital
Bristol
UK

Foreword

It has been almost two decades since the publication of a 'problem-based' paediatric anaesthesia book. In the 1980s there were two excellent books. One was *Common Problems in Pediatric Anesthesia*, edited by Linda Stehling. This book presented very short scenarios of difficult clinical situations. The other book was *Anesthesia and Uncommon Pediatric Diseases*, edited by Katz and Steward. It detailed the paediatric background of various uncommon paediatric diseases. *Problems in Anaesthesia: Paediatric Anaesthesia* is a combination of these two books: that is, clinical situations are discussed along with the pathophysiology, as well as the anaesthetic management.

This book should prove to be a treasure, not only for trainees, but for those clinicians in practice who come upon the rather infrequent diseases that are discussed herein. The authors are nationally and internationally recognised, and come from a very broad spectrum of institutions in the United Kingdom and the United States. The chapters in this book give the pathophysiology of the various conditions along with the issues that need to be considered by the clinician. The editors have done a wonderful job of putting together a spectrum of frequent and infrequent problems and the contributors have provided the reader with knowledge and thoughtful consideration. This book is like having a consultant on the bookshelf.

Fritz Berry
Professor
Anesthesiology and Pediatrics
University of Virginia

Preface

This book presents a spectrum of real and interesting case histories and their subsequent anaesthetic management. It is not intended to be a comprehensive textbook of paediatric anaesthesia. We have selected cases to illustrate a range of problems that may be encountered by anaesthetists caring for children in a general or teaching hospital, as well as the specialist centre.

The contributing authors are clinicians with local, regional, national and international expertise. The case studies outline a safe approach to the anaesthetic care of each child presented. Neither the editors, nor the contributors, offer these recommendations as the sole way to manage the child; there may be other equally acceptable anaesthetic techniques. The one chosen is not only based on the characteristics of the patient and the available evidence from the literature, but also by the preference and experience of the anaesthetist, surgeon and the institution they practise in. Each chapter is meant to stand alone, and therefore problems common to each clinical situation may be repeated.

We would like to thank all the authors for the considerable time and effort they devoted to writing their chapters and also Robert Peden and Julian Evans from Dunitz for ensuring that the book was finally completed.

Pete Stoddart and Gill Lauder
Bristol Royal Hospital for Children
October 2003

1

Anaesthesia for closure of gastroschisis/exomphalos

Dylan Parry Prosser

Introduction

Gastroschisis and exomphalos (omphalocoele) are both congenital conditions which are characterized by the herniation of viscera through a 'defect' in the anterior abdominal wall. In gastroschisis (incidence 1 in 30,000 live births), the viscera herniate through a 'true' defect in the abdominal wall (Figure 1.1), which is to the right and at the base of the umbilicus, whereas in exomphalos (incidence 1 in 6–10,000 live births) the viscera herniate into the base of the umbilical cord (Figure 1.2). The incidence of gastroschisis has been increasing on a worldwide basis since the late 1980s.[1] Both types of defect should be repaired promptly because of the increased risk of gut ischaemia and infection leading to sepsis. The anaesthetic management of both conditions is essentially the same.

Case history

A 6-hour-old, 2.13-kg baby presented for surgical repair of gastroschisis. The diagnosis was made antenatally by ultrasound scan at 20 weeks' gestation. The baby was delivered vaginally at 36 weeks' gestation following spontaneous rupture of membranes. Oropharyngeal suction was performed on delivery of the head. Apgar scores were 9 and 10 at 1 and 5 minutes, respectively. The abdominal defect was enclosed in a polyethylene 'body bag' (Figure 1.3) and the baby was transferred to the neonatal intensive care unit (NICU) breathing spontaneously in air. On arrival on the NICU the baby looked pale and poorly perfused. Venous blood gases were pH = 7.15, P_aCO_2 = 7.0 kPa, BE = −10.5 mmol.l^{-1}. The baby was given 40 ml 4.5% human albumin solution and a size 8 nasogastric tube was passed to decompress the stomach.

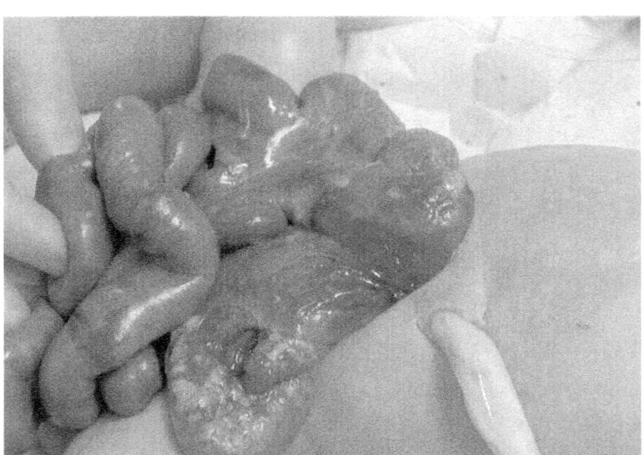

Figure 1.1
Gastroschisis.

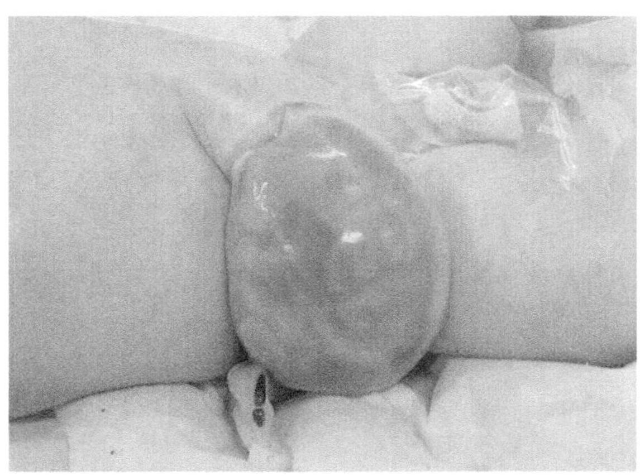

Figure 1.2
Exomphalos.

Following appropriate resuscitation and pre-operative evaluation (Table 1.1), the baby was transferred directly into theatre (ambient temperature 26 °C, relative humidity 50%) from the portable incubator. A radiant heater was positioned overhead and the baby laid onto a warm air blower mattress on the operating table. The nasogastric tube was aspirated as the baby was turned through 360 degrees, firstly to the left lateral then to the right lateral position before being turned prone and finally back to the supine position. The 24g cannula in situ, in the dorsum of the right hand, was flushed with 1 ml 0.9% saline and non-invasive monitoring (SaO_2, BP, ECG) was established. Anaesthesia was induced with 8% sevoflurane in 100% O_2, 2 µg fentanyl and 2 mg atracurium. The trachea was intubated with a size 3.0 uncuffed uncut endotracheal tube (fitted with an Ohmeda RSP low deadspace neonatal airway adapter) which was secured at 9 cm at the lip.

The endotracheal tube was secured across the forehead with adhesive fabric tape and connected to a T-piece circuit, via a heat and moisture exchange filter. The baby was ventilated to an end-tidal CO_2 4.6–5.3 kPa with a Penlon Nuffield 200 series ventilator set to an inspired time of 0.6–0.7 seconds, expired time 1.0 second and flow rate adjusted to deliver peak pressures no greater than 20 cmH_2O. Anaesthesia and analgesia were maintained with 1–1.5% isoflurane oxygen in air and 50 µg incremental boluses of morphine titrated to effect and neuromuscular blockade was maintained with 1-mg boluses of atracurium.

A 22g cannula was sited in the right long saphenous vein for intraoperative fluid replacement and a sialastic percutaneous neonatal long line was threaded 20 cm up the left long saphenous vein for postoperative parenteral nutrition.

Heart rate, capillary refill and rectal–toe temperature gradients were used to monitor the baby's state of hydration and perfusion. Maintenance fluid requirements (8 $ml.h^{-1}$ 10% dextrose) were supplemented with 20-ml boluses of Gelofusine® as dictated by capillary refill time and heart rate.

The baby was hand-ventilated prior to, during and after the replacement of the viscera back into the abdomen in order that changes in lung compliance as a result of this manoeuver could be fully appreciated by the anaesthetist and surgeon.

Following the primary closure of the defect the baby was returned to the NICU where she remained fully sedated, paralysed and ventilated with morphine (10–20 $\mu g.kg^{-1}.h^{-1}$) and vecuronium (60 $\mu g.kg^{-1}.h^{-1}$) infusions. She developed a postoperative metabolic acidosis and hyponatraemia which resolved over a period of 48 hours following boluses of human albumin solution, adjustments to ventilation, and sodium supplements. The antibiotics and vecuronium were stopped after 3 days and she was extubated on the fourth postoperative day having SaO_2 of 97% in air. Her morphine infusion was stopped on the sixth postoperative day and she was prescribed rectal paracetamol on a 'pro re nata' basis. She developed an

Preoperative medications	Penicillin 65 mg tds, netilmicin 8.5 mg od, metronidazole 16 mg bd, vitamin K 1 mg i.m. Intravenous fluid 10% dextrose 8 $ml.h^{-1}$
Preoperative examination	*Respiratory system* – SaO_2 100% in air; mild intermittent grunting; chest clear *Cardiovascular system* – HR 164 min^{-1}; normal heart sounds and pulses; normal fontanelle; capillary refill time 2 seconds *Abdomen* – large defect to right of umbilical cord; stomach, small intestine and proximal large intestine herniated through defect; bowel moderately thickened and oedematous
Preoperative investigations	Hb = 18.0 $g.dl^{-1}$, Plt = $201 \times 10^9\ l^{-1}$, WBC = $15.5 \times 10^9\ l^{-1}$ Capillary blood gas pH = 7.3, CO_2 = 6.4 kPa, BE = −3.8 $mmol.l^{-1}$ C-reactive protein = 13 $mg.l^{-1}$, Na = 129 $mmol.l^{-1}$, K = 5.1 $mmol.l^{-1}$ Urea = 3.7 $mmol.l^{-1}$, Creatinine = 76 $\mu mol.l^{-1}$ Chest X-ray and ECG were normal

Table 1.1
Preoperative evaluation

	Gastroschisis	*Exomphalos*
Birthweight	Low	Normal or high
Associated anomalies	<5%	50–60%
Mortality	0–10%	30–50%
Sac	Absent	Present
Site	To side of cord	Central
Incidence	Increasing	Decreasing
Gastrointestinal dysfunction	Present	Absent
Mother's age	Young	Average

Table 1.2
The clinical differences between gastroschisis and exomphalos (modified from Spicer[2])

ileus on the tenth postoperative day which delayed her enteral feeding programme for a further 8 days. She continued to receive parenteral nutrition until the 24th postoperative day and was discharged from the NICU on the 28th postoperative day.

At an outpatient clinic visit 8 weeks later the patient was reported to be doing extremely well having gained 1 kg in weight. This put her on the 9th centile which corresponded favourably with her birth weight centile.

Discussion

The clinical differences between gastroschisis and exomphalos are outlined in Table 1.2.

Although rare in gastroschisis, associated congenital anomalies can occur in up to 60% of infants with an exomphalos. These anomalies can be wide-ranging in nature (see Table 1.3), and of varying significance to the anaesthetist.

In approximately one in 13,000 live births exomphalos is associated with the Beckwith–Widemann syndrome. The anaesthetic management of these patients may be complicated by the presence of abnormal airway anatomy (macroglossia), congenital heart disease, organomegaly, giantism and severe hypoglycaemia (related to hyperplasia of the pancreatic islets) which needs particular attention pre- and perioperatively.[3,4]

The gestational age, lung maturity and the presence of associated anomalies, namely cardiac and craniofacial, are of greater importance to the anaesthetist than the nature of the anatomical defect itself.

Preoperative management

The primary concerns are for heat and fluid loss, trauma to herniated viscera and the development of sepsis. This is particularly true for gastroschisis, and those cases of exomphalos where the peritoneal sac has ruptured.

Heat and evaporative losses are reduced by enclosing the neonate's lower limbs and abdomen in a clear polythene 'body bag' (Figure 1.3).

Gastrointestinal tract	Malrotation of intestine, Meckel's diverticulum, intestinal atresia, colonic agenesis, biliary atresia, imperforate anus
Cardiovascular system	Tetralogy of Fallot
Genitourinary system	Bladder extrophy
Craniofacial	Harelip, cleft palate, jaw and tongue tumours, haemangiomas

Table 1.3
Congenital anomalies associated with exomphalos

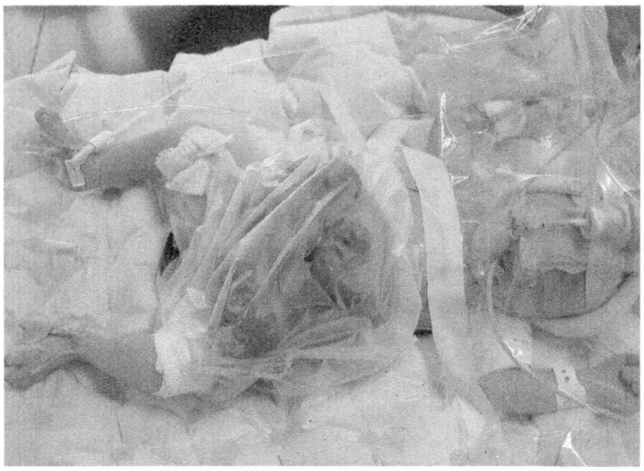

Figure 1.3
Abdomen enclosed within polythene 'body bag'.

Where spontaneous respiration is satisfactory a naso- or orogastric tube is passed to decompress the stomach thereby reducing abdominal distension and the potential for diaphragmatic splinting. This manoeuver also reduces the likelihood of regurgitation, pulmonary aspiration and further bowel distention. Broad spectrum antibiotics should be administered early.

Meticulous attention should be paid to intravenous fluid replacement, because the combination of extravasation of fluid into the bowel, peritonitis, oedema and ischaemia, can lead to hypovolaemic shock and a consequent worsening metabolic acidosis. It is not unusual for these neonates to require up to four times ($300\,ml.kg^{-1}.day^{-1}$) their normal amount of maintenance fluid in the first 24–48 hours of life.

The adequacy of the preoperative resuscitation can be assessed by monitoring capillary refill, core–peripheral temperature gradients; evidence of correction of acid base disturbance and urine output ($1–2\,ml.kg^{-1}.h^{-1}$).

Because large amounts of replacements fluid are being administered attention should be focused on electrolyte imbalances (particluarly hyponatraemia), haemodilution and the acid base status. These are best monitored by either direct arterial or venous blood sampling.

Perioperative management

Although primary closure of the defect is surgically preferred, it is not always feasible with the larger defects because there is a risk of placing the closed abdominal contents under excessive pressure. The major problems associated with an increase in intra-abdominal pressure are twofold. Firstly, splinting of the diaphragm may result in significant lung compression which can compromise ventilation and secondly, a reduction in venous return and consequent fall in cardiac output can lead to tissue hypoperfusion and its sequelae i.e. postoperative bowel ischaemia and renal failure.

Some authors advocate the measurement of intragastric and central venous pressures as a means of predicting the feasibility of a primary closure.[5,6] They noted that increases in intragastric pressure greater than 20 mmHg and increases in central venous pressure of greater than 4 mmHg were frequently associated with reductions in venous return and cardiac output, which required surgical decompression of the abdomen.

In the majority of cases the anaesthetist and surgeon can come to a joint decision as to whether or not a primary closure is feasible based simply on the observed changes in lung compliance, cardiovascular stability and gut perfusion at the time of the attempted closure of the defect.

Where primary closure of a larger defect is not possible (tight abdomen with shiny overlying skin, cardiovascular instability and decreased lung compliance) a two-stage repair is undertaken. At the first operation a sialastic or polyvinylchloride pouch or 'chimney' prosthesis is sutured over and around the edge of the defect to enclose it (Figure 1.4). This is suspended above the abdomen and its contents allowed to settle into the abdominal cavity, under gravity, over a period of 5–6 days. At the second operation the prosthesis is removed, again under general anaesthesia, and the defect's edges are opposed as per primary closure.

Postoperative management

The majority of these babies are returned to the NICU intubated. They are electively paralysed and ventilated for between 1 and 7 days until either any abdominal distension has resolved following a primary closure of the defect, or until the bowel has settled back into the abdomen under the influence of gravity in readiness for secondary closure of the abdominal wall defect.

Parenteral nutrition is often required for 3–4 weeks postoperatively in all gastroschisis patients and a large proportion of exomphalos major patients until the ileus has resolved and the gut is absorbing normally.

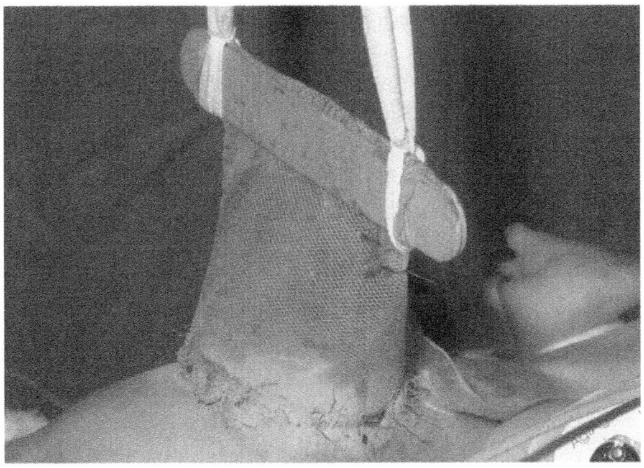

Figure 1.4
'Chimney' prosthesis enclosing viscera.

Paracetamol is administered rectally to supplement analgesia. Its morphine-sparing effect helps reduce the requirement for the opioid infusion which can result in accumulation and a consequent effect upon gut motility after several days. Muscle relaxation is facilitated, where indicated, with either boluses of pancuronium or an atracurium infusion. Antibiotics tend to be stopped after 72 hours providing septic markers (white cell count, C-reactive protein and platelets) are normal.

Outcome

Patients with gastroschisis generally do well in the long term unless they have other problems associated with their prematurity, e.g. respiratory distress syndrome, necrotizing enterocolitis, sepsis and intraventricular haemorrhage whereas the outcome for exomphalos is almost entirely dependent on the associated anomalies. Because there is a high incidence (30–50%) of mortality associated with exomphalos major defects more pregnancies are being terminated early and the incidence of children being born with this defect is decreasing. In contrast the increase in incidence of gastroschisis remains unexplained.

Learning points

- Both conditions are associated with the herniation of abdominal viscera through a defect in the anterior abdominal wall.
- Up to 60% of neonates with exomphalos will have other associated anomalies (cardiac, craniofacial and renal) which may have an impact upon anaesthesia. It is imperative that they undergo echocardiography.
- Gestational age, lung maturity and the presence of the above anomalies are often of greater importance to the anaesthetist than the nature of the anatomical defect itself. The anaesthetic management of these conditions is essentially the same.
- Both types of defect should be repaired promptly because of the increased risk of gut ischaemia and sepsis.
- Fluid resuscitation may be required prior to surgery depending on the nature and size of the defect. The neonate may be hypovolaemic, dehydrated and acidotic.
- Heat and water losses tend to be greatest from gastroschisis defects and exomphalos defects where the sac has ruptured.
- Primary closure of a defect is influenced by the size of the defect in relation to the abdominal cavity, changes in lung compliance and cardiovascular stability. Where there is doubt a two-stage procedure is preferred because there is a realistic expectation that the bowel will become more oedematous over 48–72 hours further worsening abdominal distension.
- Prolonged parenteral nutrition is required following gastroschisis repair because the bowel becomes thickened and abnormal having been exposed to urine and amniotic fluid in utero. It may take weeks or even months before it resumes normal function.
- The prognosis for patients with exomphalos is almost entirely dependent on the nature of the associated anomalies whereas the prognosis for gastroschisis depends mainly on the condition of the bowel.

References

1. Di Tanna GL, Rosano A, Mastroiacovo P. Prevalence of gastroschisis at birth: retrospective study. *BMJ* 2002; 325: 1389–1390.
2. Spicer RD. Neonatal surgical disorders of the gastrointestinal tract. *Curr Paediatr* 1994; 4: 21–26.
3. Gurkowski MA, Rasch DK. Anesthetic considerations for Beckwith–Wiedemann syndrome. *Anesthesiology* 1989; 70: 711–712.
4. Suan C, Ojeda R, Garcia-Perla JL, Perez-Torres MC. Anaesthesia and the Beckwith–Wiedemann syndrome. *Paediatr Anaesth* 1996; 6: 231–233.

5. Yaster M, Buck JR, Dudgeon DL et al. Hemodynamic effects of primary closure of omphalocoele/gastroschisis in human newborns. *Anesthesiology* 1988; 69: 84–88.
6. Yaster M, Scherer TL, Stone MM et al. Prediction of successful primary closure of congenital abdominal wall defects using intraoperative measurements. *J Pediatr Surg* 1989; 24: 1217–1220.

Further reading

Motoyama EK, Davis PJ. Smith's Anesthesia for Infants and Children, 6th edn. St Louis, Mo: Mosby, 1996.

Stehling L. Common Problems in Pediatric Anesthesia, 2nd edn. St Louis, Mo: Mosby, 1992.

2

Anaesthesia for repair of oesophageal atresia and tracheo-oesophageal fistula

Angus McEwan

Introduction

Oesophageal atresia occurs in 1:3000–1:4500 live births. In the majority of cases (85%) a fistula exists between the trachea and distal oesophagus but less common arrangements also occur. Oesophageal atresia or tracheo-oesophageal fistula may occur alone. One-third of babies affected are born prematurely. The following case history outlines the anaesthetic management of a typical case.

Case history

A 1-day-old female infant weighing 3.6 kg was referred to the paediatric surgical team from a district general hospital with a presumed diagnosis of oesophageal atresia. The baby was born at term +10 days to a 32-year-old woman. No antenatal problems had been noted and in particular ultrasound scans had been reported as normal and there was no polyhydramnios. The baby was born by a normal vaginal delivery; there was no meconium but there was a large volume of liquor.

The apgar scores at delivery were 5 at 1 minute and 10 at 5 minutes. Immediately after delivery the baby was apnoeic and required a short period of bag and mask ventilation. Two unsuccessful attempts to pass a nasogastric tube were made. After the second attempt the nasogastric tube was left in situ and a chest X-ray taken showed it to be coiled up in the oesophagus; in addition gas was noted in the stomach. The infant was given vitamin K, made 'nil by mouth' and intravenous fluids were started. A transfer to a specialist paediatric surgical centre was then arranged which took place later the same day.

On arrival that evening at the paediatric centre the infant was admitted to the neonatal intensive care unit (NICU). She was alert and active with no dysmorphic features noted. She was pink, warm with good peripheral perfusion and arterial blood saturation of 99% in air. The chest was clear and there were no murmurs. All peripheral pulses were palpable, the abdomen was soft with no palpable masses and there was a little meconium in the nappy. A replogle tube was passed through the nose into the upper oesophageal pouch and a chest and abdominal X-ray were repeated. A cardiac echocardiogram was performed to exclude cardiac disease and confirm a left-sided aortic arch. A renal ultrasound was normal as were the full blood count and urea and electrolytes. In addition there was no evidence of any hemivertebrae. Blood was cross-matched and after review by the surgical team surgery was scheduled for the following day on the designated emergency operating list.

Prior to anaesthesia and surgery the child was reviewed by the anaesthetist. The history, physical examination and investigations were noted. Maintenance fluid of 10% dextrose infusion was continued at 10 $ml.hr^{-1}$ via an indwelling intravenous cannula. No premedication was prescribed.

After transfer to the anaesthetic room monitoring equipment was applied. This included pulse oxymetry, ECG and non-invasive blood pressure cuff. Anaesthesia was induced using a mixture of nitrous oxide, oxygen and sevoflurane. The airway was easy to maintain and gentle ventilation proved easy. Suxamethonium 8 mg was given and ventilation was taken over by mask and airway. 100% oxygen was now given with isoflurane 1%. The infant was intubated using a 3.5-mm uncuffed endotracheal tube; 3 cm were passed through the cords and the tube was taped at 11 cm at the lips. Atracurium 2 mg was then given. An overhead radiant heater had been used from the outset and at this stage a temperature probe was passed and a paracetamol suppository 60 mg was given. The child was hand-ventilated while checking that there was bilateral air entry in the chest and no distension in the abdomen. The eyes were taped shut and a second 22G intravenous cannula was sited. The infant was transferred to the operating room, placed on a warm air mattress, reconnected to all the monitors and ventilated using a circle system. The overhead radiant heater was now repositioned over the child.

A rigid oesophagoscopy was then performed which showed a blind-ending upper oesophageal pouch. There was no evidence of a fistula originating from this upper pouch. The baby was then turned to the left lateral position and was prepped and draped in preparation for a right thoracotomy. The endotracheal tube position was rechecked to ensure bilateral air entry in the chest and no distension of the stomach. The 10% glucose infusion from the NICU was continued. Prior to skin incision fentanyl was given in a dose of $5\,\mu g.kg^{-1}$. Ventilation was in 28% oxygen, nitrous oxide and isoflurane 0.5–1.0%. Antibiotics, gentamicin, benzylpenicillin, and metronidazole were given. The infant's blood sugar was $4.5\,mmol.l^{-1}$.

A right lateral thoracotomy was then performed using the 4th intercostal space. An extrapleural approach was used. The fistula from the lower oesophageal pouch to the trachea was easily identified and ligated. The upper oesophagus was then anastamosed to the lower oesophagus over a size 6 feeding tube and as there was a good length of both the upper and lower pouches there was no residual tension on the anastamosis. The baby remained well throughout the procedure with a low oxygen requirement and little need of extra fluids. A total of $5\,ml.kg^{-1}$ of Gelofusine® was given during the surgery. Although there was no surgical reason to keep the baby ventilated a decision was made to send the child back ventilated to NICU. 10% dextrose was continued at $60\,ml.kg^{-1}.day^{-1}$, triple antibiotics were prescibed (gentamicin, benzylpenicillin and metronidazole), a morphine infusion was started and paracetamol was given.

The baby had a stable night and was extubated the following morning. However, immediately after extubation the baby developed postextubation stridor which was treated with dexamethasone ($0.25\,mg.kg^{-1}$) and some humidified head box oxygen. The stridor resolved over the next 1–2 hours and the baby then maintained good saturations in air and later that day she was discharged back to the surgical ward. By this time she had been started on milk feeds through the feeding tube. The baby continued to make good progress on the ward and was discharged home 1 week later.

Discussion

Clinical presentation

Oesophageal atresia (OA) occurs in 1 : 3000–1 : 4500 live births and is associated with a tracheoesophageal fistula (TOF) in the majority of cases. OA or TOF may also occur alone but this is much less common. Polyhydramnios is common in cases of OA and prematurity is associated with both OA and TOF.

In the most common form of TOF/OA (87%) there is a blind-ending upper oesophageal pouch with a fistula from the lower oesophagus to the trachea (Figure 2.1, Type 1). Ideally this is diagnosed by identifying the 'mucousy baby' at birth and confirmed by the inability to pass a nasogastric tube. However, it is sometimes diagnosed after the first feed when the baby chokes. A chest X-ray then shows the nasogastric tube coiled in the upper pouch and air is present in the stomach. Contrast media should not be used as this increases the chances of lung damage from aspiration. OA alone is the second most common condition, occurring in 8% of cases (Figure 2.1, Type 2). Again a nasogastric tube cannot be passed but in this case there is no air in the stomach on X-ray and there is a scaphoid abdomen. Choking with possible aspiration occurs when feeding is attempted if the diagnosis has not previously been made. The gap between the two ends of the oesophagus may be long on these occasions making surgical repair more difficult. The H-type fistula occurs in about 4% of cases and the diagnosis may be more difficult to make and may be delayed for days or weeks as the child develops repeated chest infections and bouts of coughing. The fistula may be difficult to find and demonstrate even if contrast is given or if oesophagoscopy or bronchoscopies are used.

Babies with TOF/OA frequently have other associated abnormalities. Congenital heart disease is common and occurs in about 20% of cases. The most common conditions being ventricular septal defect, patent ductus arteriosus, tetralogy of Fallot, atrial septal defect and coarctation of the aorta. Musculoskeletal abnormalities include vertebral anomalies, radial dysplasia and polydactyly. Gastrointestinal anomalies include imperforate anus, duodenal atresia and pyloric stenosis. There may also be renal or genitourinary abnormalities and cleft lip and palate are also more common. TOF/OA has also been linked with two associations, the VATER and VACTERAL associations. The VATER association is vertebral defects, anal atresia, TOF, oesophageal atresia

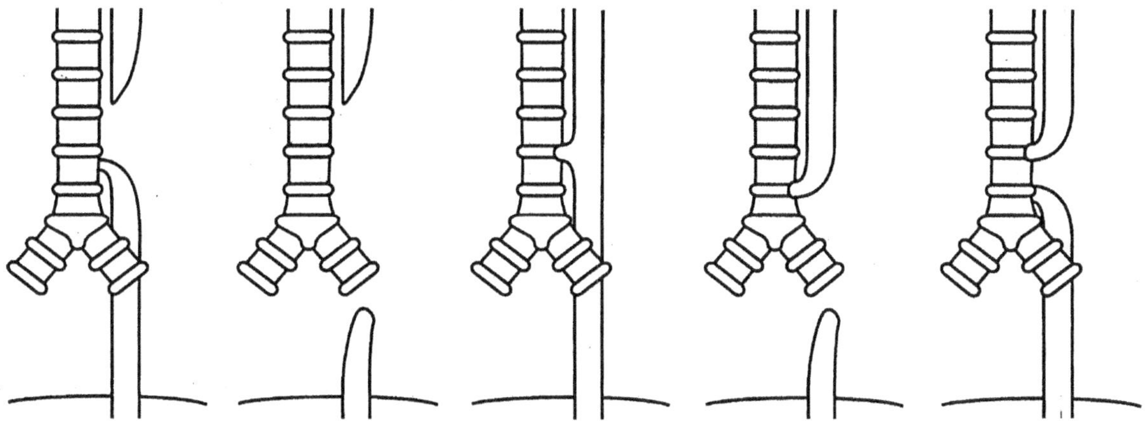

Figure 2.1
The five types of tracheo-oesophageal fistula.

and renal dysplasia or radial anomalies. The VACTERAL association has in addition cardiac and limb defects.

Anaesthetic management

Specific anaesthetic problems:
1) Lung disease from aspiration or prematurity
2) Prematurity or low birth weight
3) Associated congenital anomalies
4) Difficult intubation due to subglottic stenosis or inadvertant intubation of the fistula
5) Difficult ventilation due to gas loss through fistula or because of surgical lung retraction

The initial surgical repair depends on the size, prematurity and general medical condition of the infant. Primary repair with ligation of the fistula and repair of the oesophagus is undertaken if the anatomy and medical condition of the child allow. If this is not deemed feasible then a staged repair is undertaken. This involves ligation of the fistula and formation of a gastrostomy at the first operation and a later repair of the oesophagus. The following discussion relates more to the primary repair.

To prevent aspiration of secretions in the preoperative period oral feeds are discontinued, the upper oesophageal pouch is placed on constant suction and the baby is nursed in a semi-upright position. A careful assessment of the respiratory status is made because of the risk of respiratory distress syndrome and aspiration with associated atelectasis. Preoperative ventilation will sometimes be necessary. Delay of the surgery is seldom justified in the hope that the lungs will improve as the respiratory status will often only improve after surgical correction. Babies with severe lung disease and high airway pressures are at risk of gastric distension and/or rupture resulting in a pneumoperitoneum and require early ligation of the fistula. With the high incidence of cardiac anomalies in these patients, an echocardiogram should be performed preoperatively and if necessary a cardiology opinion sought. Babies should be kept warm preoperatively and also during transport to the operating theatre.

Opinion about the safest technique for induction and intubation in these children remains controversial because of the risk of intubating the fistula and thus being unable to ventilate adequately. Some would advocate awake intubation while others would advocate induction of anaesthesia prior to intubation either with a gaseous induction or an intravenous induction. The other point of contention is the use of either suxamethonium or long-acting muscle relaxant. The author's preferred technique is as follows. After arrival in the anaesthetic room the baby is placed under an overhead radiant heater and the appropriate monitors are connected. A gaseous induction is performed using nitrous oxide, oxygen and sevoflurane. As anaesthesia is deepened, ventilation is gently taken over ensuring that gastric distension does not take place. After changing to 100% oxygen and isoflurane, suxamethonim 2 mg.kg^{-1} is given and the baby intubated with an appropriate tube. A careful assessment of ventilation is now done to check for equal bilateral air entry and to check that no gas is entering the stomach. If all is satisfactory a longer-acting muscle relaxant is given and positive pressure ventilation at the lowest acceptable pressure is started and anaesthesia is continued with air, oxygen and isoflurane or sevoflurane. If the fistula is intubated it is sometimes possible to reposition the tube correctly by changing the angle of the bevel by rotating the tube. An additional problem is that the fistula frequently arises very close to the carina so that if the endotracheal tube is beyond the fistula it is likely to be very close to the carina or in one or other of the main bronchi. A long-acting muscle relaxant should not be given until ventilation is satisfactory. If it is not possible to secure adequate positive pressure ventilation, spontaneous ventilation should be used with some gentle assistance until the chest is open and in this situation the fistula should be ligated as soon as possible.

All the standard monitors should be employed and in addition an arterial line may be helpful in sick babies for blood gas, blood sugar and haematocrit monitoring as well as blood pressure monitoring.

Some consideration at this stage should be given to postoperative pain relief. If it is likely that the infant can be extubed at the end of the procedure, which should be possible in the majority of well babies with a short oesophageal gap, an epidural catheter can be placed to provide excellent intraoperative and postoperative pain relief. Thoracic epidural catheters can reliably be placed from the caudal space or lumbar intervertebral space. Thoracic epidurals using a thoracic intervertebral space are not used in our hospital. If however it is thought that a period of ventilation postoperatively is likely then fentanyl can be used in a dose of 5–10 µg.kg^{-1} and a morphine infusion continued postoperatively. Regular paracetamol can be added to the analgesic regime. If an epidural is not to be used and the patient is to be extubated a smaller dose of fentanyl should be used 1–3 µg.kg^{-1} and a nurse-controlled analgesia (NCA) pump can be set up postoperatively. Intercostal nerve blocks at the time of surgery placed by the surgeon are very effective if NCA is to be used postoperatively.

The surgery is performed through a right thoracotomy and thus the baby is placed in a left lateral position. It may however be necessary to perform a rigid oesophagoscopy prior to this to determine the length of the upper pouch and to determine the position and size of the fistula. Hand ventilation is sometimes advocated and indeed advantageous but in uncomplicated cases mechanical ventilation is adequate. Lung retraction can compromise ventilation and it is important from the outset that the endotracheal tube is not too small because if the leak is too great the lung retraction will make ventilation very awkward.

Preoperative maintenance fluids which are often 10% dextrose should be continued during the surgery. Additional replacement fluid is also required but the amount and type is determined by the extent and duration of the surgery and on the amount of bleeding. Initially replacement can be with Hartmann's solution and this is to take account of third space and evaporative losses. Blood loss is best replaced with a colloid such as a gelatin, although some would use human albumin solution. Serial haematocrit measurement will determine when blood is required. This is usually if the haematocrit has fallen below 30%. Temperature monitoring and maintenance is very important and it is also important to monitor blood glucose. The patient who is well, warm, haemodynamically stable, has no respiratory complications and whose oesophageal anastamosis is not under tension can be extubated. However, if there are any concerns about the ability of the patient to tolerate spontaneous ventilation then the patient should remain ventilated postoperatively.

Early postoperative complications include oesophageal leak which can lead to mediastinitis and sepsis. Swallowing can remain a problem postoperatively with aspiration continuing, in which case intensive chest physiotherapy will be required. Late complications include diverticulum of the trachea, tracheomalacia, oesophageal stricture and gastro-oesophageal reflux. Prognosis after repair depends on the maturity and birthweight of the child, on the severity of the associated anomalies and on pulmonary complications. There is an 82–100% survival in those infants with no other life-threatening congenital anomalies.

Learning points

- Oesophageal atresia occurs in 1 in 3000 to 1 in 4500 live births. In 85% of cases there is a fistula between the lower oesophagus and the trachea.
- Neonates with oesophageal atresia may have other congenital anomalies which must be investigated and excluded.
- One-third of neonates born with oesophageal atresia are born prematurely and are therefore of low birth weight.
- Various different anaesthetic techniques can be employed to secure the airway. This must be achieved without intubating the fistula and also without insufflating the stomach.
- Hand ventilation is recommended until the fistula has been ligated.
- Postoperative analgesic regimes vary but include paracetamol, intercostal nerve blocks, morphine infusion/NCA or thoracic epidurals.
- One essential of postoperative care is to prevent the chance of re-intubation and tension on the oesophageal anastosmosis.
- Survival is high when there are no associated congenital anomalies.

Further reading

Hatch D, Sumner E. The Surgical Neonate. London: Edward Arnold, 1995: 148.

Morray JP, Krane EJ. Anaesthesia for Thoracic Surgery. In: Gregory GA (ed.). Paediatric Anaesthesia. New York: Churchill Livingstone, 1989: 920.

Steward, D (ed.). Manual of Pediatric Anesthesia. 4th edn. Place: Churchill Livingstone, year: 227.

3

Anaesthetic management for pyloromyotomy in a district general hospital

Alison S Carr

Introduction

Congenital hypertrophic pyloric stenosis is one of the most common surgical conditions in small babies, occurring in approximately one in 400 live births.[1] Pyloric stenosis usually affects first-born boys between the ages of 2–8 weeks old. The pathology is hypertrophy of the longitudinal and circular muscle of the pyloric muscle associated with oedema of the pyloric mucosa. This results in obstruction of the passage of gastric contents into the duodenum. Classically, the baby presents with non-bilious projectile vomiting. Treatment is by surgical pyloromyotomy, where the pyloric muscle is split down to the mucosa to relieve the obstruction.

Case history

A 6-week-old baby boy presented to a large district general hospital (DGH) with a 1-week history of vomiting. Initially the vomiting episodes were only twice a day but for 2 days prior to admission he had vomited all feeds. Sometimes the vomits had projected across the room. The vomits did not contain bile. The baby was breast-fed. He was hungry and fed again immediately after vomiting. Occasionally the second feed was retained. The baby had not gained weight for 2 weeks. There had been fewer wet nappies in the last 24 hours. There was no pyrexia or diarrhoea. Further history, examination findings and results of investigations are shown in Table 3.1 below.

The baby was kept 'nil by mouth' and intravenous fluids were given. A large-bore nasogastric tube was inserted, kept on free drainage and aspirated regularly. The baby was assessed to have a moderate dehydration and preoperative fluid resuscitation and correction of electrolyte abnormalities were commenced.

Dehydration was assessed to be approximately 7–8% of the baby's weight. The fluid deficit and the normal maintenance fluids were calculated. The fluid and the electrolyte imbalances were corrected over 24 hours by an intravenous infusion of half-strength normal saline in dextrose, both for replacing deficit and for maintenance. Supplemental potassium was added to all intravenous fluids infused. Stomach washouts were performed via the nasogastric tube preoperatively to attempt to remove all traces of milk from the stomach. After 24 hours the resuscitation was reassessed. The patient was alert, pink and well-perfused with good urine output. Repeat capillary gas analysis revealed a pH of 7.43, pO_2 of 7.2 kPa, pCO_2 of 4.3 kPa, HCO_3^- 26 mmol.l^{-1}, BE −2.7, and chloride 105 mmol·l^{-1}. The baby was scheduled for pyloromyotomy the following morning after informed consent was obtained from the mother.

The following morning the patient was transferred to the operating room. The patient was connected to ECG, non-invasive blood pressure and oxygen saturation monitors. The in situ cannula was flushed to ensure patency. The nasogastric tube was aspirated immediately before induction of anaesthesia with the baby in the right lateral, supine and left lateral positions, to remove any traces of gastric contents (Figures 3.1a–c). A rapid sequence induction with preoxygenation was performed (Figure 3.2).

Atropine 10 µg.kg^{-1}, thiopentone sodium 4 mg.kg^{-1}, and suxamethonium 2 mg.kg^{-1} were injected intravenously. Cricoid pressure was applied as soon as the baby shut its eyes. Tracheal intubation was performed with a size 3.5 oral endotracheal tube. Anaesthesia was maintained by inhalation of sevoflurane 2–3% in oxygen and air. A short-acting non-depolarizing muscle relaxant, atracurium 0.5 mg.kg^{-1} IV was injected to maintain muscle relaxation. An oesophageal temperature probe was inserted and prophylactic

Past medical mistory	Born at term by elective Caesarean section for breech presentation, no neonatal problems	
ASA grade	I	
Family history	An uncle had undergone pyloromyotomy as a baby, no known problems with general anaesthesia	
Medications	None	
Allergies	None known	
Examination	Alert and hungry Pink Normal airway Dry mouth Chest clear, SaO_2 95% in air Normal heart sounds, pulse 160 bpm Capillary refill time 3 seconds BP 70/40 mmHg Sunken anterior fontanelle, sunken eyes	
Investigations	*Weight*	4.6 kg
	FBC	Hb 13.1 $g.dl^{-1}$, Plat 375 × 10^9 l^{-1}, WBC 10.2 × 10^9 l^{-1}
	U&Es	Na^+ 138 $mmol.l^{-1}$, K^+ 3.1 $mmol.l^{-1}$, urea 7 $mmol.l^{-1}$, creatinine 49 $\mu mol.l^{-1}$, chloride 89 $mmol.l^{-1}$
	Capillary gas	pH 7.5, pO_2 7.8 kPa, pCO_2 5.06 kPa, HCO_{3^-} 30 $mmol.l^{-1}$, BE +4.6
	Test feed	Visible peristalsis after 5 minutes Projectile vomit after 10 minutes Olive-shaped mass felt in epigastrium
	Abdominal ultrasound scan	Confirmed presence of thickened pylorus

Table 3.1
History, examination and investigation findings

antibiotics were given intravenously (30 $mg.kg^{-1}$ co-amoxiclav). 120 mg of rectal paracetamol was administered. The patient was placed on a warming mattress. The infant's blood sugar was 5.0 $mmol.l^{-1}$. The pyloric tumour was located (Figure 3.3) and the muscle incised down to but not including the mucosa.

Air was injected through the nasogastric tube to confirm the absence of a mucosal leak at the pylorus before closing the abdomen. The wound site was infiltrated with 4.5 ml of 0.25% plain bupivacaine. At the end of surgery, muscle relaxation was reversed with neostigmine 50 $\mu g.kg^{-1}$ and glycopyrrollate 10 $\mu g.kg^{-1}$. The endotracheal tube was removed in the left lateral position as soon as the baby was fully awake. The nasogastric tube was removed prior to transfer to the recovery ward (postanaesthesia care unit).

Postoperative analgesia was provided with regular doses of paracetamol 15 $mg.kg^{-1}$ for 24 hours (maximum 60 $mg.kg^{-1}.day^{-1}$). The baby was monitored on the ward for 12 hours postoperatively with an oxygen saturation and apnoea monitor. No apnoeas occurred during this time. There were no symptoms or signs of leakage from the pyloromyotomy and feeds were re-commenced 12 hours after surgery. The baby made an uneventful recovery.

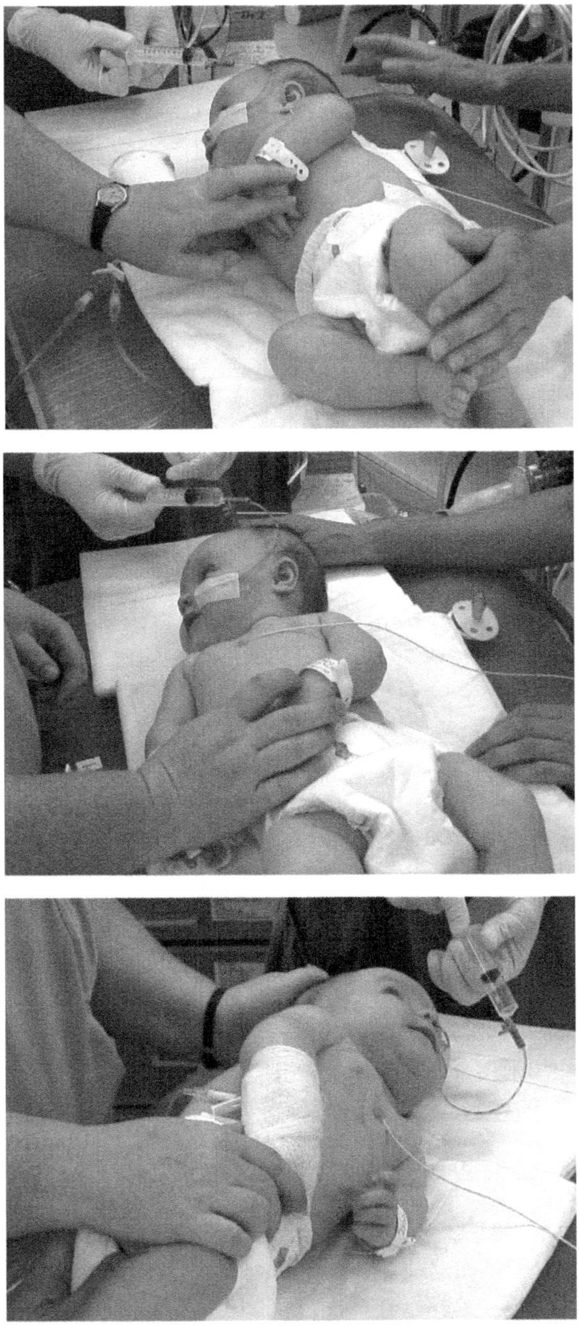

Figure 3.1(a–c)
Illustrates how gastric suction is attempted immediately prior to induction of anaesthesia in a baby with congenital hypertrophic pyloric stenosis in the right lateral, supine and left lateral positions.

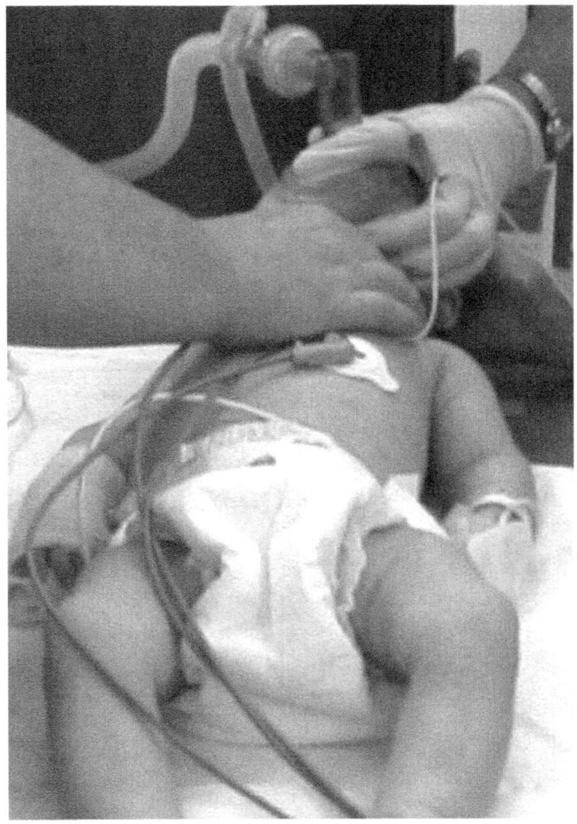

Figure 3.2
Shows the rapid sequence induction technique with cricoid pressure employed prior to pyloromyotomy.

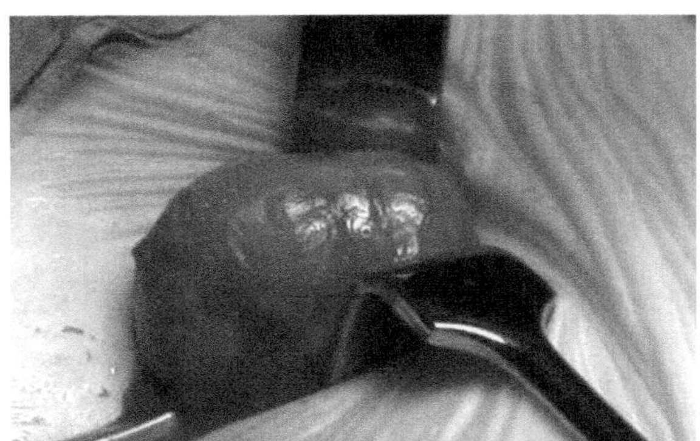

Figure 3.3
Shows the 'pyloric tumour' causing pyloric obstruction.

Discussion

Congenital hypertrophic pyloric stenosis is a common surgical condition. It mainly affects first-born males and tends to run in families, 15% of patients have a positive family history. Siblings of patients with pyloric stenosis are 15 times more likely to get pyloric stenosis. The aetiology of the condition is unknown but several theories have been proposed.[2] There are usually no associated conditions. However, elevated levels of conjugated bilirubin occur in 17% and other associated anomalies are rare occurring in 13%. There are a number of potential problems which may occur in a baby presenting with pyloric stenosis; these are outlined in Table 3.2. Pyloric stenosis is considered a medical emergency, not a surgical emergency and the baby must be fully resuscitated prior to surgery. Mortality from this condition relates to inadequate resuscitation, aspiration of stomach contents and difficult intubation. Failure to correct alkalosis can result in postoperative apnoeas. It is therefore important to address these issues prior to anaesthetic induction and surgical correction.

Vomiting in pyloric stenosis leads to loss of water, hydrogen ions, sodium ions, chloride ions and potassium ions causing the classical dehydration and hypokalaemic hypochloraemic alkalosis. Attempted compensation by the lungs involves hypoventilation and retention of carbon dioxide. There is a net increase in plasma bicarbonate concentration. In the initial stages of the disease the kidney excretes the excess bicarbonate. In the face of extracellular volume depletion the kidney attempts to conserve sodium by stimulation of aldosterone release. This attempts to conserve

Problem List	
Preoperative	Hypokalaemic hypochloraemic alkalosis Dehydration Full stomach risk Difficult intubation Elevated levels unconjugated bilirubin in 17% Associations occurring in only 13% include: Smith–Lemli–Opitz syndrome Pierre Robin Trisomy 21 Oesophageal atresia Anorectal anomalies Inguinal hernias
Peroperative	Problems associated with infant anaesthesia Securing airway in presence of full stomach risk Potential hypothermia Potential hypoglycaemia Mucosal perforation
Postoperative	Apnoeas Wound infection Wound dehiscence Incisional hernia Continued vomiting

Table 3.2
The potential problems associated with pyloric stenosis

salt and water, resulting in an increased loss of potassium and hydrogen ions by the kidney and retention of bicarbonate ions. Plasma sodium concentrations are usually maintained in the normal range. Total body potassium is low because of loss from the stomach, renal loss and extracellular to intracellular shifts because of plasma alkalosis. Plasma concentrations of potassium may be normal.

The degree of dehydration needs to be carefully assessed and the fluid replacement instituted following appropriate guidelines.[3] Severe dehydration requires a bolus of 20 $ml.kg^{-1}$ of normal saline or a colloid (for example Gelofusine®) and re-assessment. Moderate dehydration requires assessment of the fluid deficit which is added to the normal maintenance fluid requirements. 5% glucose and 0.45% saline (with 10 mmol of potassium chloride per 500 ml bag) can then be infused at the predetermined rate. Nasogastric losses should be replaced ml for ml with 0.9% normal saline. In mild dehydration 4% glucose and 0.18% saline (with 10 mmol of potassium chloride per 500 ml bag) can be used for maintenance. Regular assessment of capillary gases should be used to guide therapy and surgery should not be planned until the HCO_3^- and Cl^- levels are normal.

Who should be operating on and anaesthetizing this group of small babies has been a controversial issue for sometime. This is a common non-urgent surgical procedure and the Royal College of Surgeons have published guidelines stating that a specialist paediatric surgeon must perform the pyloromyotomy if the baby is less than 44 weeks postconceptional age. In the United Kingdom these surgeons are usually located in specialist children's centres and therefore neonates requiring pyloromyotomy should be transferred to these hospitals.[4] Pyloromyotomy may be performed in a well-organized DGH with a reasonable caseload of babies over 44 weeks postconceptional age. Only surgeons with appropriate training and experience should operate on babies. However no specific number of cases have been described as the minimum for continued surgical experience in babies.

The anaesthetist must have appropriate training and continued experience. Again there has been some debate about this with Lunn suggesting that the anaesthetist should be anaesthetizing at least one baby less than 6 months old every month.[5] In 1994 it was clear that this level of experience was not the norm.[6] However, the hospital should also provide adequate facilities and staff (including consultant and resident trainee paediatricians, paediatric nursing staff, a paediatric radiologist, suitable equipment and intensive care facilities). Operating department practitioners or anaesthetic nurses, with training and experience in working with children, should assist the anaesthetist. If any of these conditions are not fulfilled, the baby should be transferred to a hospital where they can be provided.[4]

In the theatre all equipment likely to be needed must be prepared and ready to hand, including a range of endotracheal tubes and laryngoscopes, and an introducer. Particular attention should be given to maintaining normothermia by, for example, increasing the ambient temperature and humidity (to 25 °C and 50% relative humidity), covering the baby in warm gamgee, using an overhead heater and warming blanket or a forced air warming system, and warming intravenous fluids.

Although methods are employed preoperatively to minimize the volume of gastric contents, Cook-Sather et al found the stomach often contained milk despite good preparation (including stomach washouts). Furthermore, nasogastric suction preoperatively did not substantially reduce the large volumes of gastric fluid found. 'Blind' aspiration before induction provided a reliable estimate of the volume of gastric fluid for most babies, although occasionally some gastric fluid was still retained.[7] How important this is clinically is not certain.

Cricoid pressure has been shown to effectively prevent aspiration of gastric contents in babies[8] and should be applied during induction of anaesthesia in a baby with a full stomach. However it should be remembered that the incorrect application of cricoid pressure might distort anatomy and make intubation difficult. In this case report, a rapid sequence intravenous induction with cricoid pressure was chosen. Several frequently used techniques of facilitating intubation are preferred by other anaesthetists.[5] These include the use of a non-depolarizing muscle relaxant to facilitate intubation (e.g. atracurium 0.5 $mg.kg^{-1}$, cisatracurium 0.1 $mg.kg^{-1}$) or 'deep' anaesthesia with sevoflurane. These methods avoid the use of suxamethonium, advocated by some where there may be a risk of an undiagnosed myopathy. Although more common in boys, the incidence of a myopathy is rare and so the small risk is considered by many anaesthetists to be outweighed by the real risk of aspiration of gastric contents in these circumstances. Advocates of these alternative techniques rely on preoperative preparation to minimize gastric contents. Pyloric stenosis is considered by many to be a special case of 'the full stomach' since once empty, the stomach is protected from aspiration of bile and bowel contents by the thickened pylorus.

The anaesthetic technique chosen should enable the baby to recover from anaesthesia quickly, avoiding postoperative ventilation. This is generally achieved by using a volatile agent with a rapid offset; usually no, or a single small dose of a short-acting opioid, and a small dose of a short-acting muscle relaxant. Other anaesthetic agents may be used when anaesthetizing a baby with pyloric stenosis. Although not licensed in the UK for small babies, many anaesthetists prefer the induction characteristics of propofol and routinely use propofol 3–4 $mg.kg^{-1}$ in place of thiopentone sodium. Maintenance of anaesthesia may alternatively be with isoflurane 0.5–1%, halothane 0.5–1% or desflurane 4–8%, in nitrous oxide/oxygen or air/oxygen.

Apnoea has been reported in term babies after pyloromyotomy and they should be monitored on the ward with an apnoea monitor for a minimum of 12 hours postoperatively.[9]

Learning points

- Pyloric stenosis mostly affects first-born males and occurs in 1 in 400 live births.
- Projectile non-bilious vomiting in a hungry baby is a typical presentation.
- Dehydration and electrolyte anomalies may be significant and must be fully corrected prior to planned anaesthesia and surgery.
- Pyloric stenosis is a medical emergency, not a surgical emergency.
- Surgery should be performed electively when fluid and electrolyte balance is normal.
- Good preparation in advance of the baby's arrival in theatre is essential.
- A baby with pyloric stenosis must be assumed to have a full stomach.
- The anaesthetic technique chosen should enable the baby to quickly recover from anaesthesia.
- Surgeons usually allow the babies to feed by about 12 hours after surgery, in the absence of any signs of pyloric perforation.
- Babies should be monitored on the ward with an oxygen saturation and apnoea monitor for a minimum of 12 hours postoperatively.

References

1. Jones PF. 'The general surgeon who cares for children.' *BMJ* 1986; 2: 1156–1158.
2. Ohshiro K, Puri P. Pathogenesis of infantile hypertrophic pyloric stenosis: recent progress. *Paediatr Surg Int* 1998; 13: 243–252.
3. Advanced Paediatric Life Support. The practical approach. 3rd edn. Advanced Life Support Group. *BMJ* Books.
4. The Senate of Surgeons of Great Britain and Ireland. The Provision of General Surgical Services for Children. London: 1998
5. Lunn J. 'Implications of the National Confidential Enquiry into Perioperative Deaths for paediatric anaesthesia.' *Paediatr Anaesth* 1992; 2: 69–72.
6. Stoddart PA, Brennan L, Hatch DJ, Bingham R. Postal survey of paediatric practice and training among consultant anaesthetists in the UK. *BJ Anaesth* 1994; 73: 559–563.
7. Cook-Sather SD, Tulloch HV, Liacouras CA, Schreiner MS. 'Gastric fluid volume in infants for pyloromyotomy.' *Can J Anaesth* 1997; 44: 278–283.
8. Salem MR, Wong AY, Fizzotti GF. Efficacy of cricoid pressure in preventing aspiration of gastric contents in paediatric patients. *BJ Anaesth* 1972; 44: 401–404.
9. Andropoulus DB, Heard MB, Johnson KL, Clarke JT, Rowe RW. Postanesthetic apnea in full-term infants after pyloromyotomy. *Anesthesiology* 1994; 80: 216–219.

4

Herniotomy in the *'ex-premie'*

Jane M Peutrell

Introduction

With advances in obstetric and neonatal intensive care, more premature infants with lower gestational ages and lower birth weights are surviving.[1] This leads to more of these infants requiring anaesthesia for surgery, including the repair of their inguinal hernias, a condition associated with increased prematurity.[2] Although this may appear to be a simple procedure it actually presents a significant challenge to the health care service, clinicians and the infant itself. These are highlighted in the following case history.

Case history

A 3-month-old baby presented for repair of bilateral inguinal hernias in a district hospital. He had been born by emergency Caesarean section for abruption of the placenta at 30 weeks' gestation, weighing 1200 g. He required mechanical ventilation initially for 10 days and then again at 4 weeks of age in association with sepsis. He had eventually been weaned to continuous positive airways pressure and supplementary oxygen after a short course of dexamethasone and was receiving 0.5 l of oxygen through nasal prongs until 3 weeks ago. He suffered recurrent apnoea and bradycardia (treated with theophylline) until 4 weeks ago.

He had been at home for 2 weeks and now weighed 2.4 kg. He was given iron and vitamin supplements, but no other medication.

Positive findings on examination included slight tachypnoea (48/minute), moderate subcostal and intercostal recession but no 'head-bobbing' or nasal flaring, and some crackles on auscultation. SpO_2 breathing air was 94%.

Discussion

Preoperative considerations

Institution

Babies should be managed by consultant anaesthetists and surgeons with adequate training and sufficient continuing clinical practice, in hospitals with adequate facilities and trained personnel. If the local hospital cannot meet these standards the baby should be transferred to one that can. Often this means babies must be transferred to the regional specialist centre. The general requirements for a competent surgical service for babies are given in Table 4.1.[3–5]

Surgeons and anaesthetists should not undertake 'occasional paediatric practice' because outcomes relate to the experience of the clinicians involved.[4] For anaesthesia, Lunn suggested that a 'children's anaesthetist' should manage a minimum of 12 babies aged < 6 months each year to obtain adequate experience.[6] However, anaesthetizing only one small baby per month is probably insufficient to maintain competence caring for ex-premature babies because these are the more difficult cases. Recommendations for the training and continuing experience of clinicians are given in Table 4.2.[6,7]

Preoperative assessment

At the preoperative assessment, the anaesthetist should determine the baby's weight, gestational and postnatal ages, perinatal course, and current medical condition, specifically identifying problems commonly associated with prematurity (summarized in Table 4.3).

- Suitably trained consultants in surgery and anaesthesia should be nominated to be responsible for organizing the surgical and anaesthetic services for children.[a]
- The consultant surgeon and anaesthetist responsible for the baby's immediate care should have adequate training, sufficient continuing clinical experience, and expertise in urgent surgery for babies.[a] Surgeons and anaesthetists should not undertake 'occasional paediatric practice' and 'must keep up to date and competent'.[4]
- Nurses or operating department assistants assisting the anaesthetist or providing care in recovery should have special paediatric training and skills. Appropriate paediatric equipment must be available in theatre and recovery.[5]
- The hospital services and levels of children's nurse staffing should meet the standards set out in the document *'The Welfare of Children & Young People in Hospital'* (Department of Health, 1991).[a]
- Adequate paediatric medical cover should be available.[a]
- Appropriately staffed and equipped high-dependency care for babies must be available with facilities for, and staff expert in the management of, tracheal intubation and intermittent positive pressure ventilation if required. In some large hospitals this may be best provided within the special care baby unit.
- The hospital should have support services e.g. paediatric radiology, pharmacy and laboratories (biochemistry, haematology) able to process specimens of small volume.

a Modified from the British Paediatric Association.[3]

Table 4.1
Requirements for a surgical service for babies

Postoperative apnoea

Babies born before 37 weeks' gestation are at risk of apnoea after general anaesthesia because of immaturity of central control mechanisms. Apnoea is generally defined as 'cessation of breathing for 15 seconds or for a shorter period if associated with bradycardia or oxygen desaturation'. This is in contrast to 'periodic breathing' in which there is a regular pattern of progressively increasing and then decreasing tidal volume with brief cessation of breathing lasting 2–10 seconds. Periodic breathing is common in neonates and pre-term babies, especially during rapid eye movement (REM) sleep, is not associated with dramatic changes in heart rate, and is not pathological.

The incidence of prolonged apnoea after general anaesthesia ranges from nil[8] to 81%[9] but most authors report around 30%.[10–12] Seventy-three percent are central, 6% obstructive and 21% mixed.[12] They first occur within 12 hours of surgery (and usually within 2 hours) but may then persist for up to 48 hours.[10] The incidence of apnoea is greatest in babies with the lowest postconceptional ages (postconceptional age = gestational plus postnatal age), and there is an inverse relationship with both gestational and postconceptional ages. Apnoea is particularly common until 44 weeks postconception[10,13] but the risks after general anaesthesia for inguinal herniotomy remain ≥1% until much later (54 weeks postconception for otherwise fit babies born at 35 weeks' gestation, 56 weeks for those born at 32 weeks).[13]

Apnoea may be clinically apparent or detected only at review of data recorded electronically. Many authors have used techniques of recording and subsequent data retrieval as surrogate measures of the risk of cardiorespiratory arrest although the precise relationship is unknown and most episodes of apnoea resolve without intervention.[14] However, clinically significant disturbances of breathing and life-threatening apnoea after surgery are undoubtedly more frequent in babies born prematurely.

Training

General surgery

Full-time paediatric surgeon
Holder of intercollegiate specialty examination, FRCS Paed
Holder of certificate as Provider of *'Advanced Paediatric Life Support'*

Surgeons with a substantial commitment to paediatric surgery
A minimum of 12 months in a centre accredited by the Specialist Advisory Committee for specialist training in paediatric general surgery
Holder of certificate as Provider of *'Advanced Paediatric Life Support'*

District general hospital consultants
A minimum of 6 months in a centre accredited by the Specialist Advisory Committee for specialist training in paediatric general surgery
Holder of certificate as Provider of *'Advanced Paediatric Life Support'*

Anaesthesia [a]

Consultant with a significant paediatric workload
'...individuals would be advised to obtain an additional 6 months' training in a paediatric centre (in addition to the minimum 3 months required for the Certificate of Completion of Specialist Training)'

Consultant in a specialist children's hospital
'...an additional 12 months' training in a paediatric centre (in addition to the minimum 3 months required for the Certificate of Completion of Specialist Training) would be essential'

Adequate *'continuing experience'*

General surgery

'...paediatric workload should be of adequate volume to maintain a high level of surgical competence. Typically this would equate to a minimum of one paediatric operating session each fortnight.'

Anaesthesia

Recommended minimum clinical experience each year for a *'children's anaesthetist'*:
12 babies aged <6 months
50 babies and children aged 6 months to 3 years
300 children aged >3 years

[a] Advice given by the Association of Paediatric Anaesthetists to the Royal College of Anaesthetists.

Table 4.2
Recommendations for new appointments in paediatric surgery or anaesthesia

Many authors report little correlation between apnoea and systemic disease[10,14] but this is probably because most included small numbers, and sometimes very diverse groups, of babies. However, babies with neurological impairment may be at particular risk and for much longer[10,11,15] and the incidence of apnoea decreases less quickly with age in those who are anaemic.[13] Some authors report that a clinical history of apnoea correlates with postoperative apnoea[14] but this is not supported by others.[10] Preoperative pneumography does not predict postoperative complications.[11,12]

Respiratory disease
Postoperative apnoea
Chronic lung disease
irritable airways
oxygen dependency
'stiff' lungs and increased work of breathing
ventilation: perfusion mismatch
Tracheal injury
Subglottic stenosis
Tracheomalacia
Intracranial pathology
Intraventricular haemorrhage
hydrocephalus
neuro-developmental handicap
Hypoxic brain damage
hypotonia
feeding difficulties
seizures
Anaemia
Difficult venous access

Table 4.3
Anaesthetic implications of prematurity in babies presenting for inguinal herniotomy

Chronic lung disease

Pulmonary fibrosis may occur after positive pressure ventilation for severe hyaline membrane disease, meconium aspiration or pneumonia producing chronic lung disease or 'bronchopulmonary dysplasia' (BPD). There are no precise diagnostic criteria for BPD, but clinical features include oxygen dependency, tachypneoa, intercostal recession, hypoxia and hypercarbia, and radiological changes such as hyperinflation, irregular mottling and pulmonary cystic change. Ten percent to 20% of premature babies ventilated for respiratory distress syndrome require oxygen for more than 28 days and 2–5% remain dependent beyond term. Five percent of 'very low birth weight' babies have persisting chronic lung disease at 6 months of age.

The causes of BPD are multifactorial and include hyperoxia, barotrauma, inflammation, and increased susceptibility to damage because of immaturity. The effects of pulmonary air leaks, infection, fluid overload, or left to right shunting through a patent ductus arteriosus may contribute to its development. Pathologically, there is interstitial fibrosis, which is often patchy, airway oedema, and smooth muscle hypertrophy. In severe disease (fortunately now less common) there may also be emphysema and varying degrees of obliterative bronchiolitis. The clinical effects of chronic lung disease include increased work of breathing, ventilation : perfusion mismatch, increased airway reactivity, susceptibility to pulmonary infection, and increased risk of postoperative ventilatory failure. Severe pulmonary fibrosis may also cause persistent pulmonary hypertension and right heart failure.

Tracheal injury

Subglottic stenosis

Subglottic stenosis, with narrowing of the cricoid cartilage, affects between 1% and 8% of premature babies. The aetiology includes using inappropriately large tracheal tubes, traumatic or repeated intubation, and prolonged ventilation.

Tracheomalacia

High intrathoracic pressure during mechanical ventilation may cause secondary tracheomalacia with widening of the membranous part of the tracheal ring and deficiency of the cartilage. The tracheal wall becomes weak and collapses easily. Clinical features include a 'seal-like' cough, expiratory stridor, wheeze, and airway obstruction (particularly if the baby is upset). Symptoms often become worse immediately after extubation of the trachea.

Intracranial haemorrhage and brain damage

Intraventricular haemorrhage

Intraventricular haemorrhage (IVH), resulting from rupture of the microvasculature into the cerebral ventricles, is the commonest central nervous system lesion in neonates. IVH is more prevalent in babies < 34 weeks' gestation (20% in those with birth weights < 1500 g), particularly if they have a stormy clinical course. The aetiology is probably multifactorial. Sick or immature babies may have impaired cerebral autoregulation allowing changes in blood pressure (e.g. secondary to clinical interventions) to directly affect cerebral blood flow and volume. Cerebral blood flow is also increased by hypercarbia, hypoxia, or increased local metabolism (e.g. during seizures). Raised central venous pressure (because of high airway pressure, poorly co-ordinated invasive positive pressure ventilation, rapid infusion of

IV fluids, patent ductus arteriosus, pneumothorax, etc.) may also rupture the fragile microvasculature. Other factors include increased osmolality (e.g. hypernatraemia, hyperglycaemia) and coagulopathy. Clinical signs of significant bleeds present within 3 days but minor degrees of haemorrhage are asymptomatic.

IVH is a common cause of neonatal hydrocephalus in which blood clot or debris obstructs the flow of cerebrospinal fluid (CSF) at the aqueduct between the 3rd and 4th ventricles or impairs absorption across the arachnoid villi. The obstruction often resolves but a small number of babies will need a ventriculoperitoneal shunt to treat increased intracranial pressure. Others can be managed medically with drugs that reduce the production of CSF, such as isosorbide, acetazolamide or frusemide. Some babies with ventriculomegaly develop intracranial hypertension several months after discharge from hospital. Moderate to severe IVH is frequently associated with neurodevelopmental impairment.

Birth asphyxia

Birth asphyxia is associated with cerebral infarction and intracranial haemorrhage. Both lesions may cause profound cerebral injury with persistent seizures, hypotonia, and feeding difficulties.

Anaemia

Premature babies often have a low haemoglobin (about 8 g.dl^{-1} at 48 weeks' postconception) because of the combined effects of the 'physiological anaemia of infancy' and frequent venesection during the first weeks of life.

Difficult venous access

Peripheral venous access may be difficult in babies born prematurely, particularly those with a difficult postnatal course.

Investigations

Specific preoperative investigations are determined by the condition of the baby (e.g. chest X-ray for pulmonary infection, cranial ultrasound or computed tomography for suspected hydrocephalus) and any medication prescribed (e.g. urea and electrolytes if receiving acetazolamide or frusemide for hydrocephalus). In addition to routine observations, a full blood count and SpO_2 should be obtained in all babies.

Perioperative management

Fasting

Prolonged fasting increases the risks of dehydration and hypoglycaemia in babies and should be avoided. If a regional anaesthetic technique is chosen, hunger can also make them difficult to manage during surgery. Breast milk leaves the stomach almost twice as fast as formula feed and fasting guidelines generally differ between the two. In many hospitals, babies are allowed breast milk until 3 hours, or bottled milk until 4 hours, before surgery. Clear fluids, such as glucose solution, can be given for up to 2 hours before the induction of anaesthesia without increasing the volume of gastric contents. An intravenous infusion should be started if the time of surgery is difficult to predict.

Premedication

Sedative premedication is unnecessary. Topical anaesthetics, such as EMLA® or Ametop®, can be applied if IV induction is planned. Uptake across the skin depends upon the maturity of the stratum corneum, which is determined by postnatal, rather than postconceptional age. EMLA® is safe in babies > 3 months if no more than 2 g, spread over < 16 cm^2, is applied for less than 4 hours (although it does not have a product licence for babies < 12 months). Ametop® is licensed for full term babies older than 4 weeks. If a regional technique is chosen, a small amount of topical anaesthetic can be applied over an appropriate area of the lower back.

Some anaesthetists prescribe atropine (20 µg.kg^{-1}) orally to reduce airway secretions and the vagal effects on the heart. Others prefer to give atropine IV at induction or only if clinically indicated.

Anaesthesia

General principles

The anaesthetic plan must take account of the general principles of anaesthesia for any small baby, such as having appropriate equipment and personnel, consideration of age-related physiology and pharmacology, preventing hypothermia, and so on. Steroid cover is not required.

Caffeine

Caffeine 10 mg.kg^{-1} IV at induction reduces the risk of apnoea after general anaesthesia for inguinal herniotomy in otherwise healthy preterm babies.[9]

General anaesthesia

The older agents used for general anaesthesia are associated with increased incidence of apnoea compared with regional techniques (see below). Authors have found no correlation with particular drugs (except for ketamine) probably because their studies involved small numbers of babies. Although the incidence of apnoea associated with the newer agents (sevoflurane, desflurane) is not fully known, their pharmacological characteristics make them attractive. Desflurane is associated with a much quicker recovery compared with isoflurane after pyoloromyotomy. Wolf et al also reported that none of the babies given desflurane (n = 9) had any apnoeic episodes in the immediate period after extubation compared with three of the 11 given isoflurane.[16]

Tracheal intubation and positive pressure ventilation of the lungs are usual because the airway is difficult to control with a facemask, laryngeal mask airways are often unreliable in small babies, and gas exchange is easily compromised by general anaesthesia (because of the effect of immaturity and chronic lung disease).

Anecdotally, newborn or premature babies are sensitive to opioids and local anaesthetic techniques should be used in preference for postoperative pain control. A regional block sited before surgical incision reduces the requirement for volatile agents and is associated with more rapid recovery.

A common general anaesthetic technique is to induce anaesthesia with sevoflurane in oxygen, and facilitate intubation with an intermediate-acting relaxant, such as atracurium. Light general anaesthesia, maintained with desflurane in air/oxygen, is then combined with a caudal block. Muscle relaxation is reversed at the end of surgery and the tracheal tube removed only when the baby is wide awake and breathing regularly.

Regional techniques

Regional techniques (e.g. subarachnoid or caudal block) without general anaesthesia or sedation are associated with a much lower incidence of postoperative apnoea compared with general anaesthesia using older agents such as halothane.[17,18] However, there may be few advantages compared with modern anaesthetics. The preliminary results of a small study suggest that clinical recovery from light general anaesthesia with sevoflurane (combined with a caudal block) or subarachnoid block was similar, while subarachnoid anaesthesia had a failure rate of 28%.[19] Trying to decrease the rate of failure by using routine sedation during surgery is not advisable. Sedation, particularly with ketamine, is also associated with postoperative apnoea,[17] eliminating the major advantage of regional block.

I now use regional anaesthesia only in those babies with significant medical disease, usually chronic lung disease. Babies with large hernias may be particularly difficult to manage using a regional technique, and general anaesthesia may be a better option.

Hypotension is not usually a feature of central blockade in babies and vasopressors or preloading with IV fluids are not usually required.

Subarachnoid block

Subarachnoid anaesthesia produces a rapid and dense sensorimotor block with a variable and limited duration, which rarely exceeds 45 minutes. For a given dose, the height of block differs widely between babies. The technique is often unreliable, even with experienced clinicians. General anaesthesia is required in about 10% of babies, usually because the subarachnoid space cannot be identified or the height or duration of block is inadequate. A further 10% require additional anaesthetic or analgesic supplements (sedation or infiltration with local anaesthetic), often during deep dissection of the hernial sac or traction on the peritoneum or spermatic cord. Subarachnoid block provides little postoperative analgesia, so it is useful to infiltrate the wound at the end of surgery, keeping the total dose of local anaesthetic used during anaesthesia within the accepted maximum ($2.5\,mg.kg^{-1}$ for bupivacaine).

Technique

The ECG should be monitored but blood pressure and SpO_2 measurements are often unreliable before the block is established because of movement. The volumes of local anaesthetic are relatively small compared with those for caudal block and some practitioners insert the IV cannula in the foot once the block is effective.

Subarachnoid block should be an aseptic technique. The baby can be held either sitting (the 'Buddha' position) or in the left lateral position with the back and hips flexed. The neck should be kept reasonably extended to prevent oxygen desaturation. The spinal cord terminates at L3 in newborns and an interspace below this should be chosen. Sacral interspaces can also be used because the ligaments of the sacrum do not start ossifying until 18 years of age. A small volume of lignocaine should be infiltrated into the deeper dermis to improve the analgesia obtained from topical anaesthetics. A short-bevelled needle with a solid obturator is then advanced slowly at right angles to the skin. A 'pop' is usually felt as the tip penetrates the dura at about 0.5–1.0 cm. The position of the needle within the subarachnoid space is confirmed by aspiration of CSF and an appropriate volume (Table 4.4[20,21]) of local anaesthetic injected slowly. The volumes used are generally large, probably because the volume of CSF in babies and children is twice that of adults.

Amethocaine (tetracaine) is the agent of choice in North America and has a longer duration of action than bupivacaine.

Babies often sleep during surgery, probably because of the effects of sensory de-afferentation. Those who are awake can be comforted with a 'dummy' dipped in glucose solution. It is advisable to monitor the blood pressure from a cuff on the leg so the baby is not disturbed during measurement.

Complications

The height of block for a given volume of local anaesthetic varies considerably between patients and a high block, characterized by weak cry and ventilatory compromise, can occur unpredictably. A high block associated with a hyperbaric solution has also occurred when a baby's legs were inadvertently raised to site a diathermy plate.

Although the incidence of postoperative apnoea is reduced, it is not eliminated and life-threatening apnoea has been reported. Postoperative supervision and monitoring should be consistent with the standards used after general anaesthesia.

Caudal block

Caudal block is an alternative, but in my experience, less satisfactory technique. The onset of a block adequate for surgery is slow (approximately 14 minutes), motor block is incomplete, and the baby's legs often need to be restrained during the operation.

Technique

Preparation, monitoring, and postoperative care are the same as for subarachnoid anaesthesia. An IV cannula should be sited before the block because of the larger doses of local anaesthetics used and the risks of intravascular injection.

The baby can be held, with its hips flexed, securely over an assistant's shoulders or more usually lying in the left lateral position. The sacral hiatus lies at the apex of an equilateral triangle formed with the posterior superior iliac spines. The needle should be inserted

Isobaric:[20] $1\ mg.kg^{-1}$ of 0.5% *or*	
body weight.kg^{-1}	*volume.ml*$^{-1}$
<2	0.25
2–5	0.75
5	1.0
Hyperbaric:[21] $0.06\ ml.kg^{-1}$	

Table 4.4
Volumes of bupivacaine 0.5% for subarachnoid block in babies

towards the apex of the sacral hiatus because this is the position of the greatest anterior–posterior diameter of the caudal space. The sacrum is relatively flat compared with older children and adults, so the angle of approach with the needle should be more shallow, about 15–20°. A 20g or 22g IV cannula is ideal. It provides a positive 'give' as the shoulders penetrate the sacrococcygeal membrane and the needle acts as an obturator. Once sited, the cannula can be advanced over the needle into the caudal space with little risk of vascular or dural penetration, reducing the likelihood of displacement during injection and allowing local anaesthetic to be given at a higher segmental level. After negative aspiration for blood or CSF, $1\ ml.kg^{-1}$ of 0.25% bupivacaine should be injected slowly. An epidural catheter can also be threaded and used to give further doses of local anaesthetic to extend the duration of block (maximum of $0.25\ mg.kg^{-1}.h^{-1}$).

Complications

Reported problems include a 'total spinal', intravascular injection of local anaesthetic, and penetration of the sacrum. A 'total spinal' is characterized by apnoea, loss of consciousness, and dilated pupils, but haemodynamic variables tend to remain very stable. The airway and ventilation should be supported, but it is usually unnecessary to postpone surgery. The block resolves within a few hours. As for subarachnoid block, the risks of postoperative apnoea are probably reduced but not eliminated.

Postoperative care

General care

Babies born prematurely should be observed closely after surgery and nursed on a high-dependency or intensive care unit with staff trained in advanced life support and facilities for positive pressure ventilation. In a large district hospital, care could be provided either in a side room of the special care baby unit or an appropriately staffed and equipped cubicle of the general intensive care unit.

Monitoring

The baby should be monitored using an apnoea alarm, SpO_2, and ECG for a minimum of 12 hours after surgery or the last recorded apnoeic episode. Most techniques for detecting apnoea monitor chest or abdominal wall movements, either by impedence pneumography (through the ECG electrodes) or changes in pressure in a pad attached to the abdomen, and will not identify obstructive causes.

Eighty per cent of apnoeic episodes are missed by nurses and 60% are not detected by pulse oximetry although the clinical significance of this is not known. In the study by Bell et al, both nursing observations and oximetry alerted staff to a problem in the single baby needing treatment.[14]

Analgesia

In general, paracetamol given regularly for 24 hours provides satisfactory analgesia in combination with a caudal block or wound infiltration with local anaesthetic. Anderson et al suggest $40\,mg.kg^{-1}$ as a loading dose rectally, and then $30\,mg.kg^{-1}$ given 12 hours rectally or $20\,mg.kg^{-1}$ orally every 8 hours.[22]

Fluids

Intravenous fluids (e.g. glucose 5% with saline 0.45%) should be continued at maintenance rates of $4\,ml.kg^{-1}.hour^{-1}$ until the baby is feeding satisfactorily.

Learning points

- Babies should be managed by consultant anaesthetists and surgeons with adequate training and sufficient continuing clinical practice, in a hospital with adequate facilities and trained personnel. If the local hospital cannot meet these standards the baby should be transferred to one that can.
- Ex-premature babies up to 60 weeks' postconceptional age are at risk of life-threatening apnoea after anaesthesia.
- Ventilatory stimulants, such as caffeine, given at induction reduce the incidence of postoperative apnoea.
- Regional techniques may reduce, but not eliminate, the risk of postoperative apnoea.
- Ex-premature babies should be monitored (electrocardiograph, SpO_2, apnoea alarm) for a minimum of 12 hours after surgery or the last recorded apnoea episode, in a ward with the equipment and personnel immediately available to provide advanced life support and institute positive pressure ventilation.

References

1. Draper ES, Manktelow B, Field DJ, James D. Prediction of survival for preterm births by weight and gestational age: retrospective population based study. *BMJ* 1999; 319: 1093–1097.
2. Peevy KJ, Speed FA, Hoff CJ. Epidemiology of inguinal hernias in preterm neonates. *Pediatrics* 1986; 77: 246–247.
3. British Paediatric Association. The Transfer of Infants and Children for Surgery. 1993.
4. Campling EA, Devlin HB, Lunn JN (1990). The report of the National Enquiry into Peri-operative Deaths (1989).
5. Royal College of Anaesthetists. Guidelines for the Provision of Anaesthetic Services. 1999.
6. Lunn JN. Implications of the National Enquiry into Peri-operative Deaths for paediatric anaesthesia. *Paediatr Anaesth* 1992; 2: 69–72.
7. Royal College of Surgeons. Children's Surgery – a First Class Service. England.
8. Welborn LG, Ramirez N, Oh TH et al. Postanaesthetic apnea and periodic breathing in infants. *Anesthesiology* 1986; 65: 658–661.
9. Welborn LG, Hannallah RS, Fink R et al. High-dose caffeine suppresses postoperative apnea in former preterm infants. *Anesthesiology* 1989; 71: 347–349.
10. Malviya S, Swartz J, Lerman J. Are all preterm infants younger than 60 weeks postconceptional age at risk for postanesthetic apnea? *Anesthesiology* 1993; 78: 1076–1081.
11. Kurth CD, Spitzer AR, Broennle AM, Downes JJ. Postoperative apnoea in preterm infants. *Anesthesiology* 1987; 66: 483–488.
12. Kurth CD, LeBard SE. Association of postoperative apnea, airway obstruction, and hypoxaemia in former premature infants. *Anesthesiology* 1991; 75: 22–26.
13. Cote CJ, Zaslavsky A, Downes JJ et al. Postoperative apnea in former preterm infants after inguinal herniorrhaphy. *Anesthesiology* 1995; 82: 809–822.
14. Bell C, Dubose R, Seashore J et al. Infant apnea detection after herniorrhaphy. *J Clin Anaesth* 1995; 7: 219–223.
15. Liu LMP, Cote CJ, Goudsouzian NG et al. Life-threatening apnea in infants recovering from anesthesia. *Anesthesiology* 1983; 59: 506–510.

16. Wolf AR, Lawson RA, Dryden CM, Davies FW. Recovery after desflurane anaesthesia in the infant: comparison with isoflurane. *Br J Anaesth* 1996; 76: 362–364.
17. Welborn LG, Rice LJ, Hannallah RS et al. Postoperative apnea in former preterm infants: prospective comparison of spinal and general anesthesia. *Anesthesiology* 1990; 72: 838–842.
18. Krane EJ, Haberkern CM, Jacobson LE. Postoperative apnea, bradycardia, and oxygen desaturation in formerly premature infants: prospective comparison of spinal and general anesthesia. *Anesth Analges* 1995; 80: 7–13.
19. William JM, Stoddart PA, Williams SA, Wolf AR. Post-operative recovery after inguinal herniotomy in ex-premature infants: comparison between sevoflurane and spinal anaesthesia. *Br J Anaesth* 2001; 86: 366–371.
20. Mahe V, Ecoffey C. Spinal anaesthesia with isobaric bupiracaine in infants. *Anesthiology* 1988; 68: 601–603.
21. Gallagher TM, Cream PM. Spinal anasthesia in infants born prematurely. *Anaesthesia* 1989; 44: 434–436.
22. Anderson BJ, Holford NHG, Woollard G. Paracetamol kinetics in neonates. *Anaesth Intens Care* 1997; 25: 721–722.

Further reading

Sims C, Johnson CM. Postoperative apnoea in infants. *Anaesth Intens Care* 1994; 22: 40–45.

Welborn LG. Post-operative apnea in the former preterm infant: a review. *Paediatr Anaesth* 1992; 2: 37–44.

5

Anaesthesia for the Kasai procedure (portoenterostomy)

Miguel Plaza-Barrera and David William Green

Introduction

Extrahepatic biliary atresia (EHBA) occurs in newborn infants and is the end result of a destructive inflammatory process of unknown aetiology resulting in the absence of patent extrahepatic bile ducts. It is the leading cause of cholestasis in infants younger than 3 months and the leading indication for liver transplantation in children.

It is characterized by worsening cholestasis (jaundice, direct hyperbilirubinaemia, dark urine and acholic stools), hepatic fibrosis and cirrhosis leading to portal hypertension and a decline in hepatic synthetic function.[1]

The incidence of EHBA is 6 per 100,000 births in the UK and slightly more common in females (1.2 : 1). It is a progressive inflammatory/sclerotic process divided into two types, fetal or embryonic and perinatal. The former is associated in 20% of cases with other structural abnormalities such as polysplenia, preduodenal portal vein, situs inversus, absent inferior vena cava, cardiac defects, anomalous hepatic artery supply and intestinal malrotation. In the latter, the bile ducts are patent at birth with early progression to cholestasis.[2]

The aetiology of EHBA remains unclear and early diagnosis and treatment remains the key for survival. Several factors have been implicated. These include perinatal viral infections (reovirus and rotavirus),[3,4] genetic factors,[5–8] autoimmune disorders[9,10] and defects of morphogenesis (ductal plate malformation).[11] EHBA presents with three main types of obstruction (Figure 5.1): type 1, with atresia of the common bile duct; type 2, with additional atresia of the common hepatic duct, but residual patency of the right and left ducts; and type 3, atresia of the whole extrahepatic duct system.[12]

Complications of EHBA include cholangitis, portal hypertension, nutritional issues and pruritus (Table 5.1).[2]

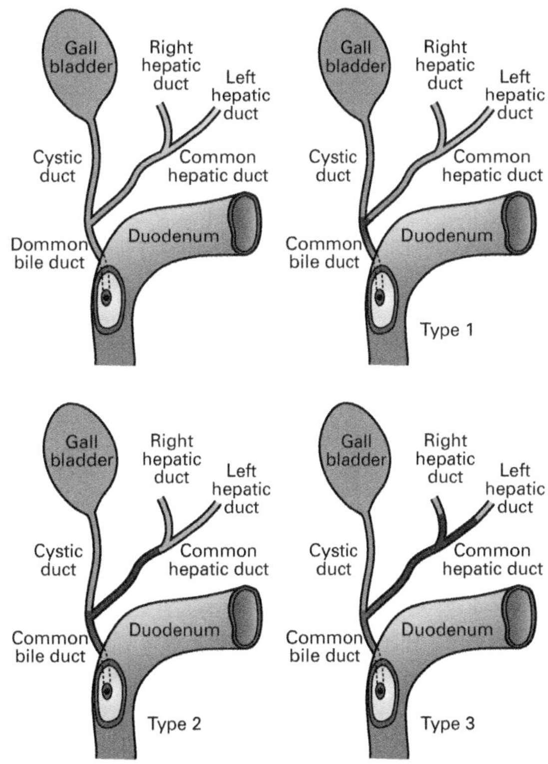

Figure 5.1
Different types of extrahepatic biliary atresia. See text for details.

Kasai portoenterostomy may restore bile flow and if successful achieve a 10-year survival of 90% with a native liver.[13,14] Before this operation the disease was uniformly fatal. It remains the standard first-line intervention.

Complication	Frequency rate (%)	Current treatment options
Cholangitis	40–60	Prophylactic antibiotics (oral neomycin) Bile acid treatment Steroids (1–2 weeks)
Portal hypertension	35–75	Prophylactic sclerotherapy Endoscopic variceal band ligation β-blockers Octreotide/somatostatin Vasopressin/terlipressin
Nutritional problems Growth failure Fat-soluble vitamin deficiency		Medium-chain triglyceride formulas nasogastric feed Fat-soluble vitamin supplements
Pruritus		Ursodeoxycholic acid Rifampicin Nalmefene

Table 5.1
Complications following portoenterostomy (Kasai procedure), in order of frequency, and current treatments

Success depends on two factors, the centre performing the operation and the age at which the surgical procedure is performed. Centres performing > 5–10 Kasai procedures/year achieve a 20% increase in survival and primary success.[14] As for the age at which the surgical procedure is performed, success rate decreases as age increases (86% success rate when performed before 8 weeks, 36% when before 12 weeks).[15] The reason for survival being less dependent on age at operation is due to improved professional education, early referral and the fact that liver transplantation is now available for the so called 'failed procedure'. Nowadays the Kasai procedure is performed before 90 days and only in selected cases thereafter.[16] Death before 2 years of age is inevitable without hepatic portoenterostomy. Primary failure of this operation is the leading indication for paediatric liver transplantation worldwide.[17]

Differential diagnosis of jaundice in the newborn

The differential diagnosis of persistent 'pathological' jaundice in the infant includes EHBA, choledochal cyst, neonatal hepatitis, intrahepatic biliary hypoplasia, and inspissated bile syndrome (Table 5.2). The first two are the two conditions most commonly requiring surgery.

- Liver function tests: serum bile acids, bilirubin, gamma glutamyl transpeptidase, urinary bile acids, stool colour cards
- Biliary scintigraphy
- Duodenal bile aspiration
- Abdominal ultrasound (90% sensitivity/ specificity)
- Liver biopsy
- Endoscopic retrograde cholangiography (ERCP)
- Magnetic resonance cholangiography
- Laparoscopy with directly visualized percutaneous cholangiogram

Table 5.2
Clinical, laboratory and radiological tests used for selection of patients for exploratory laparotomy in EHBA

Choledochal cyst is a congenital abnormality of the pancreatico–biliary system of unknown origin manifested by jaundice, abdominal mass, and if uncorrected, cholangitis and cirrhosis. It presents at any time from the perinatal period to adulthood and the anaesthetic sequence in the infant is similar to that of EHBA although the underlying hepatic function is normal, apart from the obstructive jaundice.[1] Other conditions that mimic EHBA include Alagille syndrome, cystic fibrosis and alpha 1 antitrypsin deficiency.

Definitive diagnosis is by demonstration of a fibrotic extrahepatic biliary tree at exploratory laparotomy. Selection of candidates for laparotomy include several invasive and non-invasive procedures (Table 5.2).[2] None of them are 100% sensitive or specific for EHBA.

Surgery

Combined therapy of early hepatic portoenterostomy and hepatic transplantation where cure is not possible have greatly improved the prognosis of EHBA with a 10-year survival of 90%.[13,14] Repeated revisions, except for obvious mechanical failure, should not be undertaken and, at the first sign of failure, the child should be urgently referred for hepatic transplantation assessment.[18] Hepatic artery resistance index measured by Doppler ultrasound is an early predictor of rapid deterioration and death in children with EHBA, with a resistance index of > 1.0 indicating a very high risk of early mortality.

Having confirmed the diagnosis by laparotomy, the surgical procedure involves three stages:[12,13,19]

1. Liver mobilization and dissection of atresic bile ducts (up to the liver capsule) at the porta hepatis;
2. preparation of a Roux-en-y loop of jejunum; and
3. anastomosis of the Roux-en-y loop to the prepared area at the porta hepatis which is then used as the conduit for bile drainage.

Some centres construct a valved conduit in an attempt to reduce subsequent incidence of cholangitis due to reflux of intestinal bacteria.

Anaesthesia

All considerations of neonatal anaesthesia apply. Anaesthetic problems include:

- Impaired hepatic function (especially in older children); drug metabolism is relatively unimpaired
- Hypoprothrombinaemia and impaired coagulation (older children)
- Blood loss is minimal but can be extensive; administration of gelatins/fresh frozen plasma (FFP) for volume replacement is common
- Hypotension due to surgical manipulation of the liver
- Heat loss due to extensive exposure of intra-abdominal contents.

Preoperative

Haemoglobin and clotting factors are checked, but significant coagulopathies (platelets < 100,000, INR > 1.5 : 1) are rarely seen. Vitamin K, 1 mg i.m., is administered for at least 4 days preoperatively.[20] One unit of blood and FFP are available for transfusion although this is rare as blood loss is usually minimal.

Clear fluids are administered for 24 hours preoperatively and the patient starved for 4 hours prior to surgery. An infusion of 10% glucose is usually commenced in the ward.

Oral neomycin (50 mg.kg^{-1}) is given for 24 hours at 4-hour intervals for gut sterilization in order to reduce the incidence of ascending cholangitis.

Atropine 0.05–0.1 mg (either i.m. or oral) can be given as premedication 30–60 minutes before surgery although more frequently is given intravenously at induction of anaesthesia.

Perioperative

Prior to induction of anaesthesia the patient is attached to monitoring (ECG, non-invasive blood pressure and pulse oximetry). The operating room is kept warm (26–28 °C) and the baby is placed on a thermostatically controlled warming blanket. Other methods of heat conservation are used during surgery (Bair Hugger®, fluid warmer, heat and moisture exchanger humidifier, warm irrigating fluids for intra-abdominal cavity and minimizing exposure of intra-abdominal contents).

Following preoxygenation, induction of anaesthesia is usually by inhalation of sevoflurane although intravenous induction with thiopentone can be used. Atropine is usually given i.v at induction as well as antibiotics (gentamicin 2.5 mg.kg^{-1} and cefoxitin

30 mg.kg^{-1}). A suitable uncuffed tube is inserted after muscle paralysis is achieved, usually with atracurium (0.5 mg.kg^{-1}). This, together with cis-atracurium, is the muscle relaxant of choice in patients with uncertain hepatic function.[19] A nerve stimulator is used to ensure adequate levels of muscle relaxation and subsequent doses are given on visual reappearance of the first twitch of the 'train-of-four'. A nasogastric tube (size 8 or 10-Fr) and a rectal or oesophageal temperature probe are inserted following intubation. The lungs are mechanically ventilated with humidified gases with end-tidal carbon dioxide maintained at approximately 3.5–5%.

The child usually comes to the operating room with a reliable i.v. cannula and a 10% dextrose infusion. This infusion is sometimes changed to glucose saline for maintenance with control of blood glucose in order to avoid hypoglycaemia. Maintenance fluids are kept at a fixed rate for weight (4 ml.kg^{-1} standard formula for first 10 kg weight). Blood loss is minimal and blood replacement unusual. Blood loss is replaced with warmed blood if it exceeds 10% of the estimated blood volume. Colloids 10–20 ml.kg^{-1} (gelatins or FFP) are used for third space losses and for maintenance of perfusion pressures (measured after the insertion of a central venous catheter) especially prior to liver manipulation. All fluids must be warmed. This usually keeps adequate filling pressures. Ascites is not usually a prominent feature in these cases, but if it is, 4.5% albumin in 0.9% sodium chloride can be used to replace losses. Should an inotrope be needed, dopamine or dobutamine (15 mg.kg^{-1} in 50 ml 5% dextrose at a rate starting 1 ml.h^{-1} = 5 µg.kg^{-1}.min^{-1}) are the inotropes of choice. The use of inotropes is extremely rare as judicious fluid replacement allows reversal of surgical hypotension in most cases. Urine output is not formally assessed in all cases.

Most centres institute invasive monitoring as this allows monitoring of blood gases and tight control of perfusion pressures, but other centres only use non-invasive monitoring unless it is a re-do procedure. This consists of an arterial cannula (either radial or femoral) and central venous pressure monitoring with a triple lumen catheter size 5-Fr (internal/external jugular or femoral). Cannulas sited at the upper part of the body are preferred to the femoral location as intra-abdominal compression during surgery makes them slightly less reliable, as inferior vena cava (IVC) compression generates a back pressure in the lower half of the body that does not reflect the transient hypotension generated in the upper half while the compression persists, but they are certainly useful when difficulties arise in achieving placement in the upper part. Sudden hypotension can occur due to IVC compression during surgical manipulation of the liver. This can be minimized by placing the infant in a slightly head down position, by lightening anaesthesia or by judicious fluid loading.

Maintenance of anaesthesia is achieved with a mixture of sevoflurane/air/oxygen (FiO_2 of approximately 0.4). Nitrous oxide is avoided to decrease gut distension during and after the procedure. All gases are humidified and end-tidal carbon dioxide maintained to normal levels of 3.5–4.5% (5–6 kPa).

Analgesia intraoperatively is provided with morphine (0.1 mg.kg^{-1}) or fentanyl (0.03–0.05 mg.kg^{-1}) as required.

At the end of the operation residual muscle paralysis can be reversed with neostigmine and glycopyrrolate, although in the majority of cases this is not needed, and the infant is extubated in the operating room.

Postoperative

The infant is returned to a paediatric high-dependency unit spontaneously breathing with humidified oxygen. Continuous monitoring (ECG, non-invasive blood pressure, temperature and pulse oximetry) is maintained, and i.v. fluids and blood given as required. Non-blood abdominal drainage loss is replaced with colloid, usually FFP. Nasogastric drainage is continued until bowel activity is restored.

Intravenous antibiotics are continued for 5–7 days to reduce the incidence of ascending cholangitis (pyrexia, increasing bilirubin levels). Long-term prophylaxis with oral antibiotics is usually unsuccessful in preventing recurrent cholangitis; however, oral neomycin is useful in some cases.[21]

Pain assessment is difficult in this age group. A simple 5-point behavioural assessment can be used. A morphine infusion is prepared by weight in kg of baby as mg of morphine (e.g. a 4-kg baby has 4 mg of morphine) diluted in a 50-ml syringe of saline. No loading dose is needed if the baby has received morphine intraoperatively. The infusion rate is then set at 0.5–2 ml.h^{-1}, i.e. to a maximum of 1 mg.kg^{-1} per day.

Despite derangement of hepatic function tests, drug doses need little modification as hepatic synthetic and metabolic functions are relatively unimpaired.

Postoperative problems include ascending cholangitis, portal hypertension with oesophageal varices and hepatic fibrosis in 30% of cases.[22] Hepatic failure or progressive hepatic dysfunction requires liver transplantation.

References

1. Green DW, Howard ER, Davenport M. Anaesthesia, perioperative management and outcome of correction of extrahepatic biliary atresia in the infant: a review of 50 cases in the King's College Hospital series. *Paed Anaesth* 2000; 10: 581–589.
2. Narkeewicz MR. Biliary atresia: an update on our understanding of the disorder. *Curr Opin Pediatr* 2001; 13: 435–440.
3. Tyler KL, Sokol RJ, Oberhaus SM et al. Detection of reovirus RNA in hepatobiliary tissue from patients with extrahepatic biliary atresia and choledochal cysts. *Hepatology* 1998; 27: 1475–1482.
4. Riepenhoff-Talty M, Gouvea V, Evans MJ et al. Detection of group C rotavirus in infants with extrahepatic biliary atresia. *J Infect Dis* 1996; 174: 8–15.
5. Smith BM, Laberge JM, Schreiber R et al. Familial biliary atresia in three siblings including twins. *J Pediatr* 1991; 26: 1331–1333.
6. Gunasekaran TS, Hassal EG, Steinbrecher UP et al. Recurrence of extrahepatic biliary atresia in two half sibs. *Am J Med Genet* 1992; 43: 592–594.
7. Danesino C, Spadoni E, Buzzi A. Familial biliary atresia. *Am J Med Genet* 1999; 85: 195.
8. Shim WK, Kasai M, Spence MA. Racial influence on the incidence of biliary atresia. *Prog Pediatr Surg* 1974; 6: 53–62.
9. Silveira TR, Salzano FM, Donaldson PT et al. Association between HLA and extrahepatic biliary atresia. *J Pediatr Gastroenterol Nutr* 1993; 16: 114–117.
10. Jurado A, Jara P, Camarena C et al. Is extrahepatic biliary atresia an HLA-associated disease? *J Pediatr Gastroenterol Nutr* 1997; 25: 557–558.
11. Mazziotti MV, Willis LK, Heuckeroth RO et al. Anomalous development of the hepatobiliary system in the Inv mouse. *Hepatology* 1999; 30: 372–378.
12. Howard ER. Biliary atresia: aetiology, management and complications. In: Howard ER, Stringer MD, Colombani PM, eds. Surgery of the Liver, Bile Ducts and Pancreas in Children. London: Arnold, 2002: 103–132.
13. Kasai M, Suzuki S. A new operation for 'non-correctable' biliary atresia: hepatic portoenterostomy. *Shujitsu* 1959; 13: 733–739.
14. McKiernan PJ, Baker AJ, Kelly DA. The frequency and outcome of biliary atresia in the UK and Ireland. *Lancet* 2000; 355: 25–29.
15. McClement JW, Howard ER, Mowat AP. Results of surgical treatment for extrahepatic biliary atresia in United Kingdom 1980–2. Survey conducted on behalf of the British Paediatric Association Gastroenterology Group and the British Association of Paediatric Surgeons. *Br Med J (Clin Res Ed)* 1985; 290: 345–347.
16. Chardot C, Carton M, Spire-Bendelac N et al. Is the Kasai operation still indicated in children older than 3 months diagnosed with biliary atresia? *J Pediatr* 2001; 138: 224–228.
17. Beath S, Pearmain G, Kelly D et al. Liver transplantation in babies and children with extrahepatic biliary atresia. *J Pediatr Surg* 1993; 28: 1044–1047.
18. Corbally MT, Heaton N, Rela M et al. Emergency liver transplantation after Kasai portoenterostomy. *Arch Dis Child* 1994; 70: 147–148.
19. Suruga K, Miyano T, Arai T et al. A study on hepatic portoenterostomy for the treatment of atresia of the biliary tract. *Surg Gynecol Obstet* 1984; 159: 53–58.
20. Yanofsky RA, Jackson VG, Lilly JR et al. The multiple coagulopathies of biliary atresia. *Am J Hematol* 1984; 16: 171–180.
21. Simpson DA, Green DW. Use of atracurium during major abdominal surgery in infants with hepatic dysfunction from biliary atresia. *Br J Anaesth* 1986; 58: 1214–1217.
22. Mones RL, DeFelice AR, Preud'Homme D. Use of neomycin as the prophylaxis against recurrent cholangitis after Kasai portoenterostomy. *J Pediatr Surg* 1994; 29: 422–424.

6

Anaesthesia for repair of cleft palate

Judith Dunnet

Introduction

Cleft lip and/or palate is the most common congenital craniofacial malformation with an incidence of around 1 in 700 live births.

Although cleft lip/palate occurs most frequently as an isolated anomaly, it is well recognized that it may be associated with other congenital defects. A recent review[1] of 616 babies with cleft lip/palates showed that 79% of these had isolated defects. Of these isolated cases, 85% of bilateral cleft lips and 70% of unilateral cleft lips were found in combination with a cleft palate.

The aetiology of cleft lip/palate is multifactorial.[2] No single gene abnormality is responsible, but there is a familial predisposition, especially for subsequent pregnancies after an affected child. Maternal teratogens including phenytoin, sodium valproate and methotrexate have also been implicated.

Case history

A 6-month-old male infant weighing 7 kg was admitted for repair of a cleft palate. In the past medical history, it was noted that the child had been born at term and had experienced respiratory problems which required nasal continuous positive airway pressure for a period of 3 weeks. A clinical diagnosis of Pierre–Robin sequence was made. There were no other significant congenital abnormalities.

Examination revealed a healthy well nourished child with an obvious retrognathia. Haematological and biochemical investigations were normal. The plan for general anaesthesia was discussed with the parents.

Antisialogue premedication of 20 $\mu g.kg^{-1}$ of atropine was given orally 1 hour prior to surgery. Anaesthesia was induced by inhalation of oxygen, nitrous oxide and sevoflurane and direct laryngoscopy performed under deep anaesthesia, after intravenous access had been secured. The epiglottis and the posterior commissure of the vocal cords were visible with anterior external pressure on the larynx. After neuromuscular relaxation with atracurium 0.5 $mg.kg^{-1}$, intubation was performed using a RAE™ tube with a gum elastic bougie passed through it to give greater length and a more anterior direction to the tube. Anaesthesia was maintained with oxygen, nitrous oxide and isoflurane with 3 $\mu g.kg^{-1}$ of fentanyl given intravenously. Paracetamol 40 $mg.kg^{-1}$ was administered rectally, in the anaesthetic room.

Surgery proceeded uneventfully. Blood loss was estimated at 40 ml and the baby received 150 ml of 2.5% dextrose/0.45% saline and 50 ml Gelofusine®. He was extubated awake and after some initial difficulty because of blood in the airway, settled with good oxygen saturations and was transferred to recovery. A small amount of blood oozing from the child's mouth was noted. This persisted over the next hour and the baby was noted to be swallowing fairly frequently. It was decided to take the baby back to theatre for an examination under anaesthesia. Digital pressure was applied to the hard palate. Fifty ml of Gelofusine® was given. A haemoglobin estimation (HaemoCue®) gave a result of 7.8 $g.dl^{-1}$. Seventy ml of blood was administered and inhalation induction of anaesthesia performed in theatre with full monitoring. Tracheal intubation was carried out and a suction catheter passed into the stomach to irrigate and remove as much blood as possible. Examination revealed a small bleeding point at the site of the palatal repair which was coagulated with diathermy. The child was then turned on his side and extubated when awake. He was observed in the recovery room for an hour and then returned to the ward.

Discussion

The potential anaesthetic problems when dealing with surgery for cleft palate repair are shown in Table 6.1.

The presence of other congenital abnormalities (including cardiac and renal defects) should always be considered, especially in children with isolated cleft palate. More than 150 syndromes associated with clefting have been described, but fortunately all are rare.[3]

Most babies with associated congenital abnormalities will have been seen by the relevant paediatric specialist who may be able to advise on any possible implications for anaesthesia. The commonest requirement is for perioperative antibiotic prophylaxis against endocarditis.

More of a problem to the anaesthetist are those children with syndromes known to be associated with a difficult airway, particularly Pierre–Robin sequence, Treacher–Collins and Goldenhar syndromes. Klippel–Feil syndrome can present problems because of abnormalities of the cervical spine.

Assessment of the airway before surgery should include seeking a history of any difficulties with breathing in the past, sleeping position and difficulties with feeding. The paper by Gunawardana[4] which reported on 200 children having cleft lip and palate surgery, showed that virtually all the difficult laryngoscopies occurred in children with bilateral clefts or retrognathia. As both of these can be observed at the bedside, this compensates for the lack of applicability of those methods conventionally used for assessing the adult airway. For children, a method of radiological assessment was described in 1980.[5] This is based on the measurement of the maxillo–pharyngeal angle on lateral X-ray. If this angle, which is normally greater than 100°, is less than 90°, it implies that the larynx will not be visible at direct laryngoscopy.

Associated conditions	
Airway	– intubation – extubation
Bleeding	– intraoperative – postoperative
Postoperative analgesia	

Table 6.1
Anaesthetic problems during cleft palate surgery

The management of a suspected 'difficult intubation' is covered elsewhere in the book. There are several case reports in the literature of alternative strategies for intubation, including fibreoptic intubation through a laryngeal mask airway,[6] retrograde techniques and the use of a laryngeal mask airway alone.[7] These have very limited application in small children needing elective surgery. It should always be remembered that the timing of cleft palate repair can be deferred for some months and airway problems can improve with age, especially in those babies with Pierre–Robin sequence.

Much emphasis is placed on difficulties with intubation but extubation after surgical repair, in a baby with pre-existing airway problems can be much more hazardous. The vast majority of babies who come to surgery for cleft palate repair are easy to intubate, but immediately after surgery the airway is much more at risk. They may develop tracheal oedema following intubation. There will be blood in the airway and this bleeding may continue during the recovery period. Surgery itself, by correcting the defect in the hard palate, reduces the airway and this is worst in the first 24 hours postoperatively because of oedema. It is not, therefore, surprising that, in the presence of these additional insults, the baby with pre-existing airway problems is likely to have difficulty maintaining its airway. These children are usually managed with elective ventilation until the surgical oedema has settled and the likelihood of postoperative haemorrhage has diminished.

For those other children whose airway problems are thought to be shortlived and self-limiting, the decision 'when to extubate' can be difficult. The ideal situation is a baby with no respiratory depression, full return of laryngeal protective reflexes, no blood in the airway and perfect analgesia. The reality is often somewhat different. Extubation under 'deep anaesthesia' has its advocates but assessing adequate depth particularly with the newer inhalational agents, is notoriously difficult. Laryngospasm as the child lightens can also be a problem especially if there is any bleeding. In this situation the incidence of laryngospasm is said to be 20%.[8] An awake child can at least cough and thus protect the trachea.

One of the main goals of anaesthesia is the provision of effective, safe analgesia in the perioperative period. Good analgesia is important in cleft palate repair to minimize distress and crying which can increase the likelihood of postoperative bleeding. The general principle of using simple methods with minimum side-effects first, then progressing to more complex techniques, is important. The hazards of combining respiratory depression with potential respiratory obstruction must be remembered.

A local anaesthetic technique would be useful but unlike cleft lip repair where an infraorbital nerve block provides good analgesia, there is no comparable block for cleft palate repair. Many surgeons infiltrate the palate with local anaesthetic and a vasoconstrictor to minimize bleeding during surgery but it is doubtful how much, if any, analgesia this provides in the postoperative period. The mainstay of analgesia is still paracetamol given in a loading dose of $30\,mg.kg^{-1}$ orally or $40\,mg.kg^{-1}$ rectally either preoperatively or intraoperatively. The total recommended daily dose is $90\,mg.kg^{-1}$ and there is currently much discussion as to whether the loading dose should be included in this amount.

Early feeding is encouraged as this provides both calories and comfort. Nursing by the parents is also to be encouraged.

The use of additional analgesics is another area of controversy. Standard practice would be to add a non-steroidal anti-inflammatory drug (NSAID) such as ibuprofen. However, a recent survey[9] of anaesthetic practice showed that this group of drugs was used by approximately 50% of anaesthetists, who are regularly dealing with cleft palate repair. The main potential problem stated was concern regarding increased blood loss intra- and postoperatively. The theoretical risks are well known, although documented clinical problems with bleeding are rare. It is also not clear that NSAIDs confer any additional benefit when combined with paracetamol, if the increased doses of paracetamol, now recommended, are used.

If NSAIDs are not used, the alternatives are opiates such as codeine phosphate given intramuscularly or orally, or morphine which can also be given by the rectal route. The active constituent of codeine is morphine and it is probably more logical to give morphine directly. The oral or rectal route is also more acceptable to many paediatric nurses. The dose of morphine given orally is $1.2\,mg.kg^{-1}.24h^{-1}$ and given rectally is $1\,mg.kg^{-1}.24h^{-1}$. There is a risk of direct systemic absorption with the rectal route of delivery and the individual dose should therefore not exceed 1 mg in a child under the age of 1 year.

Intravenous infusions of opiates can be used but in the previous survey this was not a widely used option – only two units in the United Kingdom used this as a method of analgesia. It is also essential that the child is monitored appropriately for side effects such as bleeding or respiratory depression when these drugs are used.

Blood loss during and after surgery can be a problem for these babies. Uncomplicated surgical repair in a well nourished baby does not usually require a blood transfusion. If there is any doubt a haemoglobin check should be carried out immediately. Fluid balance should be maintained as babies do not tolerate hypovolaemia. In the postoperative period, blood loss may be difficult to assess as some blood will be swallowed and visible losses may be mixed with saliva. The importance of regular observations and monitoring cannot be overemphasized and experienced nursing care is essential.

Learning points

- Most babies presenting for cleft palate surgery are non-syndromic.
- Airway management may require specialized techniques.
- Extubation is often more problematic than intubation.
- Good postoperative analgesia is important.
- Bleeding may be persistent and occult.

References

1. Milerad J, Larson O, Hagberg C, Idberg M. Associated malformation in infants with cleft lip and palate; a prospective population-based study. *Paediatrics* 1997; 100: 180–186.
2. Cockell A, Less M. Prenatal diagnosis and management of orofacial clefts. *Prenatal Diagnosis* 2000; 20: 149–151.
3. Lees M. Genetics of cleft lip and palate. In: Management of Cleft Lip and Palate. In press.
4. Gunawardana RH. Difficult laryngoscopy in cleft lip and palate surgery. *Br J Anaesthes* 1996; 76: 757–759.
5. Deleque L, Rosenberg-Reiner S, Ghnassia MD. L'intubation tracheale chez les enfants atteints de dysmorphie craniofaciales conigenitales. *Anesthes Analges Reanimation* 1980; 37: 133–138.
6. Dubreuil M, Ecoffey C. Laryngeal mask guided tracheal intubation in paediatric anaesthesia. *Paediatr Anaesth* 1992; 2: 344.
7. Beveridge ME. Laryngeal mask anaesthesia for repair of cleft palate. *Anaesthesia* 1989; 44: 656–657.
8. Hartley M, Vaughan RS. Problems associated with tracheal extubation. *Br J Anaesth* 1993; 71: 561–568.
9. Dunnet JM, Lauder G. Analgesia in the peri-operative period for cleft palate surgery. Proceedings of the Association of Dental Anaesthetists. Vol. 15. 1997; ISBN 0267-2723.

7

Muscle biopsy in the 'floppy' infant

Jennifer E O'Flaherty

Introduction

Although neuromuscular disease in infants is rare, it is not uncommon for these infants to come to the operating theatre for a muscle biopsy. Also, as these children get older, other surgical procedures (particularly orthopaedic procedures) are often indicated. Neuromuscular disease may present as 'floppiness' (hypotonia) in infancy. Hypotonia may result from a wide variety of neuromuscular diseases and occasionally from some non-neuromuscular disorders. Although diagnostic information may be gathered from the presenting signs, the physical exam, the family history, biochemical studies and electromyography (EMG), a muscle biopsy is often required for definitive diagnosis.

Case history

JL, a 5-month-old boy presented for muscle biopsy because of a history of hypotonia. He had been born at 37 weeks' gestation to a 32-year-old gravida 4, para 3 woman whose previous obstetric history included the delivery of a 30-week gestation baby which had exhibited decreased movement *in utero*, and had died shortly after birth from respiratory failure. Two other siblings, aged 6 and 10 years, were normal. JL appeared normal at birth, but from 3 months of age had exhibited progressive loss of head control, loss of the ability to elevate his trunk when placed in a prone position, and floppy extremities. He had no history of reflux or aspiration pneumonia. On physical examination, his weight was 5.2 kg, temperature 36.7 °C, BP 85/55 mmHg, HR 110, and RR 38. He smiled and interacted with the examiner. Respirations appeared relaxed, but he displayed some abdominal breathing. There was global hypotonia and some evidence of muscle wasting. Deep tendon reflexes were absent. Biochemical studies were normal. The EMG showed neurogenic atrophy. The ECG was normal.

JL had been nil by mouth for over 10 hours. No intravenous access was in place preoperatively. He was taken to the operating theatre for a mask induction with nitrous oxide and sevoflurane in oxygen. Routine monitoring was applied. After induction, a 24-gauge IV catheter was placed in the left hand and a lactated Ringer's solution was begun. A forced hot air warming blanket was placed on top of the infant. Under deep sevoflurane anaesthesia, a 1.5 laryngeal mask airway was placed without difficulty. Chest rise and tidal volume appeared adequate, and JL was allowed to spontaneously ventilate. Anaesthesia was maintained with 2% sevoflurane in 50% nitrous oxide. Oxygen saturation was 97% with an FiO_2 of 50%. The surgeons infiltrated the area for muscle biopsy with local anaesthesia (0.25% bupivacaine) and made their incision for the muscle biopsy.

Within a few minutes of the start of surgery, JL's end-tidal CO_2 was noted to have risen from 6.1 kPa to 8.6 kPa. Five minutes later it was 10 kPa. The heart rate was in the 120s. The patient's temperature was noted to be slightly elevated at 37.8 °C (oesophageal). An arterial blood gas (ABG) was taken which revealed a mixed respiratory and metabolic acidosis: pH = 7.08, P_aCO_2 = 10.8 kPa, P_aO_2 = 20.4 kPa, BE = –6.0. The blood glucose level was 2.8 mmol.l^{-1}. The decision was made to intubate the patient in order to control ventilation. Laryngoscopy was attempted under deep sevoflurane anaesthesia and the patient went into profound laryngospasm with oxygen saturations falling from 97% to less than 40%. The patient's heart rate fell from 120 min^{-1} to a low of 63 min^{-1}. Atropine 0.1 mg and 3 mg rocuronium were administered intravenously. JL was then successfully intubated with a 3.5

endotrachial tube, oxygen saturation returned to 100% and the heart rate was in the 140s. A bolus of 20 ml.kg^{-1} of 5% dextrose in lactated Ringer's solution was administered. The muscle biopsy was expeditiously completed without incident, and when the incision was closed 15 minutes later the patient was not making any spontaneous respiratory effort. Neuromuscular monitoring showed the patient to have return of one twitch, so the neuromuscular blockade was reversed with 0.5 mg neostigmine and 0.1 mg glycopyrrolate.

The patient was taken to the paediatric intensive care unit where mechanical ventilation was continued. Although the neuromuscular blockade was adequately reversed, the patient was making only weak respiratory efforts and demonstrated 'paradoxical respirations'. Repeat ABG was pH = 7.38, P_aCO_2 = 5.3 kPa, P_aO_2 = 13 kPa, BE = −1.0 on FiO_2 30%. Blood glucose level was 6.1 mmol.l^{-1}. Temperature was 36.5 °C. Blood pressure remained stable. The heart rate was in the 110s. The patient was ventilated overnight and successfully extubated and weaned to room air the following morning.

Results of the muscle biopsy indicated a diagnosis of Werdnig–Hoffmann disease (spinal muscular atrophy type I).

Discussion

The 'floppy' infant poses a diagnostic dilemma for physicians, as there are many diverse causes of hypotonia. The differential diagnosis includes central hypotonia (perinatal asphyxia, hypotonic cerebral palsy), metabolic disorders, benign congenital hypotonia, disorders of the spinal cord (spinal cord injury, Werdnig–Hoffmann disease), disorders of the peripheral nerves, disorders of the neuromuscular junction (congenital myasthenia, neonatal myasthenia), infantile botulism, congenital myopathies and muscular dystrophies, mitochondrial myopathies, and the glycogenoses. Most of these patients will require a muscle biopsy as a part of their work-up.

Many causes of hypotonia are genetic, so there may be a family history of neuromuscular disease. Werdnig–Hoffmann disease is autosomal recessive. JL's premature sibling probably died of respiratory failure secondary to Werdnig–Hoffmann disease rather than respiratory failure secondary to lung immaturity. It is not uncommon for patients with Werdnig–Hoffmann disease to exhibit decreased movement *in utero*.[1]

As a general rule, muscle biopsies in infants and small children must be performed under general anaesthesia. Muscle biopsies are painful, and despite evidence of hypotonia most of these patients will have sparing of the sensory nerves. Adequate pain control is difficult to achieve with local anaesthesia alone. Furthermore, young patients are usually unable to cooperate with a regional technique.

Before general anaesthesia can be administered, a careful patient history must be taken. Infants with neuromuscular disease will often show signs of failure to thrive. At 5 months of age and 5.2 kg, JL was less than the fifth percentile for weight. A history of recurrent aspiration is not uncommon, and the anaesthetist should be aware of the potential for perioperative aspiration as well as the possibility that lung damage has already occurred secondary to recurrent aspiration pneumonia. A history of respiratory distress should be sought.

The history should be followed by a careful physical examination. These patients will have varying degrees of muscle weakness, but generally the proximal muscles are more severely affected than the distal muscles. Because of muscle weakness, many of these patients will have a reduced respiratory reserve, if not frank respiratory distress. Those patients with preoperative indicators of respiratory compromise are the most likely ones to require ventilation postoperatively. Narcotics and other respiratory depressants should be used with care in these patients. Sedative premedication increases the risk of airway obstruction in patients with significant hypotonia.

These patients are at increased risk for perioperative aspiration because of airway hypotonia, gastroesophageal reflux, and gastric hypomotility. Cardiac muscle involvement may be present, particularly in Duchenne's muscular dystrophy and the mitochondrial myopathies. Manifestations of cardiac muscle involvement include arrhythmias and congestive heart failure. Perioperatively, these patients must be positioned carefully because of ligamentous laxity secondary to hypotonia.

Many of the causes of hypotonia in infancy may be accompanied by metabolic derangement, particularly hypoglycaemia.[2] Extensive preoperative fasting should be avoided in these patients. They should be encouraged to drink clear liquids up until 2 hours prior to their anaesthetic. Although Werdnig–Hoffmann disease is not usually associated with metabolic derangement, JL's prolonged fast led to hypoglycaemia and dehydration, which resulted in a metabolic acidosis intraoperatively.

Depolarizing neuromuscular blocking agents should not be used in hypotonic infants. Although there are a few case reports which cite the uneventful use of suxamethonium in hypotonic infants,[3,4,5] there is clearly a risk of hyperkalaemia and subsequent cardiovascular collapse when suxamethonium is administered to a patient with neuromuscular disease.[6] For this reason, rocuronium rather than suxamethonium was administered when JL developed laryngospasm.

The pharmacokinetics of non-depolarizing neuromuscular blocking agents in these patients is not clearly defined. There are case reports describing the uncomplicated use of non-depolarizing muscle relaxants in these patients.[7] On the other hand, there are case reports documenting increased sensitivity to non-depolarizing neuromuscular blocking agents in infants with neuromuscular disease.[8,9] It has been hypothesized that patients with neuromuscular disease may be more sensitive to non-depolarizing neuromuscular blocking agents because of changes at the motor endplate and recruitment of extrajunctional receptors. It seems prudent to avoid the use of these agents whenever possible. If muscle relaxation is desired, a deep volatile agent should suffice. In any case, if a non-depolarizing neuromuscular blocking agent is given it should be carefully titrated using a nerve stimulator. The non-depolarizing neuromuscular blocking agent must be fully reversed prior to extubation, as these patients typically have very little respiratory reserve.

Whether or not 'floppy' infants are at increased risk for the development of malignant hyperthermia (MH) under anaesthesia is still a controversial topic.[10] Metabolic abnormalities inherent to many neuromuscular disorders (acidosis, rhabdomyolysis, elevated creatinine phosphokinase) may mimic MH, which has caused the two to be linked. Also, fatal hyperkalaemia after the administration of suxamethonium in these patients has been confused with, and ascribed to, MH. Over the years many neuromuscular disorders have been linked with MH susceptibility. However, subsequent negative or equivocal halothane contracture tests and uneventful use of triggering agents in these patients has brought this association into question. In JL's case, what might have been MH (elevated P_aCO_2, acidosis and elevated temperature) was primarily a respiratory acidosis, secondary to his inability to adequately spontaneously ventilate under general anaesthesia. The metabolic component of JL's acidosis was secondary to dehydration and hypoglycaemia after a prolonged fast, and the elevated temperature was due to overwarming with the forced hot air blanket. Currently, the only neuromuscular disease clearly associated with MH susceptibility is central core disease. Interestingly, the genetic locus for central core disease is located on the long arm of chromosome 19, and is closely linked to the genetic locus of MH.[11] At the present time there is no evidence to support the routine use of a 'non-triggering' anaesthetic regimen for 'floppy' infants. Suxamethonium should not be used for the above mentioned risk of hyperkalaemia, but volatile agents need not be discarded in favour of a total intravenous anaesthetic. Routine prophylaxis with dantrolene is not indicated, and in fact may lead to serious weakness in these already neurologically compromised patients. Dantrolene, as always, must be available for emergency use.

Finally, the 'floppy' infant should be observed closely in the postanaesthesia care unit for evidence of airway obstruction in the presence of residual anaesthetic. Postoperative respiratory failure is also common, and these patients may require postoperative ventilation. Observation of respiratory sufficiency may be indicated in an intensive care unit setting postoperatively, even in the non-ventilated patient.

Learning points

- There are many diverse causes of 'floppiness' in infancy, so generalizations are difficult to make.
- Muscle biopsies in infants are usually performed under general anaesthesia.
- 'Floppy' infants may be at risk for perioperative aspiration.
- 'Floppy' infants may have decreased respiratory reserve.
- Metabolic derangements, particularly hypoglycaemia, may occur in infants with neuromuscular disorders.
- Infants with neuromuscular disorders may have cardiac muscle involvement.
- Sedative and respiratory depressant medications must be administered with caution in 'floppy' infants because of the risk of airway obstruction and respiratory depression.
- Use of suxamethonium is contraindicated in 'floppy' infants because of the risk of lethal hyperkalaemia.
- 'Floppy' infants may exhibit increased sensitivity to non-depolarizing neuromuscular blocking agents.
- MH susceptibility of 'floppy' infants is still controversial.

References

1. Thomas NH, Dubowitz V. The natural history of type I (severe) spinal muscular atrophy. *Neuromusc Disord* 1994; 4: 497–502.
2. Keyes MA, Van de Wiele BV, Stead SW. Mitochondrial myopathies: an unusual cause of hypotonia in infants and children. *Paediatr Anaesth* 1996; 6: 329–335.
3. D'Ambra MN, Dedrick D, Savarese JJ. Kearns–Sayer syndrome and pancuronium – succinylcholine-induced neuromuscular blockade. *Anesthesiology* 1979; 51: 343–345.
4. Grattan-Smith PJ, Shield LK, Hopkins IJ, Collins KJ. Acute respiratory failure precipitated by general anesthesia in Leigh's syndrome. *J Child Neurol* 1990; 5: 137–141.
5. Heard SO, Kaplan RF. Neuromuscular blockade in a patient with nemaline myopathy. *Anesthesiology* 1983; 59: 588–590.
6. Farrell PT. Anaesthesia-induced rhabdomyolysis causing cardiac arrest: case report and review of anaesthesia and the dystrophinopathies. *Anaesth Intens Care* 1994; 22: 597–601.
7. Wiesel S, Bevan JC, Samuel J, Donati F. Vecuronium neuromuscular blockade in a child with mitochondrial myopathy. *Anesth Analges* 1991; 72: 696–699.
8. Ririe DG, Shapiro F, Sethna NF. The response of patients with Duchenne's muscular dystrophy to neuromuscular blockade with vecuronium. *Anesthesiology* 1998; 88: 351–354.
9. Tobias JD, Atwood R. Mivacurium in children with Duchenne muscular dystrophy. *Paediatr Anaesth* 1994; 4: 57–60.
10. Wappler F, Scholz J, von Richthofen V et al. Association of neuromuscular diseases with malignant hyperthermia. *Anesthesiology* 1997; 87: A861.
11. Quane KA, Healy JM, Keating KE et al. Mutations in the ryanodine receptor gene in central core disease and malignant hyperthermia. *Nat Genet* 1993; 5: 51–55.

8

Intussusception in a 6-month-old baby

JA Nolan

Introduction

Intussusception is one of the commonest causes of intestinal obstruction in infants. It occurs when there is an invagination of proximal bowel into the lumen of the distal bowel, which is then propelled distally by peristalsis. Most cases can be reduced by air enema under fluoroscopic imaging guidance but a proportion will require surgical intervention. Deaths still occur due to complications such as inadequate resuscitation, perforation and sepsis,[1] although overall mortality is low. This chapter describes a classical case of intussusception and its subsequent management.

Case presentation

A 6-month-old baby weighing 6.5 kg was admitted to the emergency department with a 3-day history of screaming episodes and bilious vomiting. For several hours prior to admission he had been becoming increasingly listless. On the morning of admission his oral intake was very poor and his stools were noted to be bloodstained. At the time of presentation he was screaming and pulling his legs up towards his abdomen. He was apyrexial with a pulse rate of 152 bpm and blood pressure of 117/63 mmHg, with saturations of 96% in air. His skin appeared mottled and his capillary refill time was 4 seconds.

An intravenous cannula was inserted and he was given 20 $ml.kg^{-1}$ of albumin 4.5%. Examination of his abdomen revealed tenderness in the right iliac fossa and he was referred for surgical review. Blood taken at the time of cannulation showed a white cell count of $19 \times 10^9 mm^{-3}$ with haemoglobin of 11.5 $g.dl^{-1}$. He was started on intravenous antibiotics and an infusion of dextrose 4%/saline 0.18% was commenced at 28 $ml.hr^{-1}$. After receiving a further 20 $ml.kg^{-1}$ bolus of albumin 4.5% his capillary refill time improved to 2 seconds. Ultrasound examination revealed an ileocolic intussusception, which was successfully reduced with an air enema under fluoroscopic monitoring, and he was taken to the ward for observation.

The following day he remained well and his intravenous maintenance was continued. On day 3 of admission he vomited and developed mild abdominal distension. An ultrasound scan at this time showed a recurrent intussusception and he was taken to theatre for laparotomy.

Anaesthesia was induced with oxygen and sevoflurane after aspirating on his nasogastric tube. He was given fentanyl 15 μg and atracurium 6 mg and intubated with a size 4.0 endotracheal tube. Cefuroxime 30 $mg.kg^{-1}$ and metronidazole 7.5 $mg.kg^{-1}$ were given after induction. Analgesia was provided with 6 ml bupivacaine 0.25% via the caudal route using a 22G abbocath. Anaesthesia was maintained with oxygen, air and isoflurane. Maintenance fluid was continued at 28 $ml.hr^{-1}$ using dextrose 4%/saline 0.18%, and deficit and third space losses managed with a total of 30 $ml.kg^{-1}$ of albumin 4.5%. An ileocaecal intussusception was readily reduced. The bowel was viable and no resection was needed.

He was sent back to the ward with dextrose 4%/saline 0.18% as maintenance fluids and a nasogastric tube on free drainage (replaced ml for ml with normal saline). A morphine infusion at a rate of 10–40 $\mu g.kg^{-1}.hr^{-1}$ and regular PR paracetamol (20 $mg.kg^{-1}$ 6-hourly, maximum 90 $mg.kg^{-1}.24\ hr^{-1}$) were prescribed for postoperative analgesia. The following morning he was crying intermittently but appeared otherwise comfortable. By midday, however, he was screaming with hunger and settled after a milk feed. His morphine infusion was stopped on day 2 and he remained comfortable on regular paracetamol. By day 5 he was tolerating a regular oral diet and on day 6 he was discharged home.

Discussion

Intussusception

An intussusception is an invagination of proximal bowel into the lumen of the distal bowel, which is then propelled distally by peristalsis (see Figure 8.1). It is the most common cause of acute intestinal obstruction in children under 2 years of age, with the peak incidence between the ages of 4 and 10 months. It can occur antenatally as a cause of intestinal atresia[2] or in the neonatal period, and is more common in boys. It is usually 'idiopathic' with the apex ('leading point') of the intussusceptum being a Peyer's patch or part of the bowel wall,[3] and is often thought to be related to viral infection (usually adenovirus) because of the common association with recent upper respiratory tract infection or gastroenteritis. Pathological leadpoints occur in 2–12% of cases and are more common outside this age range, the commonest leadpoint being a Meckel's diverticulum but others include duplication cysts, polyps and solid tumours. Intussusception may occur postoperatively after abdominal or non-abdominal surgery (1–2% of cases), usually within a week of surgery and probably by a different neurogenic mechanism, and in such cases it is usually confined to the small bowel. It can also be associated with malrotation[4] and cystic fibrosis.[5]

The commonest idiopathic type is ileocolic (85%) but colocolic or ileoileal intussusception can occur and these should make one consider a pathological leadpoint. Approximately 80% of ileocolic intussusceptions extend to the ascending or transverse colon,[6] but they may reach as far as the anal margin. Multiple short segment invaginations may occur spontaneously or after trauma and retrograde invaginations (eg. duodenogastric) have been reported as complications of gastrostomy tubes.[7,8]

In 1999 the rotavirus vaccine was withdrawn in the United States because it was thought to be associated with an increased incidence of intussusception. This has caused ongoing concern with potentially unnecessary deaths from rotavirus.[9,10]

The main concern with intussusception is bowel obstruction, which can lead to ischaemia with necrosis and perforation, but early diagnosis and treatment should result in nearly 100% survival. Acute episodes may resolve spontaneously either by reduction or sloughing with union of the bowel at the neck of the intussusception.[11]

Presentation

The clinical presentation differs according to the age of the child and the site of the intussusception. The classical presentation is one of regular episodes of colicky abdominal pain (80%) in a well child with pallor and the passage of 'redcurrant jelly' stools (60%), associated with a tender mass in the right hypochondrium or epigastrium. Vomiting occurs in about 75% and may become bilious and this may be the main presenting symptom in infants. Blood in the stools is often a late finding and may only be discovered on rectal examination. About 10% may present with diarrhoea and vomiting mimicking gastroenteritis, and progressive dehydration and strangulation with bowel necrosis may result in death within days if diagnosis is delayed. Chronic presentation with recurrent episodes of abdominal pain is more likely to be due to a pathological leadpoint.

Investigations

There are several suggestive patterns for intussusception on plain abdominal X-rays such as a paucity of gas with a soft tissue mass, or a soft tissue mass surrounded by colonic air,[12] but classical signs often occur late and X-rays are rarely diagnostic. In 50% of cases the plain X-ray is suggestive and in about 25% it is normal.[13,14] Ultrasound is now the diagnostic tool of choice and plain films should not be routinely obtained. In experienced hands ultrasound has a sensitivity and specificity of 100% for both confirming and excluding an intussusception.[15,16] The intussusception appears as a 'doughnut' or 'target' in cross-section and a 'pseudokidney' or tubular structure in longitudinal section. Ultrasound can also identify pathological leadpoints. Colour Doppler can detect any reduction in blood flow suggestive of ischaemia and necrosis, which may suggest the need for laparotomy. Air and contrast enema can also be used for diagnosis as well as treatment, but are more invasive, use radiation and are probably no more effective than ultrasound.

Assessment and resuscitation

The commonest causes of death in these children are delayed diagnosis and inadequate resuscitation. Children with intussusception are at risk of bowel perforation and peritonitis. They may also present with significant dehydration from diarrhoea and vomiting, or as a result of third space losses. It is very important that these children are adequately resuscitated prior to attempted reduction. Non-operative reduction can be attempted provided there are no signs of peritonitis or perforation, and fluid loss should be replaced with normal saline or colloid. A reduced urine output is an important early sign of dehydration, cardiovascular signs such as tachycardia not necessarily occurring until they are more than 10% dehydrated.

Treatment

Non-operative reduction

The majority of cases can be treated in this way, the only contraindications being clinical signs of peritonitis or shock and signs of perforation on an abdominal X-ray. Perforation is the main complication but occurs in less than 1% of cases.

Any attempt at reduction should be made in a specialist centre where all diagnostic and treatment options are available and facilities exist for managing failed reduction and perforation. An intravenous cannula should be in place before attempted reduction and broad-spectrum antibiotics (cefuroxime and metronidazole) should be given.

Reduction can be achieved with barium or water-soluble contrast medium using fluoroscopic guidance (hydrostatic reduction), or with air or carbon dioxide (pneumatic reduction).[17,18] Ultrasound may also be used to guide reduction and is increasingly used owing to the lack of radiation exposure. An important complication of pneumatic reduction is a tension pneumoperitoneum and this requires immediate needle decompression.

Sedation with intravenous morphine is often used for non-operative reduction but there is no evidence that it increases the reduction rate, whereas there is some evidence that Valsalva manoeuvres in non-sedated infants can increase the success rate of pneumatic reduction by increasing intra-abdominal pressure. As air is compressible a Valsalva manoeuvre during reduction may also reduce the chance of perforation because of the transmural pressure generated.

Pneumatic reduction can also be performed under general anaesthesia as relaxation of the abdominal muscles may aid reduction. Gas embolism is a potential complication although rarely encountered. Nitrous oxide may affect the volume of gas in the bowel and should probably be avoided as part of the general anaesthetic technique.

Abdominal manipulation, glucagon and antispasmodics have all been used to aid non-operative reduction but are of doubtful benefit.

Pneumatic reduction involves the application of air under pressure to a maximum of 120 mmHg (though during Valsalva manoeuvres peak pressures may be higher) through a piece of soft rubber tubing inserted into the rectum and connected to a pressure gauge. Air dissects between the intussusceptum (apex) and the intussuscipiens (outer wall) and its less viscous nature allows faster and more effective reduction than with liquid. Most reductions occur within 5 minutes and will not require more than 80 mmHg. If at any time during the reduction there is no bowel movement despite application of pressure for 3–4 minutes, the applied pressure should be discontinued for 1–2 minutes before reattempting, because of the risk of perforation.

Successful reduction is confirmed by reflux of air or contrast into the terminal ileum in association with resolution of symptoms and signs. Non-reduction in a stable child can be treated by a repeat enema after 3–4 hours when oedema has subsided.[19]

An ileocaecal valve and bowel wall thickening can be mistaken for persistent intussusception, and ultrasound can be used to identify the latter. If there is uncertainty it is safe to observe the child clinically and re-image later if symptoms do not settle promptly. Clinical deterioration, however, after an unsuccessful reduction will require a laparotomy.[20]

After successful pneumatic reduction the child can feed as soon as able but should be observed for 24–48 hours in case of recurrence. Successful reduction is less likely in those with a history longer than 24 hours and in those under 3 months or older than 2 years, and also in the presence of small bowel obstruction or a pathological leadpoint. The most important predictor of adverse outcome is the duration of symptoms, others being rectal bleeding and small bowel obstruction. These do not, however, preclude attempts at non-operative reduction.[12]

Operative reduction

This is required in the child in whom attempted non-operative reduction has failed or where perforation or peritonitis are suspected. Intussusception is rare in neonates but they have a high incidence of pathological leadpoints and irreducibility, which generally lowers the threshold for surgical reduction. Preoperative preparation involves intravenous rehydration (colloid or blood may be needed) and broad-spectrum antibiotics. Surgery should proceed within hours because of the risk of perforation or worsening sepsis. A rapid sequence induction may be indicated despite aspiration of the nasogastric tube. A transverse right-sided skin incision is usually made at the level of the umbilicus and analgesia provided with a high lumbar epidural or a morphine infusion with the aim of extubation at the end of the procedure.

Operative reduction involves 'milking' back the intussusception under sustained pressure by compressing the apex or intussusceptum. The bowel must be examined for viability and infarcted areas and irreducible intussusceptions require resection and either end-to-end anastomosis or rarely temporary stoma formation.

Postoperatively intravenous fluids are continued until feeds can be tolerated orally, and a nasogastric tube is left in place until bowel function returns. Postoperative pyrexia is not uncommon in the first 24–48 hours.

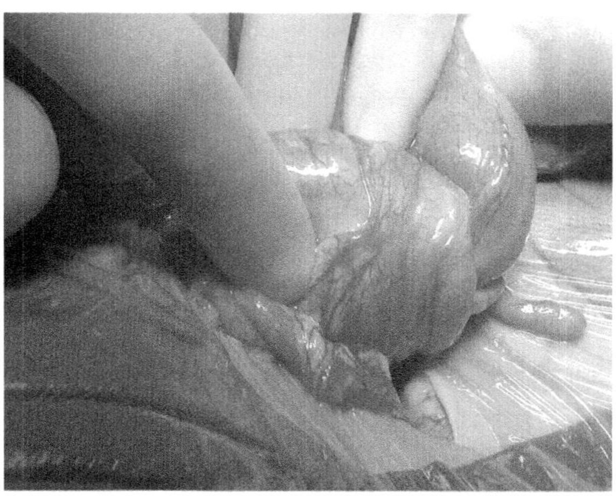

Figure 8.1
Typical appearance of an ileocaecal intussusception.

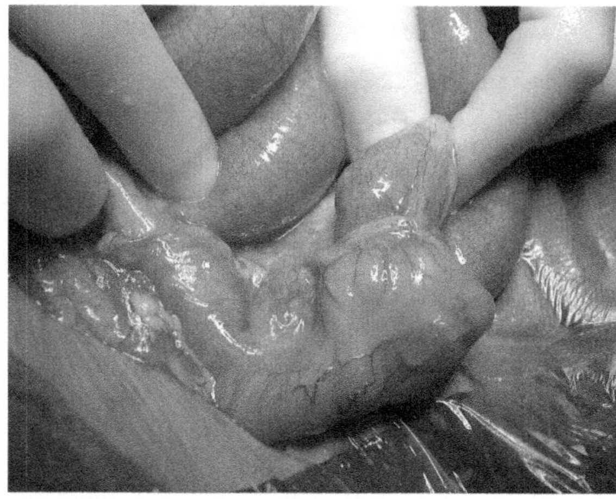

Figure 8.2
Reduction of intussusception.

Between 5% and 10% of intussusceptions will recur after either method of reduction, with recurrence being less likely after surgical reduction. One-third of recurrences occur in the first 24 hours and nearly half between 3 and 6 months. Multiple recurrences are often associated with pathological leadpoints but a first recurrence usually has no association and often reduces easily with air or contrast.[21,22] Intestinal obstruction from adhesions may occur as a late complication.

The long-term outlook is excellent for the majority of these children, even those with recurrent episodes. Vitamin B12 absorption may be impaired, however, if extensive terminal ileal resection is required. Prognosis is influenced by the underlying diagnosis. Despite the mortality of less than 1%, delayed diagnosis and inadequate resuscitation are responsible for the small but significant number of deaths in these otherwise well children.[23]

Learning points

- Intussusception is the commonest cause of acute intestinal obstruction in children under 2 years of age.
- The classical presentation is with colicky abdominal pain, vomiting and 'redcurrant jelly' stools.
- Delayed diagnosis and inadequate resuscitation are important causes of mortality.
- In experienced hands the diagnosis can be made with 100% sensitivity and specificity using ultrasound.

- Management must be in a specialist centre with appropriate resuscitation facilities.
- The success rate of non-operative reduction is 75–80%.
- Surgery is required if air enema reduction fails, perforation occurs or the child has peritonitis.
- The child should be observed for 24–48 hours after reduction as recurrence may occur.
- Mortality rate is less than 1%.

References

1. Stringer MD, Pablot SM, Brereton RJ. Paediatric Intussusception. *Br J Surg* 1992; 79: 867–876.
2. Pavri DR, Marshall DG, Armstrong RF, Gorodzinsky FP. Intrauterine intussusception: case report and literature review. *Can J Surg* 1983; 26: 376–378.
3. Ong N-T, Beasley SW. The leadpoint in intussusception. *J Pediatr Surg* 1990; 25: 640–643.
4. Ornstein MH, Lund RJ. Simultaneous occurrence of malrotation, volvulus and intussusception in an infant. *Br J Surg* 1981; 38: 440–441.
5. Holmes M, Murphy V, Taylor M, Denham B. Intussusception in cystic fibrosis. *Arch Dis Child* 1991; 66: 726–727.
6. Ravitch MM. Intussusception in Infants and Children. Springfield, IL: Charles C Thomas, 1959.
7. Oswald MP, Graviss ER, Danis RK, Silberstein MJ, Cradock TV. Duodenogastric intussusception causing gastric outlet obstruction. *J Pediatr Surg* 1982; 17: 82–83.
8. Galea MH, Mayell MJ. Gastroduodenal mucosal intussusception causing gastric outlet obstruction: a complication of gastrostomy tubes. *J Pediatr Surg* 1988; 23: 980–981.
9. Rotavirus vaccines: WHO Position Paper. *Wkly Epidemiol Rec* 1999; 74: 33–38.
10. Simonsen L, Morens DM, Elixhauser A et al. Incidence trends in infant hospitalization for intussusception: impact of the 1998–1999 rotavirus vaccination program in the United States. *Lancet* 2001; 358:
11. Robb WAT, Souter W. Spontaneous sloughing and healing of intussusception: historical review and report of a case. *Br J Surg* 1962; 49: 542–546.
12. Grier D. Radiology of gastrointestinal emergencies. In Carty H, ed. Emergency Paediatric Radiology. Springer Verlag, 1999.
13. Alford BA, McIlhenny J. The child with acute abdominal pain and vomiting. *Radiol Clin North Am* 1992; 30: 441–453.
14. Sargent MA, Babyn PS, Alton DJ. Plain radiography in suspected intussusception: a reassessment. *Pediatr Radiol* 1994; 24: 17–20.
15. Pracos JP, Tran-Minh VA, Morin DE et al. Acute intestinal intussusception in children: contribution of ultrasonography. *Ann Radiol* 1987; 30: 525–530.
16. Verschelden P, Filiatrault D, Garel L et al. Intussusception in children: reliability of ultrasound diagnosis – a prospective study. *Pediatr Radiol* 1992; 22: 741–744.
17. Shiels WE II, Maves CK, Hedlund GL, Kirks DR. Air enema for diagnosis and reduction of intussusception: clinical experience and pressure correlates. *Radiology* 1991; 181: 169–172.
18. Kirks DR. Air intussusception reduction: 'the winds of change'. *Pediatr Radiol* 1995; 25: 89–91.
19. Saxton V, Katz M, Phelan E, Beasley SW. Intussusception: a repeat delayed gas enema increases the nonoperative reduction rate. *J Pediatr Surg* 1994; 29: 588–589.
20. Pierro A, Donnell SC, Paraskevopoulou C, Carty H, Lloyd DA. Indications for laparotomy after hydrostatic reduction for intussusception. *J Pediatr Surg* 1993; 28: 1154–1157.
21. Beasley SW, Auldist AW, Stokes KB. Recurrent intussusception: barium or surgery? *Aust N Z J Surg* 1987; 57:11–14.
22. Beasley SW, Glover J. Intussusception: prediction of outcome of gas enema. *J Pediatr Surg* 1992; 27: 474–475.
23. Stringer MD, Pledger G, Drake DP. Childhood deaths from intussusception in England and Wales, 1984–9. *BMJ* 1992; 304: 737–739.

9

Anaesthesia for adenotonsillectomy in a patient with a total cavopulmonary circulation (Fontan)

Andrew R Wolf

Introduction

Recent years have seen a sharp decline in mortality in infants and children with major cardiac abnormalities, such that patients with radically altered circulation are surviving and living within the general population. These patients can then present the anaesthetist with a major challenge when they arrive at hospital for non-cardiac surgery. The key to the safe management of these children is a clear understanding of the pathophysiology of the individual lesions allowing an appropriate selection of anaesthetic technique. In this group of patients, poor understanding of the lesion and inappropriate anaesthetic management can have dire consequences. If in doubt it is essential to contact a regional paediatric centre that undertakes cardiac surgery and discuss the individual problems and pitfalls with a consultant paediatric cardiac anaesthetist. As a representative example, this chapter discusses the management of adenotonsillectomy in a child with a total cavopulmonary anastamosis.

Case history

A 4-year-old child, weighing 13 kg, presented to hospital for a routine adenotonsillectomy. She had had a series of previous operations for tricuspid atresia, which included a right modified Blalock–Taussig (BT) shunt as a neonate, a Glenn shunt (bidirectional cavopulmonary shunt) at the age of 1 year and a total cavopulmonary anastosmosis (TCPC) at the age of 2 years (see Figure 9.1). Her initial recovery after this final operation was slow and she was in hospital for 3 months with recurrent pleural effusions and ascites. She had been reasonably well for a year, but became easily tired with poor exercise tolerance. In the last year, she had recurrent throat infections, the last episode led to her developing a chest infection which necessitated a week on intensive care due to hypoxia and cardiovascular instability. There was no history of sleep apnoea. Her daily warfarin dose was titrated to maintain her INR at between 2.0 and 2.5, but this was hard to maintain in good control. The warfarin was stopped 3 days before admission. Findings on history, examination and investigation are detailed in Table 9.1.

Management

In addition to stopping warfarin 5 days before admission, captopril was discontinued the night before surgery, and on the morning of surgery EMLA® cream was applied to the hands and she was given 0.4 $mg.kg^{-1}$ of oral diazepam for premedication.

Anaesthesia was induced with ketamine 2 $mg.kg^{-1}$ and fentanyl 2 $\mu g.kg^{-1}$ and intubation facilitated with 0.2 $mg.kg^{-1}$ vecuronium. The patient was ventilated on nitrous oxide 50%, oxygen 50% and isoflurane. Prophylactic intravenous antibiotics were given: gentamicin 4 $mg.kg^{-1}$ and amoxicillin 30 $mg.kg^{-1}$. Routine intravenous maintenance fluids were commenced. The adenoidectomy was performed first using a curettage technique, and almost immediately there was a rapid loss of blood. This was packed by the surgeon and a tonsillectomy commenced. However, within a further 5 minutes, the adenoidectomy site needed to be explored and repacked due to large ongoing venous ooze. Blood loss after 15 minutes was estimated at greater than 180 ml with a large continuing loss. The adenoidectomy site was diathermied and packed and a decision made to leave the packs in overnight. The tonsillectomy was completed and although this was also associated with abnormal bleed-

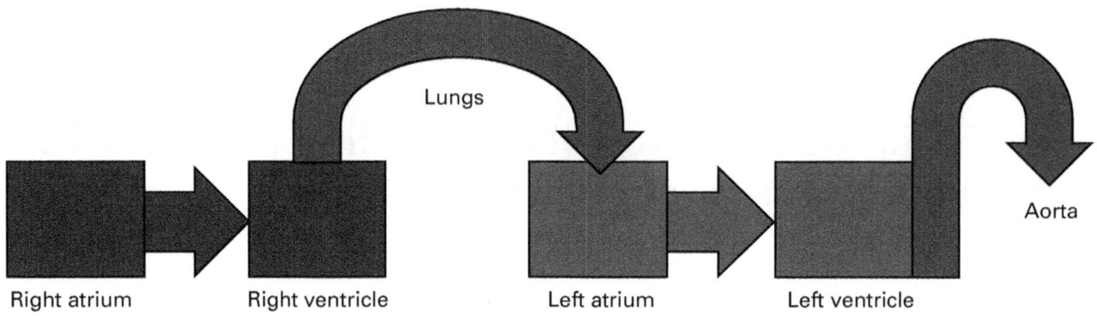

Figure 9.1a
Normal anatomy.

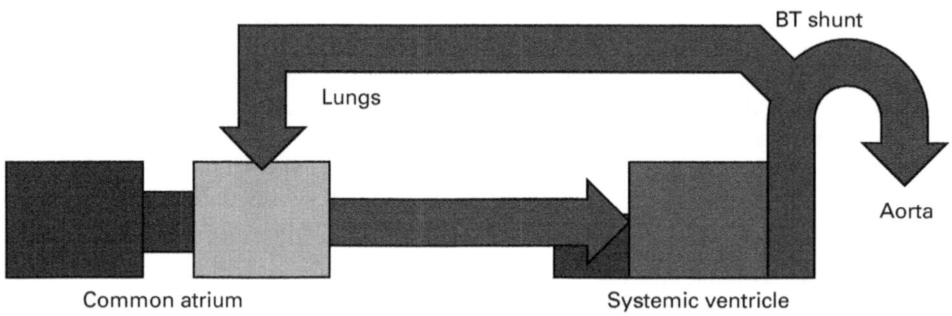

Figure 9.1b
Tricuspid atresia palliated with a BT shunt. In this situation systemic venous blood passes across a wide atrial septal defect. The right ventricle is small and connected to the left ventricle. An artificial (BT) shunt connecting a subclavian artery to the pulmonary artery has been constructed, allowing oxygenated blood into the common atrium. The patient remains cyanosed, and the systemic ventricle remains volume loaded.

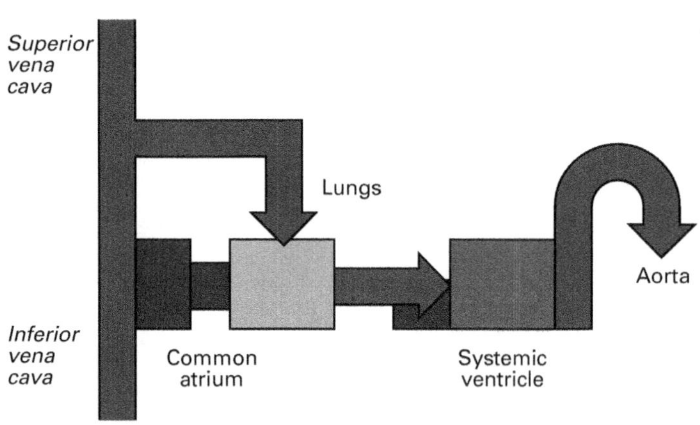

Figure 9.1c
Total cavopulmonary connection. Now desaturated blood from the systemic veins is connected directly to the pulmonary artery without mixing in the common atrium. Oxygenated pulmonary venous blood returns to the common atrium and on to the systemic ventricle. The patient should not be cyanosed and the systemic ventricle is now pumping a single cardiac output without additional shunts. Delivery of blood through the pulmonary circulation and on to the systemic ventricle is dependent on passive flow due to a gradient between the systemic veins and the common atrium.

Past medical history	Right modified BT shunt Bidirectional cavopulmonary shunt Total cavopulmonary anastosmosis Recurrent tonsillitis, no sleep apnoea Pneumonia requiring paediatric intensive therapy	
ASA grade	III	
Regular medications	Captopril 6.5 mg TDS Warfarin 2 mg daily	
Allergies	None known	
Examination	Alert, apyrexial Normal airway Chest clear, SaO_2 % in air Heart sounds Pulse 85 sinus rhythm bpm, BP 110/–75 mmHg Distended abdomen, ascites CXR large heart with clear lung fiolds Thoracotomy and sternal scars from previous surgery	
Investigations	*Weight*	13 kg
	FBC	Hb 13.0 $g.dl^{-1}$, Plat 168 × $10^9.l^{-1}$, WBC 8.5 × $10^9.l^{-1}$
	Clotting	PT time, INR 1.2, APPT s, Fibrinogen normal
	U+E's	Na^+ 138 $mmol.l^{-1}$, K^+ 4.3 $mmol.l^{-1}$, urea 6.5 $mmol.l^{-1}$, creatinine 85 $\mu mol.l^{-1}$
	ECG	Sinus rhythm
	Chest X-ray	

Table 9.1
History, examination and investigations

ing and venous ooze, adequate haemostasis was achieved. The total blood loss at the end of the procedure was 250–300 ml.

During the initial period of blood loss, blood pressure fell to 68/35 mmHg and heart rate rose from 120 to 166 beats per minute. In addition the oxygen saturation fell from 96% to 86% despite adequate ventilation. In view of the ongoing blood loss a sample was taken for urgent cross-match for three units of blood. Fluid resuscitation was commenced with Hartmann's solution and 300 ml given rapidly. Arterial access was obtained for monitoring and a femoral venous catheter inserted to monitor central venous pressure. Dopamine was commenced at 5 $\mu g.kg^{-1}.min^{-1}$ and due to continued hypotension increased to 7.5 $\mu g.kg^{-1}.min^{-1}$. The initial central venous pressure after cannulation was 1 mmHg and further fluid was infused to bring the central venous pressure up to 14 mmHg. At this point both blood pressure and oxygen saturation rose to more normal values. A blood gas taken in the middle of the resuscitation showed a low oxygen tension of 52 mmHg despite an increased inspired oxygen concentration of 80%, pCO_2 of 47 mmHg, and pH of 7.2 with a mild base deficit of –2.5. Blood, fresh frozen plasma and platelets were ordered and given over the following 12 hours to cover the ongoing blood loss.

The patient was taken to the paediatric intensive care unit, where she was electively ventilated and sedated with fentanyl 10 $\mu g.kg^{-1}.hr^{-1}$ and midazolam

50–100 µg.kg^{-1}.hr^{-1}. Paralysis was maintained over the following 24 hours with a vecuronium infusion 50–100 µg.kg^{-1}.hr^{-1}. The adenoidectomy packs were removed uneventfully the following day without further blood loss and the patient extubated. A continuous heparin infusion at 10 units.kg^{-1}.hr^{-1} was started to provide protection against spontaneous thrombus formation in the pulmonary vascular bed and this was converted to her usual warfarin regimen once she had fully recovered.

Discussion

The child with a Fontan circulation has only a single functional ventricle. In order to separate the pulmonary and systemic circulations, it is necessary for the pulmonary circulation to be supplied by passive flow from the vena cava instead of the normal arrangement of being pumped from the right ventricle. The resultant circulation is one in which the systemic venous pressure drives blood through the pulmonary vascular bed and on to the systemic ventricle (Figure 9.1). Fontan first described the original cavopulmonary shunt as a palliative treatment for tricuspid atresia in 1971.[1] The TCPC is a modified version of this original procedure and is now usually performed as the third and final operation to separate pulmonary from systemic circulations. The first stage, the modified BT shunt, allows some blood into the pulmonary artery from the subclavian artery and is effectively like an artificial ductus arteriosus.[2] The child remains cyanosed and the BT shunt is replaced with a bidirectional cavopulmonary shunt (modified Glenn shunt) at about 9 months of age or when the child outgrows the BT shunt (becomes more cyanosed). In this second operation the BT shunt is taken down, the superior vena cava is connected to the pulmonary artery, leaving the inferior vena cava continuing to drain into the common ventricle.[2] The child still remains cyanosed after this procedure (usually with an SpO_2 on air of 80–90%), and this circulation does not promote further growth of pulmonary arteries,[3] but it reduces the pressure and volume overload on the systemic ventricle, allowing adaptation before proceeding to the TCPC. Finally, the TCPC separates the two circulations and results in a child with normal arterial oxygenation and a systemic ventricle that is pumping only into a systemic circulation.

In the normal heart, systemic venous blood at a low pressure (2–6 mmHg) is pumped through the right ventricle at a systolic pressure of 25 mmHg into the pulmonary circulation. In contrast in the TCPC relatively high pressures in the vena cava (8–15 mmHg) are needed to drive blood through to the common atrium (2–5 mmHg). Clearly, an abnormally high common atrial pressure (due to a–v or aortic valve disease or systemic ventricular failure) reduces the transpulmonary gradient and can lead to failure of this circuit. Similarly, high pulmonary vascular resistance will also result in failure of the TCPC. Children with this shunt may appear reasonably well but can rapidly become sick if the delicate balance within their pulmonary circulation is disturbed. The TCPC circuit presents a variety of problems for both anaesthetist and surgeon.

Slow response to intravenous drugs

The flow through the pulmonary circuit is sluggish due to the low driving pressure. It is therefore important to give intravenous drugs slowly, and to give sufficient time for them to reach and act on their target organ.

Potential inability to cope with postural changes

Changes in posture can alter the blood flow through the pulmonary circuit and result in poor delivery to the systemic ventricle. The result will be a fall in blood pressure and oxygen saturation, which may need to be treated by returning to the original posture and giving additional fluid. If a non-invasive blood pressure monitor is used it should be switched into a rapid repeat measurement mode on induction or during postural changes.

High systemic venous pressure

This was a key feature in this case. It is also a sign that the TCPC was not running in an ideal fashion. An adenoidectomy produces a raw bed of tissue that can bleed unchecked unless it is packed carefully. Careful preoperative assessment and discussion with the paediatric cardiologist involved can give some assessment of risk. A key point is that the surgeon must be aware of the implications of the high venous pressure and have a plan to deal with excessive bleeding. The above patient lost 32% of her circulating blood volume. This degree of blood loss would be rare in a normal patient but is not unexpected in the Fontan patient. The anaesthetist needs to ensure that matched blood is available. This may prove to be difficult as the patient will have already received several blood transfusions and the incidence of incompatibility due to antibodies increases.

Dysrhythmias

Re-entry tachycardia is a common problem in older patients after TCPC (particularly supraventricular tachyarrhythmia and atrial flutter). These patients often do not cope well with atrial dysrhythmias, in that they need an atrial contraction ('atrial kick') to empty the atrium and drive blood into the systemic ventricle. An atrial contraction against a closed a–v valve which occurs during a junctional rhythm will result in a rise in pressure in the common atrium and reduction of the all important transpulmonary gradient. If dysrhythmia is present on a preoperative ECG then the operation needs to be postponed until a cardiology opinion has been given.

Poor adaptation to hypovolaemia

The above case demonstrated this problem well. As soon as venous pressure dropped due to blood loss, the TCPC circuit failed. The driving pressure through the pulmonary vascular bed was lost, resulting in inadequate blood reaching the common atrium and systemic ventricle. This needs to be treated rapidly with volume replacement but central venous pressure measurement is also needed to prevent overtransfusion.

Variable performance of the systemic ventricle

The TCPC is performed in a variety of cardiac conditions that result in there being only one functioning ventricle. In the case of pulmonary atresia (as above), the systemic ventricle is morphologically of left ventricular origin but this is not always the case. In some conditions the left side of the heart fails to develop with hypoplasia of the left ventricle and aorta (hypoplastic left heart syndrome). In this situation the systemic ventricle after a TCPC is of right ventricular morphology and may act as a poor systemic pump. Even when the morphological left ventricle is left as the systemic pump the performance may be poor, and these children may remain in cardiac failure after surgery.

Susceptibility to infection

Children who have congenital heart defects usually require prophylactic antibiotics before any surgery due to the risk of bacterial growth in either prosthetic material or on abnormal intracardiac tissue. The sick cardiac child is additionally more at risk from chest infections and other systemic infections after surgery.

Oedema and potentially low albumin and protein

The high venous pressure of the TCPC circuit is associated with pleural, pericardial effusions and ascites. These may affect pulmonary or cardiac function and need to be assessed before surgery. In some cases a protein-losing enteropathy occurs which reduces plasma proteins and can compound the problem.

Management of anticoagulation for surgery

Not all centres use warfarin to provide anticoagulation in patients with TCPC. Some use aspirin alone. There is a balance between the risks of thrombus formation in these patients against the risk of surgical bleeding in the perioperative period. In this case, despite reasonable efforts to normalize coagulation before surgery, the patient still had a major bleed during surgery. If it is essential to maintain some anticoagulation right up to the time of surgery and to have tight control on the level of anticoagulation, then warfarin should be discontinued early before the operation and replaced by intravenous heparin. The heparin is then discontinued 4 hours prior to the planned surgery.

Learning points

- Increasing numbers of patients with congenital heart disease are present in the community and will not always be referred to a regional centre for routine surgery.

- These patients have complex pathophysiology that needs to be understood before undertaking anaesthesia and surgery.
- Discussion with cardiologists or paediatric cardiac anaesthetists is necessary in these cases to avoid the pitfalls.
- In the patient with TCPC having adenotonsillectomy it is essential to have adequate blood products available before surgery, and to ensure coagulation and platelet counts are within normal limits.
- Induction of anaesthesia should avoid significant venodilation.
- Appropriate antibiotic prophylaxis must always be administered.
- Blood loss should be treated aggressively to avoid dropping systemic venous pressure.
- Invasive monitoring during surgery may need to be considered.

References

1. Fontan F, Baudet E. Surgical repair of tricuspid atresia. *Thorax* 1971; 26: 240.
2. Lake CA, Ed. Pediatric Cardiac *Anesthesia*. Norwalk, CT: Appleton and Lange, 1993.
3. Penny DJ, Pawade A, Wilkinson JL, Karl TR. Pulmonary artery size after bidirectional cavopulmonary connection. *J Card Surg* 1995; 10: 21–26.

10

Hypoplastic left heart syndrome

Hamish M Munro

Introduction

Hypoplastic left heart syndrome (HLHS), originally described by Lev in 1952 and named by Noonan and Nadas 6 years later, accounts for 1–4% of all congenital heart defects. If left untreated it is the commonest cardiac cause of death in the newborn period. Approximately 1000–1500 babies in the USA and 200 babies in the United Kingdom are born with HLHS each year. Two different treatment strategies are presently available, staged palliative reconstruction and neonatal cardiac allotransplantation. Advances in medical and surgical management over the last two decades have resulted in a significant improvement in outcome of this once uniformly fatal lesion. Five-year survival rates in excess of 70% are being consistently reported. The staged surgical management involves three separate procedures ultimately leading to a single ventricular repair with modified Fontan anatomy. The functional capacity and neurodevelopmental outcome of these children is reported to be no different to that of other children with complex congenital heart disease. This chapter will detail the case management of a neonate undergoing the first-stage reconstruction.

Case report

A 27-year-old pregnant woman was scheduled for routine prenatal ultrasound screening at 18 weeks' gestation. The scan revealed a fetus with severe aortic stenosis and the diagnosis of HLHS was confirmed with serial examinations during the course of the pregnancy. Parental counselling was initiated after the diagnosis was made and the decision to proceed with staged surgical repair was agreed. The baby was delivered at a tertiary referral centre with a paediatric congenital heart programme. The infant was born at 38 weeks' gestation weighing 3.6 kg following an uneventful labour and delivery. Apgar scores were 5 and 8 at 1 and 5 minutes, respectively. Following routine suctioning, the airway was cleared and pulse oximetry showed the oxygen saturation to be > 90% while breathing spontaneously in room air. This finding, accompanied by a high respiratory rate suggested pulmonary overcirculation and the inspired oxygen concentration was lowered by the addition of nitrogen within a hood and titrated to an oxygen saturation in the mid 80% range. Umbilical artery access was obtained and a peripheral intravenous line was inserted. Following confirmation of the anatomy by echocardiography, prostaglandin E1 at a dose of 0.03 $\mu g.kg^{-1}.min^{-1}$ was started to maintain ductal patency. An initial blood gas revealed a metabolic acidosis with a base deficit of 6. This was corrected with a fluid bolus of 10 $ml.kg^{-1}$ normal saline and 4 mEq sodium bicarbonate. The baby was allowed to breast feed and was scheduled for elective repair at 5 days of age.

On arrival in the operating room, the following monitors were placed: 5-lead ECG, pulse oximetry probes on the left hand and foot, and the existing umbilical artery line was transduced. Initial values showed a heart rate of 162 beats per min, blood pressure of 67/22 mmHg with an arterial oxygen saturation of 89% in room air. Twenty-one percent oxygen was administered by face mask prior to an intravenous induction using midazolam 0.3 mg, fentanyl 50 µg and pancuronium 0.8 mg. Cefazolin 25 $mg.kg^{-1}$ was administered intravenously for antibiotic prophylaxis. Following tracheal intubation, ventilation parameters were set to achieve a normal end-tidal CO_2 in the 40 mmHg range and the F_IO_2 was set at 0.21 to maintain arterial saturations less than 90%. A 5F 5-cm long double-lumen catheter was inserted into the left femoral vein, and following urinary catheterization, rectal and nasopharyngeal temperature probes were placed and the patient was positioned for surgery with appropriate padding. Following a negative test dose, 2 ml.kg^{-1} of aprotinin (Trasylol®) was infused over 20 minutes followed by an infusion of 2 ml.kg^{-1}.hr^{-1} for the duration of the case. Anaesthetic depth was maintained with the judicious use of isoflurane. As part of the preparation for bypass, snares were placed around both pulmonary arteries and the right snare was tightened to restrict pulmonary blood flow and increase systemic blood pressure. At this time, the F_IO_2 was increased to 1.0. Following the administration of 400 U.kg^{-1} of heparin and with an activated clotting time > 480 seconds, cardiopulmonary bypass (CPB) was initiated through a cannula in the proximal main pulmonary artery and a single cannula in the right atrial appendage. With a pump prime of 220 ml, the haematocrit was 20% on full CPB and the mean arterial pressure was maintained at approximately 25 mmHg. Ice was placed over a towel on the head (to avoid direct contact with the scalp and the risk of thermal injury) and the patient was cooled to 18 °C over 20 minutes. Mixed venous and regional cerebral haemoglobin oxygen saturation (rSO_2) were monitored continuously. The surgical plan is described below. Approximately 45 minutes of circulatory arrest was required to complete the arch reconstruction and the modified Blalock–Taussig (BT) shunt was completed during rewarming. Further doses of fentanyl, midazolam and pancuronium were administered upon rewarming. Temporary pacing wires, a direct right atrial line and chest tubes were placed, and the shunt was unclamped with a resultant 15 mmHg drop in the mean arterial pressure. Once the core temperature had reached 36 °C, and with blood gas variables within normal limits, bypass was terminated aided by a dopamine infusion of 5 μg.kg^{-1}.min^{-1} and low-dose epinephrine at 0.04 μg.kg^{-1}.min^{-1}. Initially ventilation parameters were set at an F_IO_2 of 1.0 and a tidal volume of 20 ml.kg^{-1}, the oxygen concentration was gradually lowered as the SaO_2 settled in the low 80% range. Following 15 minutes of modified ultrafiltration, protamine sulphate was administered in a dose guided by the heparin concentration. Haemostasis was aided by the use of platelet and cryoprecipitate infusions. A target haematocrit of greater than 40% was achieved with blood transfusions. The chest was left open and the sternotomy covered by a synthetic patch. The patient was returned to the intensive care unit (ICU) fully monitored. The sternum was closed in the ICU on postoperative day 2 and the baby was extubated 24 hours later. The subsequent postoperative course was uneventful.

Discussion

Definition and demographics

HLHS represents a continuum of anomalies characterized by underdevelopment of the aorta, aortic valve, left ventricle, mitral valve and left atrium. Although males are affected slightly more commonly than females, the recurrence rate for siblings is low (0.5%) and the majority of neonates with HLHS are born at term without any non-cardiac anomalies. There is a slight increase in the incidence of HLHS in Turner's syndrome, trisomy 18 and duplication of the short arm of chromosome 12.

Anatomy

There are significant differences in the anatomy of the neonatal heart in HLHS compared with normal (Figure 10.1). The underdevelopment of left-sided heart structures can result in numerous combinations of lesions. Most commonly there is aortic valve atresia with resultant hypoplasia of the ascending aorta and arch. This is frequently accompanied by atresia, hypoplasia or stenosis of the mitral valve and as a consequence, a severely hypoplastic left ventricle. Variants of HLHS occur in 25%, either in the form of aortic and left ventricular hypoplasia with double-outlet right ventricle and mitral atresia, or an unbalanced complete atrioventricular canal. The common feature is that of a non-functioning left ventricle often with concomitant hypertrophy of right-sided structures. Pulmonary venous blood returns to a small left atrium and crosses to the right atrium by means of an atrial septal defect (ASD) or patent foramen ovale. Mixing of pulmonary and systemic venous return occurs in the right atrium. Cardiac output is sustained to the body via the right ventricle and ductus arteriosus down the descending aorta. Coronary perfusion is dependent on retrograde flow through the diminutive ascending aorta (see Figure 10.1). Postnatally, the circulation is dependent on three major factors: the patency of the ductus arteriosus, the size of the interatrial communication and the relative resistance of the pulmonary and

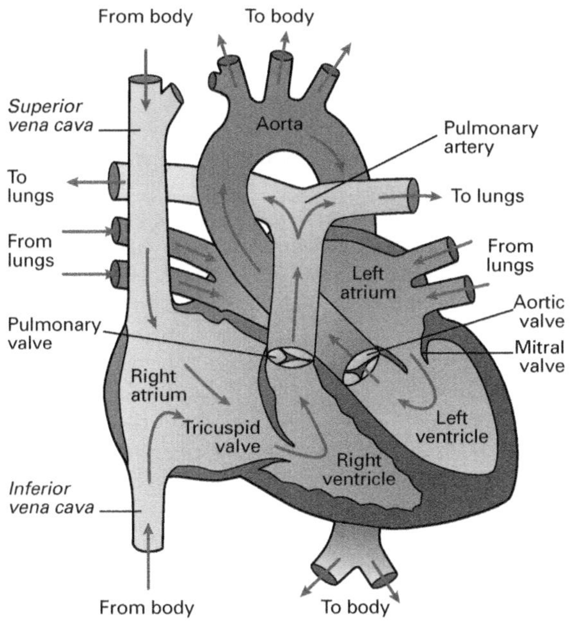

Figure 10.1
Anatomy of the normal heart.

systemic circuits. As the PO_2 increases following birth, the ductus arteriosus tends to constrict and the pulmonary vascular resistance (PVR) falls. This combination will result in a marked decrease in both systemic and coronary perfusion with resultant metabolic acidosis, myocardial ischaemia, circulatory shock and ultimately death.

Diagnosis

With the more widespread use of prenatal ultrasonography, the prenatal diagnosis of HLHS is possible. This allows for the diagnosis of extracardiac defects, provides time for the parents to receive counselling, for the delivery to be planned at a location specializing in neonatal cardiac surgery and for the various surgical options to be considered. Two-dimensional echocardiography is used to define the anatomy, evaluate pulmonary and systemic resistances, assess atrial ventricular valve competence and delineate pulmonary venous return and the degree of interatrial restriction.

Most infants with HLHS are born at full term. Cyanosis is rarely obvious at delivery, but it usually appears within hours or days. Heart failure is inevitable and tachypnoea, tachycardia, hepatomegaly and a gallop rhythm are usually present. A non-specific systolic ejection murmur at the left sternal border may be heard. Peripheral pulses may be normal, diminished or absent depending on the patency of the ductus arteriosus. Typical chest X-ray findings include moderate cardiomegaly with increased pulmonary vascular markings. Electrocardiogram features are non-specific but usually show right axis deviation and right ventricular hypertrophy. Routine cardiac catheterization is not indicated. Echocardiographic findings show the enlarged right heart structures and pulmonary arteries and the underdeveloped left heart chambers and aorta. The aortic root size and function of the mitral valve should be assessed. Transport of the patient to a tertiary referral centre can be achieved either in utero or after delivery and stabilization. Delivery at the tertiary centre avoids the risk of transporting a potentially unstable newborn and enables immediate availability of the team members specialized in the diagnosis and management of this condition.

Perioperative management

Once the diagnosis has been made, ductal patency is maintained by a continuous infusion of prostaglandin E1 (0.01–$0.05\,\mu g.kg^{-1}.min^{-1}$). Umbilical or peripheral venous and arterial access should be obtained and secured. Hypoperfusion and acidosis should be corrected with fluid resuscitation and sodium bicarbonate, respectively. Prolonged preoperative intubation is rarely required unless there is apnoea secondary to prostaglandin therapy. Further management is aimed at achieving a balance between the systemic and pulmonary blood flow (Q_P:Q_S ratio). Most neonates have a moderately restrictive interatrial communication that will allow adequate pulmonary blood flow with mild pulmonary venous hypertension without congestion. These babies are warm and well perfused with good peripheral pulses, normal systemic blood pressure and normal acid/base balance. An arterial oxygen saturation of 75–80% represents a Q_P:Q_S ratio of approximately 1.0. Neonates with widely patent interatrial communications have excessive pulmonary blood flow ('overcirculated') at the expense of systemic and coronary perfusion. Metabolic acidosis develops and the baby will hyperventilate in an attempt to compensate, the resulting reduction in $PaCO_2$ will further lower PVR and exacerbate the problem. In order to control pulmonary blood flow, two strategies can be employed. The inspired oxygen concentration can be lowered by the addition of nitrogen to the ambient air within a hood to achieve an F_IO_2 of 0.16–0.17 and maintain arterial saturations in the 80% range. Conversely, carbon dioxide (1–3%) can be added. The effect of adding CO_2 to an already hypoxic mixture may be additive. In less than 10% of cases, the infant is born with a markedly restrictive or absent interatrial communication with inadequate pulmonary blood flow and severe hypoxaemia. These babies will require tracheal intubation, volume resuscitation and inotropic support and emergent intervention in the catheterization laboratory or operating room in order to establish an adequate interatrial communication. It is our preference to allow these babies to stabilize in the ICU following this procedure before continuing with further surgical palliation.

Additional supportive measures that may be necessary prior to surgery include treatment of neonatal sepsis, inotropic support, and treatment of hepatic and renal insufficiency. These patients should be transported to the operating room fully monitored taking care to simulate ICU ventilation, with room air, as closely as possible (relative hypoventilation).

The surgical plan

The surgery involves division of the pulmonary artery, construction of a neo-aorta and the establishment of an alternative source of pulmonary blood supply. The atrial septum is excised, the main pulmonary is divided at the bifurcation and the distal end closed by a Gortex patch. The diminutive aorta is opened and anastomosed proximally to the divided pulmonary trunk and the remainder of the aorta is augmented by a patch of cryopreserved allograft. Finally a 3–3.5-mm Gortex shunt is anastomosed between the distal innominate artery and the central pulmonary artery.

As a result of these interventions, there is complete mixing of systemic and pulmonary venous blood at the atrial level. The single right ventricle pumps blood to both the body (via the neo-aorta) and the lungs (via the BT shunt) (Figure 10.2). As a consequence the baby is centrally cyanosed at the end of this procedure.

Anaesthetic technique

The goal of anaesthesia is to maintain the Q_P:Q_S ratio of 1.0 and avoid myocardial depression. An opioid-based anaesthetic in conjunction with low-dose inhalational agents is appropriate. We used fentanyl 15–25 $\mu g.kg^{-1}$ in conjunction with pancuronium and a benzodiazepine at induction and during the rewarming phase in the above case. Particular attention must be paid to ventilation to avoid excessive changes in PVR through hyper- or hypoventilation. A tidal volume of at least 10 $ml.kg^{-1}$ is set, and the respiratory rate and inspired carbon dioxide level is adjusted to maintain $PaCO_2$ at 40 mmHg. The inspired oxygen concentration is kept close to 21% to maintain saturations between 80% and 85%. The anaesthesia machine should be adapted to deliver nitrogen or carbon dioxide if required. Additional intravenous access is obtained, usually with a multilumen catheter in a femoral vein and arterial access is via an existing umbilical catheter, femoral artery or left radial artery. Venous access in the neck veins is avoided due to the risk of thrombosis, and intra-arterial cannulae in the

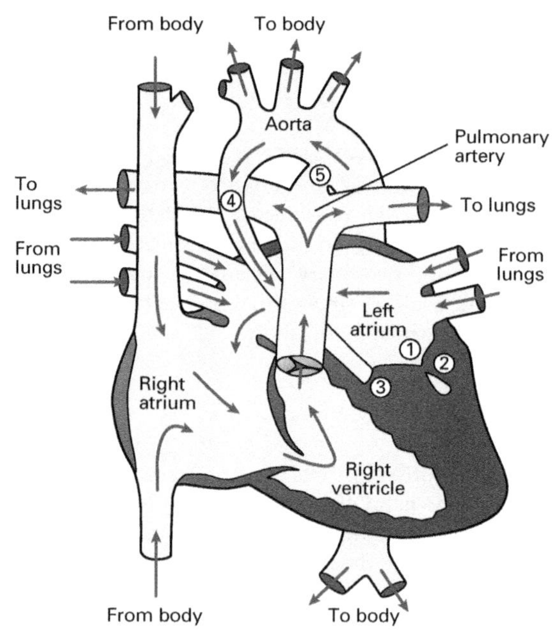

Figure 10.2
Hypoplastic Left Heart Syndrome. 1 = mitral atresia; 2 = hypoplastic LV; 3 = aortic atresia; 4 = diminutive ascending aorta; 5 = ductus arteriosus.

right radial artery should be avoided as subsequent measurements may be inaccurate after establishment of the right BT shunt.

During bypass, in addition to monitoring mixed venous oxygen saturation (a crude measure of whole body oxygen delivery), we routinely measure rSO_2 with the non-invasive INVOS Cerebral Oximeter (Somanetics Corp, Troy, MI, USA). A baseline reading is obtained shortly after induction of anaesthesia and we aim to maintain rSO_2 within 20% of that baseline value. Diminished cerebral blood flow can be the result of suboptimal cannula position, systemic hypotension or cerebral vasoconstriction. Manoeuvres to increase rSO_2 will depend on the cause with the aim to increase the supply of oxygen to the brain or reduce oxygen consumption. Strategies include increasing mean arterial pressure or the pump flow rate, increasing F_IO_2 or CO_2, raising the hematocrit, deepening anaesthesia or repositioning the cannula.

In preparation for separation from CPB, dopamine 5 μg.kg.$^{-1}$.min^{-1} is begun which has been shown to have positive inotropic effects without increasing systemic or pulmonary vascular resistance. Diastolic blood pressures should be maintained above 20 mmHg and the use of a low-dose infusion of epinephrine is useful in this regard. Sustained hypoxaemia may be the result of high PVR or inadequate pulmonary blood flow secondary to a kinked or undersized BT shunt. If the usual methods to counteract the high PVR (hyperventilation, increasing F_IO_2, correction of acidosis, increased sedation and adequate paralysis) fail, it may be necessary to load the patient with milrinone (75 μg.kg^{-1}) and infuse at 0.5 μg.kg^{-1}.min^{-1}. Inhaled nitric oxide 20–80 ppm may be beneficial in some cases. The routine use of aprotinin and fresh whole blood (< 48 hours old) in these cases has greatly improved post-bypass bleeding. Leaving the sternum open at the conclusion of the case will allow rapid re-exploration should haemorrhage or tamponade occur, as well as allowing time for myocardial oedema to resolve prior to definitive chest closure.

Postoperative care

The management of the patient in the first 24–48 hours postoperatively is crucial to the overall outcome. Balancing the pulmonary and systemic circulations to achieve an even distribution of blood flow (Q_P:Q_S = 1.0) should be the goal. The 'ideal' set of blood gases would be pH 7.40, PO_2 40 mmHg and PCO_2 40 mmHg, with an arterial saturation in the 75–80% range and mixed venous oxygen saturation 45–60%. With these parameters, adequate oxygen delivery is shown clinically by a well perfused infant with good peripheral pulses and adequate urine output in the absence of metabolic acidosis. Should the latter develop, it should be aggressively treated with sodium bicarbonate and the cause determined. The commonest causes of inadequate oxygen delivery are (1) excessive pulmonary blood flow, (2) inadequate pulmonary blood flow and (3) inadequate cardiac output. Any technical problem should be excluded or corrected. Excessive pulmonary blood flow is indicated by a raised systemic oxygen saturation (> 85%), and high PO_2 (> 45 mmHg) and can be treated by lowering the F_IO_2 to room air, decreasing the minute ventilation to allow the PCO_2 to raise and adding positive end-expiratory pressure. PVR can be further raised by the addition of nitrogen to achieve subambient oxygen concentrations, or by adding CO_2 to raise PCO_2 > 50 mmHg. Inadequate pulmonary blood flow will result in a falling PO_2 (< 25 mmHg) and systemic arterial oxygen saturations less than 60% with a mixed venous oxygen saturation less than 40%. The BT shunt (kinked, anastomotic narrowing or too small) should be ruled out as a cause, and manoeuvres to reduce PVR should be instituted. This again includes raising the F_IO_2 to 1.0, increasing the minute ventilation to lower PCO_2 to less than 30 mmHg, treating acidosis, ensuring adequate sedation/paralysis and considering treatment with inhaled nitric oxide. Inadequate cardiac output is usually manifested by a systemic oxygen saturation < 70% with a PO_2 < 30 mmHg, coupled with hypotension, oliguria and a persistent metabolic acidosis. It is important to evaluate the patient for any technical problem related to the surgery (poor myocardial protection, compromised coronary blood supply, tricuspid regurgitation or residual neo-aortic obstruction). Provided there is no 'correctable' lesion, efforts to improve cardiac output would include ensuring adequate preload, increasing the haematocrit and the use of inotropes and vasodilators. Extracorporeal membrane oxygenation (ECMO) has been used with variable success in the treatment of myocardial dysfunction following the first stage of palliative reconstruction.

The second stage surgery (bidirectional Glenn anastomosis or hemi-Fontan) is usually performed at 3–6 months of age once PVR has decreased. Cardiac catheterization is performed prior to surgery to evaluate right ventricular function, tricuspid regurgitation, pulmonary artery architecture and PVR. Contraindications to surgery include poor ventricular

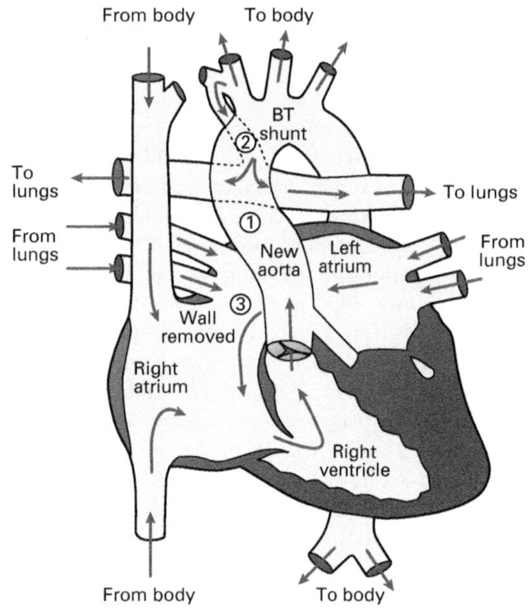

Figure 10.3
Stage 1 (Norwood procedure). 1 = neo-aorta; 2 = BT shunt; 3 = atrial septectomy.

function and elevated PVR. Surgery involves ligating the BT shunt and providing pulmonary blood flow by anastomosing the superior vena cava to the pulmonary artery (a cavopulmonary connection (Figure 10.3). This will have the physiological effect of reducing the volume load on the right ventricle and thereby lowering the end-diastolic pressure and allowing ventricular 'remodelling'.

The final stage Fontan is undertaken between 12 and 18 months of age. Again, preoperative assessment is necessary to evaluate haemodynamics, anatomy, valve function and to coil-embolize major collateral vessels that may have developed as a result of continued hypoxaemia. All systemic venous return is directed entirely to the pulmonary artery, bypassing the systemic right ventricle. This can be achieved by an intra-atrial Gortex patch or an extracardiac conduit. A small fenestration is often created to allow right to left shunting in the presence of systemic venous hypertension (Figure 10.4). This opening will often close spontaneously or may be occluded in the catheterization laboratory resulting in the final separation of the two circulations (Figure 10.5).

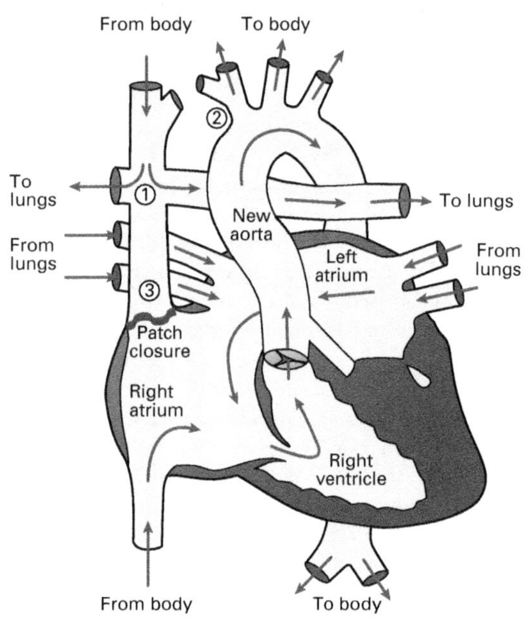

Figure 10.4
Stage 2 (bi-directional Glenn or hemi-Fontan. 1 = SVC to PA anastomosis; 2 = BT shunt ligated; 3 = patch closure to right atrium.

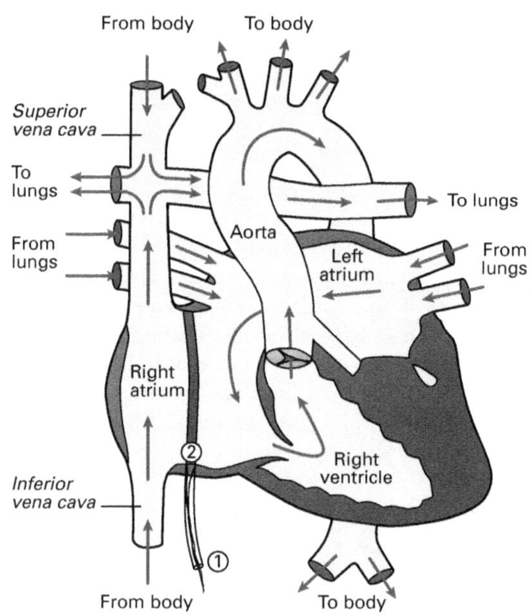

Figure 10.5
Stage 3 (Fontan). 1 = external snare; 2 = site of possible fenestration.

With over two decades of experience in the treatment of hypoplastic left heart syndrome, survival rates are encouraging, yet mortality is still highest in the newborn period. New interventional procedures in the catheterization laboratory are evolving which may reduce perioperative mortality. The care of this complex lesion is best undertaken at a few centres of excellence with a coordinated team approach involving all specialties.

Learning points

- HLHS is an underdevelopment of left-sided heart structures. Most commonly there is a severely hypoplastic left ventricle, aortic valve atresia, hypoplasia of the ascending aorta and arch, with atresia, hypoplasia, or stenosis of the mitral valve.
- Advances in the medical and surgical management over the last two decades have resulted in a significant improvement in outcome of this once uniformly fatal lesion.
- The treatment of HLHS involves a collaborative effort between cardiologists, surgeons, anaesthetists and intensive care personnel and should only be undertaken at specialized centres.
- A thorough understanding of the anatomy and physiology is essential in the perioperative management of HLHS.
- Meticulous attention must be paid to physiological parameters in order to optimize the balance between the pulmonary and systemic circulations during anaesthesia, surgery and in the postoperative period.
- The second stage surgery is usually performed at 3–6 months of age and involves ligation of the BT shunt and anastomosis of the superior vena cava to the pulmonary artery.
- The final stage Fontan is undertaken between 12 and 18 months of age. All systemic venous return is directed entirely to the pulmonary artery, bypassing the systemic right ventricle.
- Five-year survival rates following staged palliative repair are reported in excess of 70%.

Suggested reading

Bove EL. Surgical treatment of hypoplastic left heart syndrome. *Jpn J Thorac Cardiovasc Surg* 1999; 47: 47–56.

Cheatham JP, Galantowicz M, Amplatz K et al. A new era in the treatment of HLHS: transcatheter Stage I palliation and Stage III completion. *Catheteriz Cardiovasc Intervent* 2002; 56: 150.

Daubeney PEF, Smith DC, Pilkington SN et al. Cerebral oxygenation during paediatric cardiac surgery: identification of vulnerable periods using near infrared spectroscopy. *Eur J Cardiothorac Surg* 1998; 13: 370–377.

Erle AH. Postoperative management after the Norwood procedure. *Sem Thorac Cardiovasc Surg* 1998; 1: 109–121.

Goldberg CS, Schwartz EM, Brunberg JA et al. Neurodevelopmental outcome of patients after the Fontan operation: a comparison between children with hypoplastic left heart syndrome and other functional single ventricle lesions. *J Pediatr* 2000; 137: 646–652.

Jenkins PC, Flanagan MF, Sargent JD et al. A comparison of treatment strategies of hypoplastic left heart syndrome using decision analysis. *J Am Coll Cardiol* 2001; 38: 1181–1187.

Keidan I, Mishaly D, Berkenstadt H et al. Combining low inspired oxygen and carbon dioxide during mechanical ventilation for the Norwood procedure. *Paediat Anaesth* 2003; 1: 58–62.

Koutlas TC, Gaynor JW, Nicolson SC et al. Modified ultrafiltration reduces postoperative morbidity after cavo-pulmonary connection. *J Thorac Cardiovasc Surg* 1997; 64: 37–43.

Kurth CD, Steven JL, Montenegro LM et al. Cerebral oxygen saturation before congenital heart surgery. *Ann Thor Surg* 2001; 72: 187–192.

Maegawa Y, Mizobe T, Yamagishi M et al. The use of nitrogen and nitric oxide to control pulmonary blood flow in the Norwood operation. *J Cardiothorac Vasc Anesth* 2002; 16: 264–266.

Mahle WT, Spray TL, Gaynor JW et al. Unexpected death after reconstructive surgery for hypoplastic left heart syndrome. *Ann Thor Surg* 2001; 71: 61–65.

Mahle WT, Spray TL, Wernovsky G et al. Survival after palliative surgery for hypoplastic left heart syndrome: 15-year experience from a single institution. *Circulation* 2000; 102(Suppl 3): III 136–141.

Migliavacca F, Pennati G, Dubini G et al. Modeling of the Norwood circulation: effects of shunt size, vascular resistances, and heart rate. *Am J Physiol Heart Circ Physiol* 2001; 280: H2076–2086.

Nicolson SC, Steven JM, Jobes DR. Hypoplastic left heart syndrome. In: Lake C (ed). *Pediatric Cardiac Anesthesia* 3rd edn 1998. Stamford, Conneticut.

Pearl JM, Nelson DP, Schwartz SM et al. First-stage palliation for hypoplastic left heart syndrome in the twenty-first century. *Ann Thor Surg* 2002; **73**: 331–339.

Pigula FA, Nemoto EM, Griffith et al. Regional low flow perfusion provides cerebral circulatory support during neonatal arch reconstruction. *J Thorac Cardiovasc Surg* 2000; 119: 331–339.

Pizarro C, Davis DA, Healy RM et al. Is there a role for extracorporeal life support after stage I Norwood? *Eur J Cardiothorac Surg* 2001; 19: 294–301.

Poirier NC, Drummond-Webb JJ, Hisamochi K et al. Modified Norwood procedure with a high-flow cardiopulmonary bypass strategy results in low mortality without late arch obstruction. *J Thorac Cardiovasc Surg* 2000; 120: 875–884.

Tabbutt S, Ramamoorthy C, Montenegro LM et al. Impact of inspired gas mixtures on preoperative infants with hypoplastic left heart syndrome during controlled ventilation. *Circulation* 2001; 104: I-159–164.

Weinstein S, Gaynor JW, Bridges ND et al. Early survival of infants weighing 2.5 kilograms or less undergoing first stage reconstruction for hypoplastic left heart syndrome. *Circulation* 1999; (Suppl 12): 167–170.

11

Management of an adolescent with chronic knee pain and severe disability

John M Goddard

Introduction

Knee pain is very common in childhood and can be caused by a variety of conditions. Anterior knee pain, also known as patellofemoral pain, has a number of causes and accounts for a large proportion of children presenting with knee pain. Significant disability associated with knee pain is not common, but frequently results in prolonged absence from school. Some children are disabled by pain associated with a congenital, inflammatory or major traumatic condition. Other children, usually adolescents, are severely disabled by anterior knee pain, a condition that does not usually produce such severe disability. I rely upon my orthopaedic colleagues to provide a diagnosis and to be of the opinion that multidisciplinary pain management is appropriate.

History

David, a 13-year-old boy, was referred to the Paediatric Accident and Emergency Department by his general practitioner. He was accompanied by his mother. He gave a 3-week history of increasing pain affecting the medial aspect of his right knee. The pain was made worse by weight-bearing and going up and down stairs. He also complained of some swelling of his knee, and that his knee would click and give way but he would not fall. He was unable to do his physical exercise lessons and had stopped his paper round. Rest, bandaging and paracetamol had not helped his symptoms. He had been sent home from school earlier that day because of pain, had been to his general practitioner who had prescribed diclofenac and advised Accident and Emergency attendance if his pain did not improve. He was reported to have had 'clicky knees' as a toddler but no other past medical history. Physical examination demonstrated a small effusion, local tenderness and some limitation of flexion. There was no erythema or local warmth. Plain X-rays showed no bony abnormality. His knee was immobilized with a Robert–Jones bandage and he was sent home with a fracture clinic appointment.

At the fracture clinic, 3 days later, a history of his knee locking was felt to be significant; he was admitted from the clinic for an arthroscopy. Review on the ward by an orthopaedic senior registrar demonstrated full extension, limitation of flexion due to pain and no effusion. Arthroscopy was postponed and management consisted of regular diclofenac, codeine phosphate and cold compresses. He was discharged home 2 days later with crutches and an outpatient appointment in 1 week. Within 2 days he was readmitted to the ward in severe pain, his knee was immobilized in a plaster backslab and he was discharged again. David attended the orthopaedic clinic five times over the next 2 months, but remained in a backslab unable to weight-bear or co-operate with physiotherapy. School attendance was minimal. Several investigations were normal. A referral was made to a Paediatric Pain Clinic.

Investigations

The following investigations wre undertaken:

Full blood count – haemoglobin 14.2 g.dl^{-1}, WBC, 7.5 × 10^{9}.l^{-1}, normal differential count
Erythrocyte sedimentation rate – 3 mm in 1 hr
C-reactive protein – < 6 mg.l^{-1} (normal 2–10)
Plain X-rays of both knees with skyline views – normal on several occasions
Plain X-rays of both hips – normal
Rheumatoid factor – 2 IU.ml^{-1} (normal 1–8)
Isotope bone scan – very mild increased uptake around medial condyle of right femur
Magnetic resonance imaging scan of right knee – normal.

Management

Before a letter of referral had been received by the pain management service, David's mother had contacted both the nurse specialist and the physiotherapist to request an early appointment. She was very distressed that a satisfactory diagnosis had not been reached and explained to her; she intended to seek a second orthopaedic opinion.

Three weeks later David was seen with his mother in the multidisciplinary pain clinic. When his history was reviewed, the only notable addition was that the pain had been present intermittently for several months before his initial presentation. He described the pain as a dull ache that was present all the time; the backslab was very helpful and was allowing him to sleep at night. He reported that if his knee was touched or moved he would experience a severe sharp pain. On direct questioning there was no history of allodynia. He was attending school part time, unhappy that he was unable to go full time. He was upset that he was unable to do his paper round, play football, go skiing, or even go fishing. He was spending much of his time on the computer and felt isolated from his friends. He lived with his parents and elder sister, his father was in full-time employment and his mother worked part time. Limited examination of his knee did not reveal any swelling, temperature variation, colour or trophic changes. Quadriceps wasting was noticeable.

At the last orthopaedic appointment it had been explained to his mother that David's tibial tuberosities were situated quite laterally and that this could cause mechanical problems leading to a degree of chondromalacia patellae. Chondromalacia patellae is one cause of anterior knee pain. This diagnosis was discussed at length with David and his mother; it was reinforced that this condition would improve with time and that no surgical operation was appropriate. We also discussed how long-standing pain could lead to changes in the central nervous system and the development of chronic pain, and the normal psychological effects of this situation upon the individual and his family. A review of David's analgesic intake revealed that he was taking appropriate doses of diclofenac and codeine phosphate three times daily; we suggested that he should continue with both drugs but stagger their administration. Paracetamol was recommended as a rescue analgesic. David was agreeable to a trial of Transcutaneous Electrical Nerve Stimulation (TENS) and an appointment with the nurse specialist was arranged as a daycase; it was further agreed that she would show him some relaxation techniques. The process of graded exercise and rehabilitation was discussed with David and his mother; they agreed with the physiotherapist to begin by removing the splint for 2 minutes four times a day. A further meeting with the physiotherapist was arranged at the same time as his TENS assessment. It was suggested to David's mother that a future family appointment with the clinical psychologist might be helpful, to allow further discussion of the issues surrounding her son's incapacity; this offer was accepted.

Six days later David was admitted for his TENS trial. Pre-TENS he rated his severe pain as 87 and his dull pain as 40 on unmarked 100 mm visual analogue scales, post-TENS, using four pads, he rated his dull pain as 26. He thought that altering the timing of his codeine phosphate had been helpful and was proud that he had been able to remove his splint as directed. He was reviewed by the physiotherapist with a TENS machine still applied to his knee. He did not wish his knee to be touched, but was able to manage static quadriceps exercises and 10 degrees of flexion/extension after verbal instruction. He was discharged with a home exercise programme, a TENS machine and weekly outpatient physiotherapy appointments. The day after his second physiotherapy appointment, his mother rang to say that his pain was much worse and that he had needed to be collected from school early. His mother was reassured that this was not unusual and did not signify a return to 'square one'; a plan was discussed with her. David was to use an ice pack on his knee that evening, he was to return to using four TENS pads having altered to only two, the possibility of resting his leg at lunchtime in the school medical room was to be investigated, and at his next appointment the nurse specialist would coach David in relaxation and breathing exercises. On review, David was maintaining his exercise programme, and seemed to appreciate insight into the control of his breathing. He attended weekly for 6 weeks.

David and his parents met with the clinical psychologist on one occasion, 3 weeks after the pain clinic meeting. His parents took this opportunity to further express their anger and frustration at the delay and apparent confusion there had been in making a diagnosis regarding their son's condition. They were also highly critical of the apparent indifference there had been to the extreme pain he had suffered. Space was given for these feelings to be aired, and they were acknowledged before any intervention was attempted. Further explanation was given regarding the development and maintenance of chronic pain, including the role of fear and negative thoughts; strategies to gain control of the situation and empower child and family were discussed.

The family returned from a Mediterranean holiday where David did a lot of swimming. At this stage he was able to flex his knee to 90 degrees, but was unable to fully weight-bear and was still dependent on two crutches. He was no longer wearing a splint and had discontinued his analgesics except for occasional codeine phosphate. A decision was made at this stage to transfer his physiotherapy from the pain management service to the outpatient service. He continued to attend regularly over the next 4 months, weaning himself from both crutches. David was reviewed in the pain clinic 7 months after his initial appointment. He was still having regular physiotherapy, but had returned to school full time. He found his TENS machine helpful and used it mainly for his physiotherapy appointments. He was taking no medication. He was due to start basketball and a paper round soon. We arranged to meet again only if necessary.

Outcome

David continued to experience pain in his right knee. He attended physiotherapy less frequently. At an orthopaedic review a year later it was noted that he was playing basketball and, to a limited extent, football. He was unable to run long distances because of pain. His knee was thought to be clinically normal with excellent quadriceps power. He was discharged from hospital follow-up.

Discussion

Anterior knee pain, also known as patellofemoral pain, is common in adolescence. In a cohort of 446 normal schoolchildren aged 13–17 the prevalence of knee pain was 31%.[1] Of those reporting knee pain, 29% had seen a doctor and 18% had stopped sports. Anterior knee pain is a chronic disorder but does not usually cause severe disability. Sandow and Goodfellow reported on 54 female adolescents 2–8 years after presentation, none of whom had undergone an operative procedure.[2] 95% continued to experience some pain but its severity had reduced in 46% and had worsened in only 13%. 82% reported that they felt pain about once a week or less frequently and 87% used analgesics never or rarely.

We now know that the nocioceptive system functions as an active and complex integrative mechanism; neural activity initiated by tissue damage can be modified by a diverse array of physical and psychological factors. All perception of pain is affected by situational, behavioural and emotional factors; when managing children the additional factors of age, cognitive level and parental perceptions have to be considered.[3] For these reasons most paediatric clinics seeing children with chronic pain have developed with multidisciplinary involvement, as recommended by Berde et al.[4] In my opinion the initial appointment should be for at least 1 hour, thus allowing plenty of time to listen to the inevitable concerns and anxieties of the family, as well as the history of the painful problem. In addition, time allows information to be fed back to the family regarding the diagnosis, and the development and maintenance of chronic pain. At the end of this appointment it is usual to be able to agree a management plan with the child and family and to have sown the seeds of a trusting relationship.

A review of current analgesia is always appropriate. Tweaking of the dose and timing of simple analgesics is often helpful and provision needs to be made for the administration of rescue analgesia when pain is not fully controlled by regular medication. There is remarkably little data available to support the efficacy and safety of long-term drug use in children with chronic pain; most treatment is based on efficacy studies in adults. Sethna[5] has recently reviewed this topic. I find that tramadol and amitriptyline are often helpful drugs when simple analgesics are not fully effective and further drug therapy is considered appropriate.

A TENS trial is usually worth considering.[6] TENS is tolerated well by most children, has almost no side effects, and while dramatic improvement is the exception rather than the rule many children find it helpful in combination with other modalities. There is no data on its efficacy in the paediatric population, however a Cochrane review supports the use of TENS for pain control in adults with osteoarthritis of the knee.[7] In my view TENS should be introduced in a structured manner, involving assessment, training and evaluation by an experienced healthcare professional.

Psychological methods of treating pain can be very effective and are useful whether the pain is considered to be primarily of a physical or psychological origin.[8] Also as McGrath, Dick and Unruh state: 'Health professionals cannot choose to avoid using psychology to treat pain. Our choice is whether to use psychology in a conscious, constructive fashion or to leave the psychological aspect of our interventions to chance.' A positive proactive attitude to recovery should be inherent in the overall approach of the multidisciplinary team. Some psychological methods require specialized psychological skills, but others, such as control of breathing and relaxation, can be taught by nursing and physiotherapy staff.

Physiotherapy is another vital component in the management of most children with chronic pain.[6] Pain inhibits function and leads to disability. Intervention begins with a comprehensive evaluation of both the pain and its effects on activities of daily living; a programme is then developed to suit the individual child. An important aspect of this process is to gain the confidence of the family. Many children have had previous experiences of challenge to their physical status, and have become disillusioned with failure. Facilitation is required in identifying realistic goals for the child, and the pace of progress; these help the development of better motivation, a greater sense of control, and increased confidence in both themselves and the team. It can be helpful to talk in terms of rehabilitation rather than physiotherapy.

The provision of multidisciplinary care can be difficult; communication and record keeping are not always easy. I believe that a full time co-ordinator with a healthcare background is essential. A paediatric nurse usually fulfils this role, organizing and co-ordinating the team as well as providing a point of telephone contact for children and, more commonly, their parents. Hiccoughs in progress are not uncommon and catastrophe needs to be avoided; readily available contact, trouble shooting and reassurance is frequently very helpful.

Learning points

- Knee pain is a common chronic condition in childhood.
- Knee pain resulting in severe disability is unusual. Situational, behavioural and emotional factors are usually adversely affecting the perception of pain.
- School attendance is a good indicator of disability.
- A multidisciplinary approach to the management of chronic knee pain associated with disability is frequently required.
- Rescue analgesia should be discussed.
- A TENS trial is usually indicated.
- Psychological methods of managing pain should be used in a conscious, constructive fashion.
- A rehabilitation programme, tailored to the individual child, is required.
- Accessible telephone contact for families is often helpful in avoiding crises.

References

1. Fairbank JCT, Pynsent PB, Van Poortvliet JA, Phillips H. Mechanical factors in the incidence of knee pain in adolescents and young adults. *J Bone Joint Surg* 1984; 66-B: 685–693.
2. Sandow MJ, Goodfellow JW. The natural history of anterior knee pain in adolescents. *J Bone Joint Surg* 1985; 67-B; 36–38.
3. McGrath PA, Hillier LM. Modifying the psychologic factors that intensify children's pain and prolong disability. In: Schechter NL, Berde CB, Yaster M eds. Pain in infants, children and adolescents, 2nd edn. Philadelphia: Lippincott Williams and Wilkins, 2003: 85–104.
4. Berde CB, Sethna NF, Masek B et al. Pediatric pain clinics: recommendations for their development. *Pediatrician* 1989; 16: 94–102.
5. Sethna NF. Pharmacotherapy in long-term pain: current experience and future direction. In: McGrath PJ, Finley GA, eds. Chronic and Recurrent Pain in Children and Adolescents. Seattle: IASP Press, 1999: 243–266.
6. McCarthy CF, Shea AM, Sullivan P. Physical therapy management of pain in children and adolescents. In: Schechter NL, Berde CB, Yaster M, eds. Pain in infants, children and adolescents, 2nd edn. Philadelphia: Lippincott Williams and Wilkins, 2003: 434–448
7. Osiri M, Welch V, Brosseau L et al. Transcutaneous electrical nerve stimulation for knee osteoarthritis (Cochrane Review). In: The Cochrane Library, 1, 2001. Oxford: Update Software.
8. McGrath PJ, Dick B, Unruh AM. Psychologic and behavioral treatment of pain in children and adolescents. In: Schechter NL, Berde CB, Yaster M, eds. Pain in Infants, Children and Adolescents, 2nd edn. Philadelphia: Lippincott Williams and Wilkins, 2003: 303–316.

12

Management of pain in patients with sickle cell disease

Julia Ely and Anthony Moriarty

Introduction

Pain is the most common and debilitating problem associated with sickle cell disease (SCD). The episodes of pain are severe, relapsing and unforgiving in their nature and are often termed 'crises'. The management of pain in SCD has improved little over the recent years. Recent practice has highlighted the usefulness of non-pharmacological techniques such as cognitive behavioural therapies.

Case report

'Steven' is a 14-year-old boy who has had four previous hospital admissions with painful sickle cell crises. On this occasion he was admitted to our hospital with a 3-day history of abdominal pain and priapism. Steven had been managed at a district general hospital prior to transfer with a combination of non-steroidal anti-inflammatory drugs (NSAIDs) and oral morphine but his pain remained uncontrolled. Unfortunately, his priapism did not resolve and Steven required surgery to treat this condition. The operation required bilateral saphenous vein grafting to improve flow into and out of the penis. Peroperatively a lumbar epidural catheter was placed to provide analgesia and an increase in blood flow through the vessels. An epidural infusion of plain local anaesthetic was continued postoperatively for 5 days. This epidural infusion provided such good analgesia that it was continued despite full heparinization of the child. Steven made an uneventful recovery.

Discussion

- SCD occurs predominantly in persons of African and Afro-Caribbean origin and affects approximately 5000 people in the UK.[1]
- SCD is caused by a single base mutation which results in the substitution of glutamine for valine at position 6 of the β globin chain. Individuals with the abnormal gene still synthesize normal fetal haemoglobin (HbF) and so the disease does not manifest until about 6 months of age when the HbF decreases to adult levels and is replaced with the abnormal sickle cell haemoglobin (HbS).
- The oxygen-carrying capacity of the HbS is normal, but with deoxygenation it polymerizes and forms crystal-like rods. These rods then aggregate, resulting in inflexible sickle-shaped erythrocytes which become trapped during their passage through the microcirculation, resulting in obstruction of these vessels.
- This vaso-occlusion causes tissue ischaemia and infarction and sets off a cascade of further sickling and results in the recurrent painful episodes which characterize the disease.

Pain syndromes of sickle cell disease

- Severe, painful vaso-occlusive crises are the most common manifestation of SCD and are recurrent and unpredictable in their timing.
- The crises are commonly precipitated by hypoxia, infection, stress, dehydration, hypothermia, but often no cause is found.
- There is marked individual variation in the severity of the disease and the incidence of painful episodes in SCD is a spectrum, from patients who never experience any pain to those who are admitted to hospital more than 10 times per year.
- In more severe cases, vaso-occlusion may lead to infarction of organs such as the spleen

(autosplenism), lungs (part of a process referred to as acute chest syndrome), kidneys, placenta and brain (stroke). These complications are the commonest causes of death in patients with SCD.

- Pain in SCD is multivariate in presentation, although it commonly presents as skeletal pain involving long bones, back, chest and hip joints, it is also a cause of an acute abdomen and headaches.
- In younger children the pain more commonly involves extremities such as fingers and toes (dactylitis) and an episode of dactylitis presenting before the age of 1 year correlates significantly with a poorer prognosis.[2]
- In adolescents crises frequently present as abdominal, chest and lower back pain. Priapism is an unfortunate presentation in the older boys. The time scale of pain is also variable, regularly lasting between 4 and 14 days.
- Over a period of time the pain associated with SCD may become chronic, becoming physically and mentally incapacitating to the patient and their families. Although over 90% of admissions in SCD are for pain or pain-related causes, most sickle pain is minor and treated in the community.
- Pain has been reported to occur on 30% of days, with a loss of 10% of school days in children.
- Children with SCD undergo an increase in hospitalization and thus more commonly undergo painful procedures in hospital.
- This procedural pain, on a background of vaso-occlusive pain may be particularly difficult to manage.

Problems in treating the pain in sickle cell crises

Traditionally the pain of sickle cell crises had been inadequately managed. The difficulties of treating the often excruciating and underestimated pain are compounded by the problems of it being predominantly self-reported and the barriers caused by social and cultural prejudices. Accurate assessment of the severity and nature of any pain is the first step to optimal treatment and herein lies one of the biggest problems in this group of patients. The pain varies enormously not only from one individual to another, but within the course of each episode and between different episodes in the same patient. Many healthcare professionals view these patients and their reported levels of pain with scepticism, especially as the pain may not respond to conventional analgesic regimens, even in very large doses, in a predictable fashion. Some believe them to be addicted to the strong analgesics used, despite little evidence to support this concern, further hampering effective delivery of care. Many patients continue to function to a level which seems to the observer to contradict their levels of reported pain and this adds to mistrust of their symptom reporting, despite evidence that any individual's ability to cope with pain is affected not only by genetic and psychological factors, but also by a wide variety of external influences. Along with the mistrust of patient's account of their pain, healthcare providers often try to wean the doses of opiates, which can further result in manipulative 'drug-seeking' behaviour often interpreted as a sign of addiction. The key to successful pain control is involvement of the patient and their family in treatment planning and attention to not only the physical aspects of the pain, but also the psychological, social and cultural effects. Individualized therapeutic planning may be best achieved in the outpatient setting between episodes rather than during an acute phase when patients often suffer from inconsistencies in management which arise from being treated by unfamiliar doctors out-of-hours. Inadequate pain management over the years promotes adversarial relationships between patients and their caregivers and further perpetuates difficulties in working together to achieve optimal analgesia for the acute episodes which in turn fails to minimize the chronic pain which may lead on from these.

Pain is a subjective experience and its assessment relies heavily on self-reporting and the use of validated measurement tools. This is particularly challenging in children who may not have sufficiently developed means of expression to fully convey the nature and severity of their personal pain experience. Specialized pain assessment tools have been designed for use in varying ages of children.

Assessment of pain in children will be covered elsewhere, but usually rely on visual scales, such as a faces scale. The faces scale is able to be used from children aged 5 and upwards, it is also able to be used by non-English-speaking children.

Pain management

The management of pain in patients with SCD can be divided into the following categories:

- institutional protocols
- pharmacological therapies
- non-pharmacological therapies
- treatment of chronic pain syndromes.

- Basic management including warmth and adequate hydration
- A hierarchy of pharmacological techniques (see below)
- Criteria for blood transfusion as the adverse effects such as iron overload may outweigh the benefits apart from in well defined exceptions, e.g. acute chest syndrome
- A pathway of care, from outpatient to intensive care, defining responsible clinicians
- A reminder that a full medical history and examination should always be undertaken to rule out other causes of pain
- A self-report pain scale to allow individual variation in pharmacokinetics and pharmacodynamics
- The use of cognitive therapies

Table 12.1
Protocols for management of pain in SCD

Institutional protocols

Protocols are required by each institution because historically pain management of SCD has been poor. The use of such a protocol reminds healthcare workers of the nature of the disease and directs pain management to the individual. A protocol should include the items noted in Table 12.1.

Pharmacological therapies

The World Health Organization ladder for the treatment of increasing levels of pain in cancer sufferers is applicable to the management of pain in sickle cell crises.[3] Mildly painful episodes are usually managed at home and paracetamol and NSAIDs form the mainstay of treatment for these. Opiates are added with increasing severity of the pain both in oral and parenteral forms. More recently, other methods of achieving analgesia, such as epidural infusions have been employed.

Experience has shown that tackling the pain of sickle cell crises using a multimodal approach is the most successful, each patient requiring an individualized treatment plan tailored to their pain experience. Combinations of analgesics, local anaesthetics and cognitive interventions have synergistic effects and minimize the undesirable effects of using large measures of any type of therapy alone. Pre-emptive analgesia may prevent the onset of pathological responses to pain, the 'upregulation' of the nervous system and the subsequent 'pain behaviour'.

Paracetamol should form the first step in building any analgesic combination in the vast majority of patients, and further classes of drug added from the following;

- NSAIDs
- opiates
- adjunct drugs
- hydroxyurea
- local anaesthetics.

A pain management strategy is demonstrated in Figure 12.1.

Non-steroidal anti-inflammatory drugs

These can be used in oral (e.g. ibuprofen, diclofenac) or parenteral (e.g. ketorolac, tenoxicam) forms and all work primarily by prostaglandin inhibition. NSAIDS have the advantage of good analgesia without the risks of respiratory depression and dependence encountered with high-dose opiates. On the downside though, they carry the risk of gastritis and peptic ulceration, and blood loss from the gastrointestinal tract, even if insidious, may decompensate patients in precarious haemodynamic balance from chronic anaemia. Another adverse effect is a reduction in renal blood flow which can precipitate or worsen renal failure in patients already at risk from sickle cell nephropathy. Studies have shown that NSAIDS are safe in SCD patients with normal renal function[4] but should be used with more caution in those with compromised function as irreversible renal failure may occur.[5]

Opiates

Opiates are widely used in the setting of SCD and are often required to be administered for long periods and in much larger doses than in other types of acute pain. Inherent in this are the problems of tolerance and physical dependence; these are to be expected and should not be confused with psychological dependence and 'addiction'. Many patients know which opiate, in what dose and by which route works best for them and many healthcare professionals assume that their very specific requests represent addiction rather than a long and frustrating and often inconsistent treatment history that these patients have often suffered. Opioids should never be withheld for fear of producing

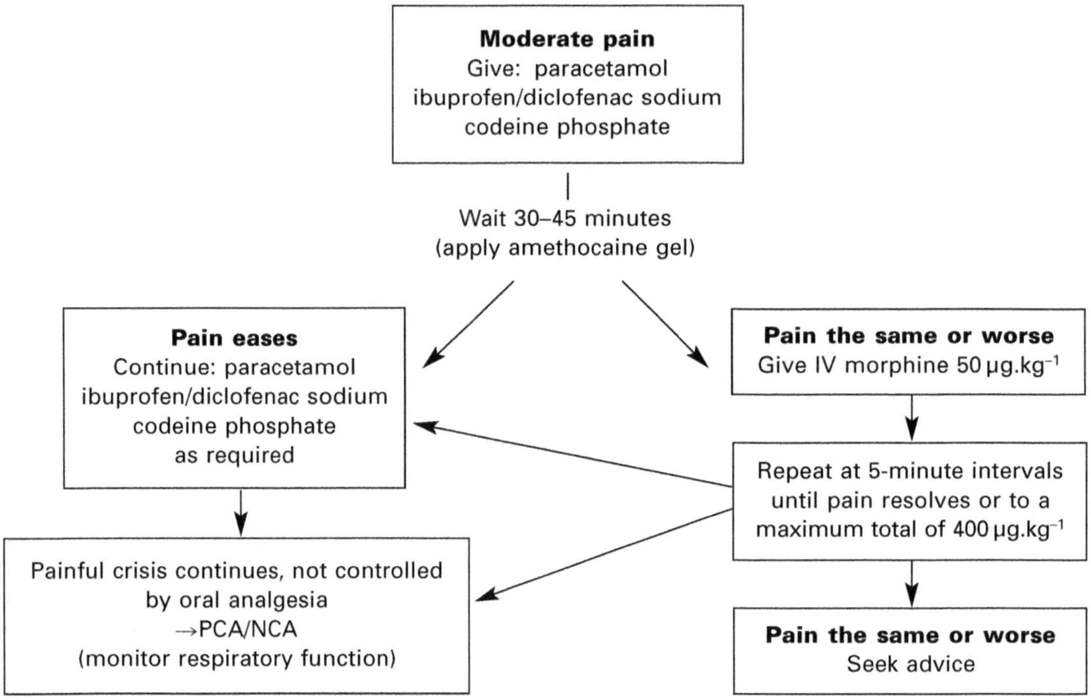

PCA, patient-controlled analgesia; NCA, nurse-controlled analgesia

Figure 12.1
Sickle cell crisis pain management strategy.

dependence. In addition, slow weaning from opiate regimens is required to prevent withdrawal syndromes.

Morphine is the most widely used of the opiates; it has the advantage of variability in delivery methods available and even moderate-severe pain can be managed out of hospital with oral opiates. In particular, oral controlled-release morphine has been shown to be a reliable, non-invasive alternative to intravenous infusions of morphine in children with SCD.[6] Improvements in technology have allowed the development of a wide range of patient-controlled devices giving patients autonomy over their own analgesia, which has therapeutic benefits in its own right, and allowing patients to titrate their dosing to their current pain level. Patient-controlled analgesia (PCA) also decreases delays associated with the procedures involved in checking and dispensing individual doses of controlled drugs and in addition has built-in safety features which reduce the risk of respiratory depression. Whether parenteral opiates are used in the form of a continuous infusion, PCA or a combination of PCA with a background continuous infusion, monitoring must be employed to detect and prevent respiratory depression, which leads to a respiratory acidosis and an increase in hydrogen ion concentration resulting in a dissociation of oxygen from haemoglobin (the Bohr effect) and further sickling, worsening vaso-occlusion. An isolated case of death following a continuous opiate infusion in SCD is reported in the literature postulated to be due to a build up of morphine-6-glucaronide, a more potent metabolite than the parent drug.[7] Significant differences have been observed in clearance rates of opiates between individual children and therefore considerable individualization of morphine dosing is necessary.[8]

Pethidine is another opiate with troublesome and potent metabolites. One of these, norpethidine, has resulted in a sharp decline in the use of pethidine in SCD because of the risk of accumulation causing seizures and dysphoria. Despite this, any patient who has been previously stabilized on a regimen of pethidine should not be changed abruptly.

Other opiates which have a place in the management of sickle cell-related pain include codeine and fentanyl. Codeine has the advantage that it can be used both orally and rectally and is useful for mild to moderate pain treated out of hospital or a part of the treatment of severe pain in the hospital setting. Some early studies have been done investigating whether the transdermal administration of fentanyl, using varying dose patches, has a role in sickle cell crises, but so far have not proved conclusive.

Adjuncts

Adjunctive drugs such as tricyclic antidepressants and anticonvulsants are so far unproven, but may have a role in the treatment of pain in SCD.

Hydroxyurea (hydroxycarbamide)

Hydroxyurea (hydroxycarbamide) is an antineoplastic drug whose mechanism is not fully elucidated. It is not licensed for use in SCD, but early studies suggest it is efficacious in children with frequent crises. There are several, as yet not fully explored, concerns including potential myelosuppression, teratogenicity and possible long-term toxicity.

Local anaesthetics

Epidural analgesia has been used in vaso-occlusive crises for the management of severe pain refractory to other interventions and, in particular, is effective in treating patients whose main manifestation is abdominal pain. In addition to the superior level of analgesia, epidurals may actually have a place in treating the vaso-occlusion itself. They can result in a favourable influence on blood flow by inducing venodilatation. Regional analgesia has the added advantage of producing pain relief without the risks of respiratory depression or precipitating or worsening acute chest syndrome.

Non-pharmacological therapies

The use of psychological and behavioural interventions is not a substitute for pharmacological therapies, but may enhance the effect of medications or help reduce their use.

- These therapies should form part of a balanced approach to acute or chronic pain in patients with sickle cell disease.
- The main objectives of cognitive behavioural therapies (CBT) are to help individuals to examine their thoughts and feelings and challenge their beliefs and to train them to use problem-solving behavioural strategies.
- Behavioural techniques include relaxation, assertiveness and activity re-scheduling.
- Inappropriate behaviours can be unlearned with the aim of the elimination of psychological distress and the enhancement of coping strategies.
- Play therapy can have a valuable place in young children where it is particularly important to instil coping mechanisms before pathological patterns of pain-behaviour become entrenched.
- Physical therapies are often useful in treating both acute or chronic sickle cell pain with the advantage of few, if any, adverse effects.
  - These strategies include hydration, heat, physiotherapy and transcutaneous electrical nerve stimulation (TENS).
  - Hydration should help improve the flow in the microcirculation, improving the vaso-occlusion as should the vasodilatation which results from heat therapies.
- Inclusion of the patient and their families in treatment planning can be therapeutic in itself and goes some way to preventing the development of adversarial relationships with healthcare professionals which hamper the optimal delivery of pain relieving treatments.

Management of chronic pain in sickle cell disease

As with the acute pain experienced by this group of patients, chronic pain in sickle cell disease is best tackled by a multimodal approach including pharmacological and non-pharmacological therapies. Drugs including antidepressants such as amitriptyline and anticonvulsants such as carbamazepine and more recently gabapentin have been employed with variable results. CBT is important as children whose functioning is impaired often display psychosocial dysfunction by adolescence.

Lessons from Steven

Steven is a child with a long history of painful SCD crises. He was treated with parenteral analgesics at a district general hospital. These did not control the pain, either because the doses of analgesics were too low, or the pain he experienced was greater than usual.

Steven demonstrates very well that routine analgesic regimens need to be modified and tailored to the individual child not the expectations of medical staff. On transfer to the children's hospital Steven was initially managed with PCA. For surgery Steven received a plain local anaesthetic epidural infusion. This produced excellent analgesia, improved blood flow to the penis (because of the vasodilator effect of epidural infusion), and prevented respiratory depression associated with opiates. The epidural infusion was continued despite full heparinization of the patient because it was considered that the effect of improving blood flow was more important than the possibility of an extradural haematoma. Steven made excellent progress and the epidural was removed after a period of cessation of heparin.

The pain of vaso-occlusive crisis in children with sickle cell disease is still not fully understood and often remains refractory to even the most advanced analgesic interventions. Unfortunately, in many cases the available knowledge in clinical practice is not well implemented due to various barriers between patients and care providers. Until advances in knowledge are achieved, the biggest improvements in analgesia for patients suffering these debilitating episodes may be making up this shortfall by changes in beliefs and attitudes.

References

1. Brozovic M, Davies SC, Brownell AI. Acute admissions of patients with sickle cell disease who live in Britain. *BMJ* 1987; 294: 1206–1208.
2. Miller ST, Sleeper LA, Pegelow CH et al. Prediction of adverse outcomes in children with sickle cell disease. *New Engl J Med* 2000; 342: 83–89.
3. World Health Organization. Cancer Pain Relief. Geneva: WHO, 1986.
4. Paydas S, Tetiker T, Baslamisli F, Kocak R. Comparison of effect of an anti-inflammatory drug and a narcotic analgesic on renal function in sickle cell anaemia. *Nephron* 1996; 73: 498.
5. Simckes AM, Chen SS, Osorio AV et al. Ketorolac-induced irreversible renal failure in sickle cell disease: a case report. *Paediatr Nephrol* 1999; 13: 63–67.
6. Jacobson SJ, Kopecky EA, Joshi P, Babul N. Randomised trial of oral morphine for painful episodes of sickle-cell disease in children. *Lancet* 1997; 350: 1358–1361.
7. Gerber N, Apseloff G. Death from a morphine infusion during a sickle cell crisis. *J Paediatr* 1993; 123: 322–325.
8. Damplier CD, Setty BN, Logan J et al. Intravenous morphine pharmacokinetics in pediatric patients with sickle cell disease. *J Pediatr* 1995; 126: 461–467.

13

Laparoscopic fundoplication in a child with cerebral palsy

Louise Aldridge

Introduction

Following the first report of paediatric laparoscopic fundoplication in the early 1990s, increasing numbers of children have reaped the benefits of this minimally invasive surgery, with an accompanying reduction of postoperative respiratory and wound complications, analgesic requirement, and duration of hospitalization.[1]

Severe gastro-oesophageal reflux is common in children with cerebral palsy. It may be associated with frequent chest infections, especially when there is recurrent aspiration because of cranial nerve weakness/bulbar palsy/poor co-ordination of laryngeal muscles.[2]

With the traditional open Nissen fundoplication the significant morbidity and even mortality are largely associated with the requirement for large doses of postoperative opiates in a vulnerable child with a 'bad chest' and a large upper abdominal wound.[3] Because of this, neurologically impaired children gain particular benefit from the laparoscopic approach.

Case report

A 10-year-old boy, weight 15.8 kg, presented for laparoscopic fundoplication and insertion of a gastrostomy tube.

Past medical history

Following his birth by emergency Caesarean section for fetal distress, he had a stormy neonatal course with perinatal asphyxia requiring ventilation and subsequent fits. Metabolic screening was normal. The cranial ultrasound findings were consistent with leucomalacia. He was microcephalic, with severe dystonic and spastic quadriplegia, severe psychomotor retardation, cortical visual impairment and myoclonic epilepsy.

A number of orthopaedic procedures including bilateral femoral de-rotation osteotomy and hamstring lengthening had been undertaken in an attempt to correct his increasing windswept posture and enable him to sit in his wheelchair.

A recurrent cough, sticky secretions and intermittent wheeze necessitated frequent courses of antibiotics. Maintaining nutritional status presented major problems and he had recently lost 2 kg due to increasing difficulty in eating. As part of the surgical assessment for fundoplication, he had more recently undergone upper gastrointestinal endoscopy and pH studies.

Medications

Medications are as follows:
Clobazam 5 mg in morning and 10 mg at night
Sodium valproate 400 mg morning and night
Lamotrigine 7.5 mg in morning and 10 mg at night
Salbutamol 100 µg twice daily
Budesonide 200 µg twice daily via a spacing device
Ranitidine 75 mg, Gaviscon® and omeprazole 20 mg daily.

Preoperative assessment

Five days prior to surgery a further chest infection had necessitated admission to the medical ward. On admission he was pyrexial, lethargic and agitated. In addition to his usual medications, he was treated with intravenous fluids, cefotaxime, nebulized salbutamol and physiotherapy. No focal lesion was seen on chest X-ray and his blood gases returned to normal over 24 hours. No organisms were cultured. He improved sufficiently to be allowed home for 36 hours prior to his surgical admission.

By the time of admission on the day prior to surgery when he was seen with his mother, his chest had returned to 'normal' or as good as could be achieved until the elimination of recurrent aspiration of feeds or refluxed gastric contents. Blood biochemistry was normal and his haemoglobin was $13.6\,g.dl^{-1}$ with a white cell count of $13.7 \times 10^9\,l^{-1}$. As he had not had any previous abdominal surgery, it was anticipated that the Nissen fundoplication would be possible laparoscopically; however, his mother was warned that reversion to the open technique was possible. Information on postoperative analgesia was given on the basis of the laparoscopic approach with the additional comment that considerably more analgesia would be required and given were a laparotomy required. A phosphate enema was administered the evening prior to surgery in an attempt to empty the transverse colon and facilitate surgery.

Surgery was scheduled for the afternoon so all his usual morning drugs were given. He was fasted 6 hours for milk/solids and 4 hours for clear fluids. EMLA® cream was applied to the dorsa of his hands.

Theatre

In the anaesthetic room his veins were not markedly visible and to minimize distress, oxygen and halothane were administered by mask. Venous access was secured and fentanyl 80 µg along with atracurium 8 mg given. He was intubated with a cuffed 6-mm endotracheal tube. A nasogastric tube was inserted to ensure the stomach was deflated. Anaesthesia was maintained with oxygen, air and isoflurane ($E_T$iso 0.6–0.9%) via a Servo 900 ventilator, fentanyl at $2\,\mu g.kg^{-1}.hr^{-1}$ and atracurium $0.5\,mg.kg^{-1}.hr^{-1}$ were administered by infusion. Ondansetron 3 mg was given; he also received a single dose of co-amoxiclar (Augmentin®) because a gastrostomy was to be performed once the fundoplication was completed.

During the procedure oxygen saturation, ECG, blood pressure, temperature, end-tidal carbon dioxide, end-tidal isoflurane, along with inspired oxygen concentration, and ventilator pressures were routinely monitored. Throughout the 2.5-hour procedure he remained haemodynamically stable with minimal blood or fluid loss, intravenous fluid replacement consisted of 200 ml of half-strength saline with 5% dextrose. The end-tidal carbon dioxide gradually rose by 1 kPa during the carbon dioxide pneumoperitoneum.

Position

The patient was placed on a warming blanket in a modified Lloyd Davis position with the surgeon standing between the abducted legs, pressure-relieving gel pads and softband padding being used to protect pressure areas. Prior to insertion of the ports, the surgeons infiltrated 10 ml of 0.25% bupivacaine with 1 in 200,000 epinephrine (adrenaline) between the five port sites to minimize bleeding. A carbon dioxide pnuemoperitoneum was created with a maximum intra-abdominal pressure of 10–12 mmHg. A 36F Maloney oesophageal bougie was inserted once the patient was positioned in theatre, and advanced and withdrawn at the request of the surgeon, enabling him to assess the tightness of the wrap during the fundoplication.

Analgesia

To ensure that the patient did not cough or have excessive abdominal movement, the fentanyl/atracurium infusion was continued until surgery was complete and all laparoscopic instruments removed from the abdominal cavity. Once the port wounds were stitched and tissue-glued, the patient was reversed with atropine and neostigmine. Paracetamol 500 mg and diclofenac 25 mg suppositories were inserted. As soon as good spontaneous respiration was established, codeine phosphate 18 mg intramuscularly was given. He was extubated virtually awake and taken to the recovery ward, where $6\,l.min^{-1}$ oxygen was delivered by face mask for approximately 40 minutes until he was fully awake, comfortable and ready to return to the surgical ward with maintenance intravenous fluids running and his gastrostomy tube on free drainage.

Postoperative

He was nursed on the general surgical ward next to the nurses' station. During the first postoperative night he required supplemental oxygen as saturations fell to the low 90s during deep sleep. Over the following 48 hours he received three doses of rectal paracetamol 240 mg and diclofenac 12.5 mg, along with three doses of dihydrocodeine 15 mg via the gastrostomy. His inhalers and his antiepileptic drugs along with ranitidine were given as usual. Gastrostomy feeds were commenced at 24 hours with his mother receiving instruction on the management of this technique. By 66 hours he was tolerating four feeds of 250 ml Nutrini® fibre a day. His mother was coping well and he was discharged home. When seen at the clinic 6 weeks later all his food and drink were delivered by the gastrostomy tube, weight was increasing and his mother reported him to be more relaxed with fewer dystonic spasms, presumably because of the reduction of stress and discomfort caused by reflux.

Discussion

Recent advances in optical systems and video equipment along with surgical instrumentation have stimulated development of endoscopic surgical techniques. In addition to the capital cost of the video system, there is the increased cost of the specialized instruments, many of which are disposable. In adult practice, however, it has been shown that these costs can be offset by the reduced hospital cost resulting from decreased hospital stay.[4] Although an increasing number of procedures are being undertaken laparoscopically in paediatric surgery, it is fundoplication which carries the greatest benefit over the open operation, with long-term success rates similar to the open technique.[5]

There is a long learning curve for a surgical team commencing laparoscopic fundoplications as a number of technical problems exist, including judging the size of the hiatus.[6,7] In consequence, operating time decreases with experience which may require postoperative care and analgesia to be adjusted.[8] There is a marked difference in analgesic requirement between the open Nissen fundoplication and the laparoscopic approach.[9] With the open procedure, the need for an intensive care unit (ICU) bed on account of respiratory complications is significant, amounting to 33% of cases when morphine infusion is used and 17% when an epidural infusion of bupivacaine/fentanyl is employed, with 20% (morphine) and 8% (epidural) requiring ventilation.[3] Postoperative ICU/HDU (high dependency unit) following the open technique is indicated in babies under 1-year-old and those with a history of apnoea.[10] In contrast there is no routine requirement for ICU/HDU admission following the laparoscopic technique. However, in very small infants (less than 6 kg or less than 6 months old) where there is a history of apnoeas, overnight admission to ICU with ventilatory support as required and respiratory monitoring is advisable.

Feeding is tolerated earlier with decreased ileus and a shorter hospital stay. The incidence of postoperative pneumonia and chest infection is reduced.[11]

Preoperative

More than half the patients presenting for laparoscopic fundoplication are neurologically impaired, many with cerebral palsy of varying degree.

Epilepsy is a frequent accompaniment and patients may be on a variety of antiepileptics, most of which are administered at breakfast time and bedtime, so that it is possible to give the morning dose early to allow for fasting. By the bedtime dose it is usually possible to use the nasogastric tube or gastrostomy tube following laparoscopic fundoplication. If this is not possible it may be necessary to change to a *per rectum* or intravenous medication depending on the frequency or severity of the fits.

Cerebral palsy can also be associated with painful muscle spasms, which are frequently treated with diazepam.

A variety of ‘chest problems’ are common in this group of patients. Muscle weakness with or without scoliosis along with chronic pulmonary aspiration because of poor co-ordination of the laryngeal muscles in a child who may, in addition, be significantly malnourished because of the feeding difficulties, make recurrent chest infections common. These patients should be optimized with preoperative physiotherapy and bronchodilators.

Premedication is optional and is dependent on the state of the child and the anaesthetist’s preference. Antacid with or without prokinetic prophylaxis is at the discretion of the anaesthetist. If intravenous induction is planned, local anaesthetic cream is applied over the vein.

Induction

Induction may be gaseous or intravenous. Many of these children have ‘difficult’ veins and a gaseous induction can be less traumatic especially in a child who may be visually impaired or who has limited understanding. Once asleep an intravenous cannula is inserted and neuromuscular relaxant given. Cricoid pressure and/or a slight head up tilt may be employed until the airway is protected by the endotracheal tube. A cuffed tube is better, especially in older children; when an uncuffed tube is used, a size permitting only a high-pressure leak is best. If there is a large leak around the endotracheal tube it is more difficult to ventilate and measure E_TCO_2 with rising intra-abdominal pressure. A nasogastric tube is passed to deflate the stomach as a distended stomach increases surgical difficulty.

Following the initial dose of relaxant, an infusion of atracurium $0.5\,mg.kg^{-1}.hr^{-1}$ or vecuronium $0.1\,mg.kg^{-1}.hr^{-1}$ is beneficial because of the length of the procedure and the inconvenience of unexpected patient movement.

Anaesthesia is maintained with a volatile agent in oxygen and air. Both isoflurane and halothane have been used successfully.[12] However, it has been reported that there is an increased occurrence of arrhythmias with halothane in spontaneously breathing adults undergoing laparoscopic procedures associated with hypercarbia.[13] Isoflurane has been associated with excessive secretions and bronchospasm.[14] Total intravenous anaesthesia (TIVA) using a propofol infusion has also been successfully employed.[15,16]

Nitrous oxide is generally not used as it can increase bowel distension, increase nausea and vomiting and increase the danger in the rare event of air embolism. An antiemetic, such as ondansetron $0.1\,mg.kg^{-1}$ (max 4 mg) is given routinely to prevent retching, which would damage the wrap.[6]

Analgesia can be bolus fentanyl $2–5\,\mu g.kg^{-1}$, followed by infusion at $2\,\mu g.kg.hour^{-1}$, with codeine phosphate $1–2\,mg.kg^{-1}$ intramuscularly, given at the end of the procedure, usually after reversal of relaxant and once adequate spontaneous ventilation has returned, or an infusion of nemifentanil 0.1–1 µg.kg–min, followed by morphine $0.1–0.2\,mg.kg^{-1}$. At the end of surgery, paracetamol 15–20 mg.kg and diclofenac $1–2\,mg.kg^{-1}$, if not contraindicated, are administered rectally.

Position

In theatre, the patient is placed in a modified Lloyd Davis position using padded leg supports with the operating surgeon standing between the legs and the assistants on either side (see Figure 13.1). However, some children with cerebral palsy have severe contractures, which restricts hip abduction and good surgical access can only be attained by placing them obliquely across the table. It is essential to avoid force on fixed

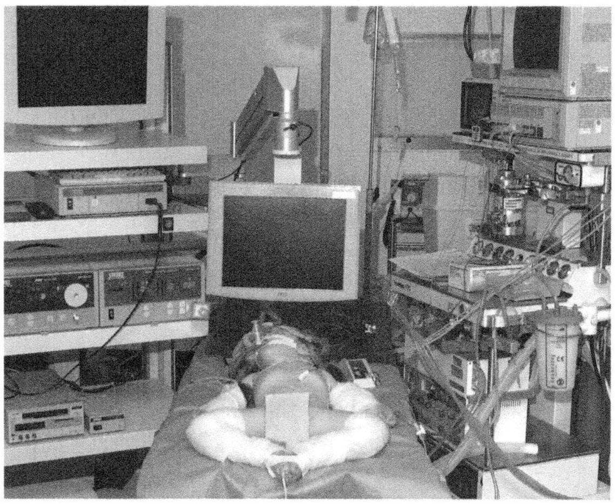

Figure 13.1
'Patient position'
This illustrates the theatre set up in a patient too small for the Lloyd Davis leg supports. The position of the legs is such as to allow the surgeon good access from the bottom of the table.

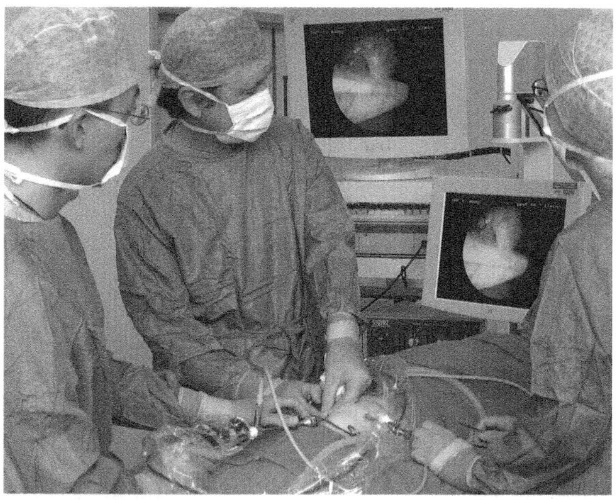

Figure 13.2
'Surgeon position'
The position of the surgeons and video monitors during fundoplication. The main operator stands at the bottom of the table facing the monitor at the patient's head with the assistants on either side of the table.

joints during positioning. The use of a warming blanket is important to counteract the effect of cold CO_2 in the peritoneal cavity. Rectal or nasopharyngeal temperature is routinely monitored. Adequate padding is of particular importance in protecting children who have deformed posture, with attention paid especially to elbows, knees, hips and heels. Laparoscopic surgical access is frequently better than the conventional open approach in children with severe skeletal deformities.[17] A slight reverse Trandelenberg tilt allows the stomach and other organs to fall away from the oesophageal hiatus, it also facilitates drainage of peritoneal fluid and blood from the surgical field.

Carbon dioxide pneumoperitoneum

Historically a number of gases have been used to facilitate laparoscopic surgery. Peritoneal gas insufflation is essential to enable exposure, visualization and manipulation of abdominal contents. Nitrous oxide has been used for diagnostic gynaecological surgery, but because of its flammable nature is unsuitable when electrocautery is required. Carbon dioxide does not support combustion and has evolved as the insufflation gas of choice for laparoscopic surgery.[13] It is a highly diffusible gas, which is absorbed across the peritoneal surface and ultimately transported via the systemic and portal venous systems to the right heart and pulmonary circulation. Carbon dioxide absorption is greater in younger children due to the physiological properties of the peritoneum, decreased thickness and increased absorptive surface relative to weight.

The cardiorespiratory effects of pneumoperitoneum in combination with the reverse Trendelenberg position employed to optimize surgical access during fundoplication, are complex.[18]

The functional residual capacity (FRC) is low in children. There is a fall in FRC additional to that induced by anaesthesia, which is related to diaphragmatic elevation, reduction in chest wall dimensions, reduction in muscle tone, and changes in intrathoracic blood volume. If the FRC falls below closing volume, there is increased pulmonary shunting and hypoxaemia.[19] However, with the supplementary oxygen given during general anaesthesia, the oxygen saturation is not affected as this occurs on the flat part of the oxyhaemoglobin dissociation curve. During the initial insufflation there is cephalad movement of the diaphragm towards the carina, which may result in endobronchial migration of a low placed endotracheal tube or bronchospasm.[14] There is a reduction in lung compliance and increase in peak inspiratory pressure during volume controlled ventilation with an increase in E_TCO_2, which may necessitate an increase in rate and minute ventilation.[7,9,15] The head up tilt mitigates against these effects.

The accuracy of end-tidal carbon dioxide (P_ECO_2) monitoring has been shown, especially in small infants, to be related to the position of the sampling port and the type of ventilator.[20,21] However, a recent study comparing end-tidal versus transcutaneous monitoring of carbon dioxide showed that both methods provided clinically acceptable estimates of arterial carbon dioxide with the transcutaneous method being only slightly more accurate in children during general anaesthesia with mechanical ventilation.[22] Reduced cardiac output, hypovolaemia and increased respiratory dead space all adversely affect E_TCO_2 accuracy.

End-tidal carbon dioxide pressure can sometimes overestimate arterial carbon dioxide during laparoscopic surgery in children.[23] Although in the author's experience the overestimation is minimal, in the region of 0.2–1 kPa, in patients with significant cardiopulmonary abnormality or if a prolonged procedure is anticipated, the insertion of an arterial line for blood gas analysis may be helpful.

Cardiovascular changes during laparoscopy are related to increase in intra-abdominal pressure, changes in arterial carbon dioxide and surgical positioning. As intra-abdominal pressures increase up to 15–20 mmHg, cardiac output is decreased by vena caval compression, which is accentuated by positive pressure ventilation and head up position while systemic vascular resistance is increased by aortic compression, hypercarbia and possibly the release of humoral factors such as vasopressin.[19,24,25] The reduction in cardiac output and rise in systemic vascular resistance caused by pneumoperitoneum during laparoscopy in children, has been confirmed using impedance cardiography and also by transoesophageal echocardiography.[26,27]

Fortunately several groups, using standard monitoring devices, have shown there is minimal cardiovascular change in paediatric laparoscopy where the peak intra-abdominal pressure is limited to 10–12 mmHg.[12,14,24,27] None the less, some patients develop hypertension and tachycardia, which may be related to the rise in systemic vascular resistance or carbon dioxide, but may also be due to inadequate anaesthesia during the particularly stimulating hiatal dissection.

In infants, E_TCO_2 increases with insufflation of CO_2 to intra-abdominal pressures of 10 mmHg and 15 mmHg, cardiac index, mean arterial pressure and heart rate remain stable, unaffected by body position. Cerebral blood flow velocity increases with increasing E_TCO_2.[28]

Complications from pneumoperitoneum include surgical emphysema around the port sites, pneumothorax, and pneumomediastinum. Trauma to viscera and blood vessels can occur but carbon dioxide embolism is extremely rare. The complications of inadvertent puncture of organs or blood vessels may be reduced if the surgeons use the open introduction technique for the first trocar and pneumoperitoneum.[29] Having a large orogastric tube or Maloney bougie down the oesophagus and passing it through the wrap during surgery when requested by the surgeon can reduce postoperative dysphagia by avoiding overly tight suturing of the wrap. At the end of the procedure it can be exchanged for a nasogastric tube to allow free drainage of air, as eructation is difficult following fundoplication.

Although there is usually minimal blood or fluid loss, hypovolaemia should be avoided as it compounds the effects of the reverse Trandelenberg position. Reflex bradycardia from vagal stimulation should be treated with atropine.

During the laparoscopic procedure one has to be prepared with a good reliable intravenous cannula for an urgent laparotomy in case of bleeding.

Monitoring

Routine monitoring of ECG, pulse oximetry, non-invasive blood pressure and temperature along with capnography that displays both values and waveform of E_TCO_2 as a function of time, E_TAAgent, F_IO_2 and peak inspiratory pressure.

Postoperative

Pain following laparoscopic surgery consists of early transient vague abdominal and shoulder discomfort due to peritoneal irritation by residual CO_2. This can be reduced if as much CO_2 as possible is released from the abdomen when the trocars are removed at the end of surgery. Pain from the trocar puncture wounds is generally mild because the wounds are small and are produced without cutting muscle fibre (Figure 13.3). A deep-seated pain relating to trauma at the surgical site can also be experienced.

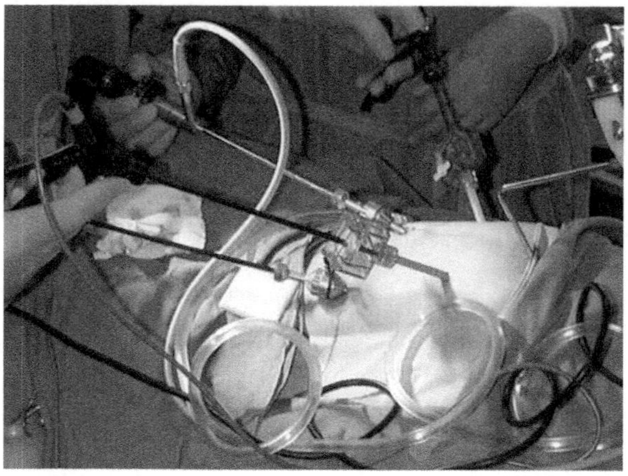

Figure 13.3
'Port sites'
Operation in progress showing the five port sites used in laparoscopic fundoplication.

Although an epidural improves the outcome following open fundoplication with reduced hospital stay, there is still a need for postoperative ICU and ventilation in a significant percentage of the patients.[3,30,31]

One study has shown that the total amount of morphine required is similar for both open and laparoscopic but the period for which analgesia was required was significantly less in the laparoscopic group.[32]

In the author's experience of over 100 laparoscopic fundoplications, the majority of patients can be managed postoperatively with oral/nasogastric/gastrostomy or rectal medications: paracetamol 15 $mg.kg^{-1}$ 6-hourly with diclofenac 1 $mg.kg^{-1}$ 8-hourly (3 $mg.kg^{-1}.24\,hr^{-1}$) and dihydrocodeine or oral morphine (Oramorph®) in standard doses. Intravenous morphine infusions are rarely necessary.[12] There is no difference in analgesic requirement between neurologically impaired and normal children (Figure 13.4). Most series report minimal opioid requirement postoperatively.

Patients who have swallowing difficulties, failure to thrive and are incapable of adequate oral nutrition may require a gastrostomy tube placement at the same time as the fundoplication.[33] This can be carried out entirely laparoscopically or it can be percutaneous endoscopically assisted. Patients undergoing gastrostomy are usually in hospital a day longer to establish feeding and to educate the child's carer in its management.[7] Fundoplication, frequently with gastrostomy, allows restoration of nutritional status, reliable administration of medication and prevention of aspiration which can

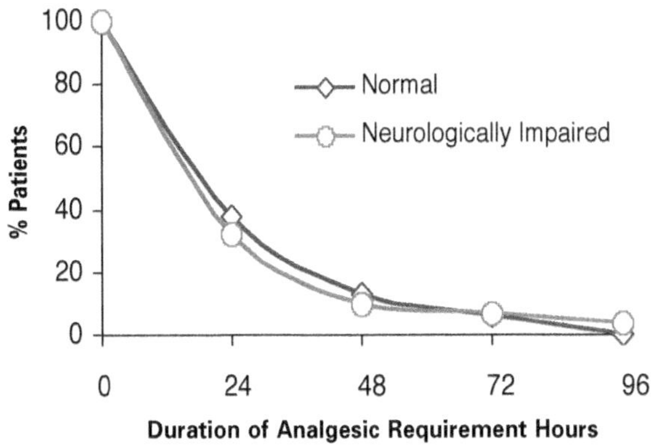

Figure 13.4
Duration of requirement for postoperative analgesia.

transform the lives of cerebral palsy children and their carers. In addition to the immediate postoperative benefits, there is a reduced incidence of bowel obstruction and wound complications following the laparoscopic technique in addition to the increased cosmetic benefit.[34]

Learning points

- Optimization of chest with physiotherapy and bronchodilators as required.
- Care with positioning of patient and use of warming blanket.
- IV infusion of relaxant.
- Routine use of antiemetic.
- Maloney bougie or large orogastric tube.
- Minimal opioid analgesic requirement.
- Analgesic requirement may reduce with increasing experience of the team.

References

1. Lobe TE, Schropp KP, Lunsford K. Laparoscopic Nissen fundoplication in childhood. *J Paediatr Surg* 1993; 28: 358–361.
2. Berquist WE, Rachelefsky GS, Kadden M et al. Gastroesophageal reflux-associated recurrent pneumonia and chronic asthma in children. *Pediatrics* 1981; 68: 29–35.
3. Wilson GAM, Brown JL, Crabbe DG et al. Is epidural analgesia associated with an improved outcome following open Nissen fundoplication? *Paed Anaesth* 2001; 11: 65–70.
4. Jones R, Canal DF, Inmam MM et al. Laparoscopic fundoplication: a three-year review *Am Surg* 1996; 62: 632–635.
5. Tovar JA, Olivares P, Diaz M et al. Functional results of laparoscopic fundoplication in children. *J Paediatr Gastroenterol Nutr* 1998; 26: 429–431.
6. Munro W, Brancatisiano R, Adams IP et al. Complications of laparoscopic fundoplication: the first 100 patients. *Surg Laparosc Endosc* 1996; 6: 421–423.
7. Rothenberg SS. Experience with 220 consecutive laparoscopic Nissen fundoplications in infants and children. *J Paediatr Surg* 1998; 33: 274–278.
8. Leggett PL, Churchman-Winn R, Ahn C. Resolving gastroesophageal reflux with laparoscopic fundoplication. *Surg Endosc* 1998; 12: 142–147.
9. Rowney DA, Aldridge LM, Munro FD et al. Laparoscopic fundoplication: anaesthesia, analgesia, and physiologic aspects. *J Pediatr Endosurg Innov Tech* 2000; 4: 25–29.
10. Dearlove OR, Fernandez P, Sharples A et al. Prediction of need for intensive care or high dependency care after Nissen fundoplication procedure. *Care Crit Ill* 1997; 13: 33.
11. Collins JB, Georgeson KE, Vicente Y et al. Comparison of open and laparoscopic gastrostomy and fundoplication in 120 patients. *J Pediatr Surg* 1995; 30: 1065–1071.
12. Rowney DA, Aldridge LM. Laparoscopic fundoplication in children: anaesthetic experience of 51 cases. *Paed Anaesth* 2000; 10: 291–296.
13. Cunningham AJ, Brull SJ. Laparoscopic cholecystectomy: anaesthetic implications. *Anesth Analg* 1993; 76: 1120–1133.
14. Sfez M, Guerard A, Desruelle P. Cardiorespiratory changes during laparoscopic fundoplication in children. *Paediatric Anaesth* 1995; 5: 89–95.
15. Manner T, Aantaa R, Alanen M. Lung compliance during laparoscopic surgery in paediatric patients. *Paed Anaesth* 1998; 8: 25–29.
16. Ivani G, Vaira M, Mattioli G et al. Paediatric laparoscopic surgery: anaesthetic management. *Paed Anaesth* 1994; 4: 323–325.
17. Schier F, Waldschmidt J. Laparoscopic fundoplication in a child. *Eur J Pediatr Surg* 1994; 4: 338–340.
18. Chui PT, Gin T, Oh TE. Anaesthesia for laparoscopic general surgery. *Anaesth Intens Care* 1993; 21: 163–171.
19. Coventry DM. Anaesthesia for laparoscopic surgery. *J R Coll Surg Edinb* 1995; 40: 151–160.
20. Badgwell JM, McLeod ME, Lerman J et al. End-tidal PCO_2 measurements sampled at the distal and proximal ends of the endotracheal tube in infants and children. *Anesth Analg* 1987; 66: 959–964.

21. Badgwell JM, Heavner JE, May WS et al. End-tidal PCO_2 monitoring in infants and children ventilated with either a partial rebreathing or a non-rebreathing circuit. *Anesthesiology* 1987; 3: 405–410.
22. Nosovitch MA, Johnson JO, Tobias JD. Noninvasive intraoperative monitoring of carbon dioxide in children: endtidal versus transcutaneous techniques. *Paed Anaesth* 2002; 12: 48–52.
23. Laffon M, Gouchet A, Sitbon P et al. Difference between arterial and end-tidal carbon dioxide pressures during laparoscopy in paediatric patients. *Can J Anaesth* 1998; 45: 561–563.
24. Tobias JD, Holcomb GW, Brock JW et al. Cardiorespiratory changes in children during laparoscopy. *J Paediatr Surg* 1995; 30: 33–36.
25. Odeberg S, Ljungqvist O, Svenberg T et al. Haemodynamic effects of pneumoperitoneum and the influence of posture during anaesthesia for laparoscopic surgery. *Acta Anaesthesiol Scand* 1994; 38: 276–283.
26. Kardos A, Vereczkey G, Pirot L et al. Use of impedance cardiography to monitor haemodynamic changes during laparoscopy in children. *Paed Anaesth* 2001; 11: 175–179.
27. Sakka SG, Huettemann E, Petrat G et al. Transoesophageal echocardiographic assessment of haemodynamic changes during laparoscopic herniorrhaphy in small children. *Br J Anaesth* 2000; 84: 330–334.
28. Rowney DA, Emery J, Kim PCW et al. The haemodynamic effects of carbon dioxide pneumoperitoneum in infants. *Paed Anaesth* 2001; 11: 760.
29. Humphrey GME, Najmaldin A. Modification of the Hasson technique in paediatric laparoscopy. *Br J Surg* 1994; 81: 1319.
30. Challands JF, Facer EK. Epidural anaesthesia and familial dysautonomia (the Riley Day syndrome). Three case reports .*Paed Anaesth* 1998; 8: 83–88.
31. McNeely JK, Farber NE, Rusy LM et al. Epidural analgesia improves outcome following pediatric fundoplication. A retrospective analysis. *Reg Anesth* 1997; 22: 16–23.
32. Dick AC, Coulter P, Hainsworth AM et al. A comparative study of the analgesia requirements following laparoscopic and open fundoplication in children. *J Laparoendosc Adv Surg Tech A* 1998; 8: 425–429.
33. Meehan JJ, Georgson KE. Laparoscopic fundoplication in infants and children. *Surg Endosc* 1996; 10: 1154–1157.
34. Thompson WR. Laparoscopic fundoplication. *J Paediatr Endosurg Innov Tech B* 1998; 2: 181–184.

14

Craniotomy for medulloblastoma

AER Young

Introduction

The incidence of paediatric brain tumours is increasing at approximately 2% per year.[1] It is the second most common form of childhood cancer with an incidence just less than or equal to that of acute lymphoblastic leukaemia, and is the third leading cause of death in children.[2,3] Approximately one-third occur in children under the age of 3 years.[4] Symptoms of increased intracranial pressure often present late in the very young child because of the increased pliability of the skull leading to delay in diagnosis. Malignant tumours predominate (75%), the most common being ependymomas and primitive neuroectodermal tumours (PNET) including medulloblastomas. Surgery for cerebral tumours in childhood aims to achieve a histological diagnosis, treat associated hydrocephalus, achieve maximum tumour reduction and neural decompression. Total surgical excision is the most important therapeutic option in several cerebral tumours of childhood including cerebellar astrocytomas,[2,5] ependymomas,[6] medulloblastomas and choroid plexus tumours.

Case history

A 28-month-old girl weighing 11 kg was admitted to the regional neurosurgical centre with a diagnosis, following computed tomography scanning, of a posterior fossa tumour. The child presented to the local hospital with signs and symptoms of raised intracranial pressure including nausea, vomiting, lethargy and ataxia. After discussion with the regional centre the child was started on intravenous dexamethasone prior to transfer.

Magnetic resonance imaging (MRI) was obtained under general anaesthesia after arrival at the regional neurosurgical centre. The child was scheduled for gross total removal of the tumour the following day. The parents were counselled by the neurosurgical team with reference to the management plan, possible intraoperative complications including haemorrhage, neurological damage and death. The possibility of postoperative bulbar problems, difficulty of weaning from the ventilator, tracheostomy and the prognosis were also discussed. The paediatric neuroanaesthetist discussed intraoperative care including blood transfusion, and the need for invasive lines, a nasogastric tube and a urinary catheter as well as postoperative care in the paediatric high dependency unit (PHDU) with the possibility of a postoperative stay in the neurointensive care unit. The paediatric oncology team discussed the requirements for postoperative chemotherapy and/or radiotherapy.

Preoperative investigations included a full blood count (FBC), urea and electrolytes (U&E) and a coagulation screen; these were all normal (see Table 14.1). The child was cross-matched for two units of blood. A cannula was in situ following anaesthesia for MRI scanning. Preoperative blood pressure was 90/60 mmHg. Availability of neurointensive care and PHDU facilities was ascertained.

On the day of surgery the child was fasted following normal preoperative guidelines and premedicated with 30 mg.kg^{-1} paracetamol orally. The child was brought to the warmed anaesthetic room on her bed, accompanied by her parents and a paediatric ward nurse. The child was quiet and lethargic. Pulse oximetry monitoring was attached before intravenous induction with fentanyl (2 µg.kg^{-1}), propofol (4–5 mg.kg^{-1}) and atracurium (0.5 mg.kg^{-1}). The child was then manually ventilated via a T-piece circuit with oxygen, air and isoflurane. After induction of anaesthesia, the paediatric nurse accompanied

	Hb ($g.dl^{-1}$)	Platelets $\times 10^6 l^{-1}$	Sodium ($mmol.l^{-1}$)	INR
Preoperative	10.5	342	136	1.0
Intraoperative	9.5	182	142	1.4
Postoperative	10.2	201	140	1.1

Table 14.1
Investigations

the parents back to the ward. Full non-invasive monitoring was then introduced.

Intubation was accomplished with an oral armoured 4.5-mm uncuffed endotracheal tube (ET). A small leak was confirmed and air entry also confirmed to both right and left lungs equally. An 8 French Gauge (FrG) nasogastric tube (NG) was inserted and correct positioning ascertained. An oral airway was inserted to aid tube security and the tube carefully taped in place with Elastoplast®. A further large piece of Elastoplast® that covered the NG tube, ET tube and airway was added. The eyelids were carefully taped, ensuring that they were fully closed under the tape. End-tidal carbon dioxide (E_TCO_2) monitoring was instituted. The child was ventilated to mild hypocapnia (32–35 mmHg) with pressure control ventilation.

After intubation, a right radial 22G intra-arterial catheter was inserted and continuously monitored. A second, larger intravenous cannula was inserted into the long saphenous vein (20G) and an 8-cm, 5 FrG triple lumen central line (to measure central venous pressure, CVP) into the femoral vein under aseptic conditions. Finally the child was catheterized, also aseptically, with an 8 FrG urinary catheter and an hourly urinary collection system attached. A rectal temperature probe was inserted. During the induction period 10 $ml.kg^{-1}$ of Hartmann's solution were infused.

The child was positioned prone on gamgee rolls. A remifentanil infusion was started at 0.4 $\mu g.kg^{-1}.min^{-1}$ and 0.3 $mg.kg^{-1}$ atracurium were given prior to positioning and paediatric head pin insertion. After positioning and pinning, all lines were checked and taped further as necessary, pressure points including knees were padded, freedom of the abdomen and eyes was carefully noted and the child's arms were positioned down the length of her body. Any undue pressure on the abdomen or the neck would lead to increased venous pressure and an increased blood loss. A small lower body Bair Hugger® was placed over the child's body and taped at the upper back. Equal air entry to both lungs was rechecked. The child was wheeled with full monitoring into theatre.

Before starting surgery, the cross-matched blood was brought to theatre and checked carefully. Five hundred ml of 4.5% human albumin solution (HAS) was placed into a warming cabinet for use later. Dexamethasone (0.25 $mg.kg^{-1}$) and cefuroxime (30 $mg.kg^{-1}$) were given intravenously before the start of surgery. Anaesthesia was maintained with oxygen, air and isoflurane with an ET isoflurane concentration of between 0.4 and 0.5 MAC. The remifentanil infusion was continued at between 0.35 and 0.5 $\mu g.kg^{-1}.min^{-1}$ with atracurium boluses (0.3 $mg.kg^{-1}$) every 30 minutes during the course of the procedure. Intraoperative monitoring included intra-arterial pressure blood pressure (BP) maintained at or near preoperative values, CVP, half-hourly urine output, core temperature, maintained at between 36 and 37°C, ECG, ET agent and E_TCO_2. An arterial blood gas was sent on a number of occasions during the procedure to reliably monitor carbon dioxide levels. Pulse oximetry was monitored with a disposable adhesive pulse oximeter to ensure reliability of placement throughout the case.

Surgical procedures included the insertion of an external ventricular drain (EVD) to allow drainage of cerebrospinal fluid (CSF) and to decompress the posterior fossa, thus making brain dissection easier. Posterior fossa craniotomy, dural opening, and preliminary exploration of the tumour then followed. Microsurgical techniques were employed using the operating microscope for dissection and an ultrasonic aspirator for tumour resection. Shortly after the start of dissection, in an attempt to decompress the posterior fossa further and to aid dissection, mannitol 0.5 $g.kg^{-1}$ (2.5 $ml.kg^{-1}$ 20% mannitol) was administered intravenously over 15 minutes.

The operation lasted 8 hours. After a gross total removal had been achieved, the dura was closed with a dural patch and the bone flap replaced. Over the course of the procedure 30 ml.kg^{-1} of Hartmann's solution, 30 ml.kg^{-1} HAS 4.5% and 20 ml.kg^{-1} packed cells were required to replace losses and keep Hb > 8.0 g.dl^{-1}. Fluid requirements were assessed using clinical criteria including heart rate, capillary refill time, intra-arterial blood pressure, CVP and half-hourly urine output. The aim was to keep the child cardiovascularly full, in order to decrease the chances of an air embolus occurring (see below). Crystalloid solutions were used with great care to ensure overinfusion of hypotonic solutions did not occur. After 20–30 ml.kg^{-1} crystalloid had been given, colloid and blood were used in preference. Care was given to ensure a normal to high sodium (Na^+) concentration and a glucose concentration that was no higher than the upper limit of normal.

Blood loss was estimated by measuring loss from the suction device (paediatric suction bottle) and the swabs. Swabs can be weighed, however both weighing swabs and measuring blood collected via the suction device can considerably underestimate blood loss in these operations because of the volume of unmeasurable blood collected on the surgical drapes. The only reliable way to assess the requirement for a blood transfusion is to maintain euvolaemia and to measure haemoglobin (Hb) concentration or haematocrit regularly. Transfusion should occur at a predetermined Hb concentration. A Haemocue® machine was used during the procedure to monitor Hb every 30–60 minutes. Total blood loss during the operation was estimated at 300 ml (approximately 1/3 blood volume).

Towards the end of the procedure blood tests were performed (see Table 14.1). A further 10 ml.kg^{-1} packed red cells were given as well as 10 ml.kg^{-1} fresh frozen plasma (FFP).

During the operation there were three episodes of hypertension with an associated bradycardia (BP increased to 130/80 mmHg and heart rate decreased from 110 to 80 bpm) for 30–45 seconds. The surgeon was informed on all three occasions, the anaesthesia deepened and the cardiovascular changes reverted to normal spontaneously. All episodes were associated with dissection of the tumour from the brain stem. Atropine (20 µg.kg^{-1}) was not required, but had been drawn up prophylactically.

A fresh tumour specimen was sent during the procedure to the neuropathologist. The result of the specimen was discussed with the neurosurgeon. The diagnosis at this stage was of a medulloblastoma.

At the end of the procedure the pins were removed, the child turned supine onto a warmed bed. Anaesthesia including the remifentanil infusion was stopped at this point, the muscle relaxation reversed with neostigmine (50 µg.kg^{-1}) and glycopyrrolate (10 µg.kg^{-1}) and the child ventilated manually on 100% O_2 until breathing was established. The child was extubated awake and alert. The NG tube was left in place. The child was transferred to the recovery room where oxygen was given via a facemask and full monitoring (arterial BP, temperature, ECG and urine output) were monitored. Neurological observations were performed every 15 minutes. The child was obeying commands shortly after arrival in the recovery room. Fentanyl 1.0–3.0 µg.kg^{-1} was titrated to effect as necessary. The arterial line and peripheral cannula were carefully bandaged in place. A morphine infusion (20 µg.kg^{-1}.hr^{-1}) was started and a 250-mg paracetamol suppository given. The neurosurgical consultant spoke to the parents immediately following surgery.

After 60 minutes in recovery the child was transferred to the paediatric HDU. The anaesthetist handed over in detail to the paediatric team caring for the child in HDU. The child was transferred awake and comfortable, neurologically intact and talking. Arterial blood pressure, ECG, temperature, hourly urine output, hourly respiration rate and hourly neurological observations were performed in HDU. One-to-one nursing was available. The paediatric registrar sent a repeat FBC, coagulation screen and U&Es at 20.00 that night and 08.00 the following day. Postoperatively the child was prescribed 2.5% dextrose/0.45% saline at 80% maintenance requirements until oral fluids were tolerated. The NG tube was kept in place until bulbar function was assessed as normal by the speech and language team the following day. Regular paracetamol (20 mg.kg^{-1} orally or per rectum 8-hourly) was prescribed on the day of surgery and ibuprofen (5 mg.kg^{-1} orally 6-hourly) the day after surgery. Non-steroidal anti-inflammatory drugs are generally avoided for 12–14 hours after surgery. Nausea and vomiting is relatively common after posterior fossa surgery and an antiemetic was prescribed regularly for the first 48 hours postoperatively. Analgesia was assessed regularly and reviewed the following day by the paediatric acute pain sister.

The EVD was placed at 10 cm above head height and drainage measured hourly. The losses were replaced with 0.9% saline ml per ml if predicted losses were greater than 10% daily maintenance fluid requirements. 0.9% saline was used as this best matches CSF composition.

An MRI was performed 48 hours later under general anaesthesia. The neurosurgical team and the paediatric oncology team visited the child and parents after this. Details of the gross total resection were explained, along with the confirmed histology and likely prognosis. The paediatric neuro-oncologist explained the plans for the future including chemotherapy. Radiotherapy was not indicated, as the child was less than 3 years of age. Transfer to the oncology ward was planned for the following week. Ongoing care was by the neurosurgical, neuro-oncology and paediatric neurology teams.

Discussion

Brain and spinal tumours in children account for 20–25% of childhood cancer cases affecting 1 : 2500 children. In the UK, 350 new cases are diagnosed each year, of which 55% survive 5 years.[7] These figures are increasing.[1] In children over 2 years of age posterior fossa tumours predominate, with supratentorial tumours predominating in the younger child. The prognosis is worst in children of less than 2 years of age. In a series from British Columbia of 137 children presenting with posterior fossa tumours, the average age of presentation was 87 months (range 2–197 months); 25% of these children had primitive neuroectodermal tumours (medulloblastoma).[8] Symptoms and signs of raised intracranial pressure (ICP) secondary to obstructive hydrocephalus were present for 1–24 months prior to presentation.

The rationale for gross total removal of posterior fossa astrocytomas, ependymomas, medulloblastomas and PNET includes the need to decrease intracranial hypertension by opening CSF pathways and relieving hydrocephalus, to lessen tumour pressure on adjacent cerebellar and brain stem structures and to decrease tumour burden thereby facilitating chemotherapy and/or radiotherapy. Depending on histology, resection alone may be curative. In certain types of malignant cerebral tumours, the extent of surgical resection is related to outcome. Childhood medulloblastoma is one example of a malignant posterior fossa tumour that benefits from maximum cytoreduction.[4] Treatment after resection consists of chemotherapy, and radiotherapy in children older than 3 years.

Intraoperative complications include haemorrhage (3/105 in one series with one death[8]), air embolism[9] (more common with the sitting position) and cardiac dysrhythmias including bradycardia (10/120 in one series[10]). Blood loss is usually not excessive in these cases, but the ability to transfuse rapidly must be achieved as complications such as transection of major vessels is always possible. Air embolus is extremely uncommon particularly in the prone position. This complication is decreased further if the child is kept well hydrated with a normal to high CVP. The best indicator of an intraoperative air embolus is a decrease in E_TCO_2. Careful setting of the alarm settings for E_TCO_2 is imperative for these procedures. Intraoperative cardiovascular instability is usually associated with tumours of the fourth ventricle, especially medulloblastomas and ependymomas. Significant problems of this type are a possible indication for postoperative ventilation. However, the best monitor of postoperative condition is an awake and neurologically intact child, therefore every effort is made to wake and extubate these children at the end of the procedure. Care in a specialist paediatric high dependency environment, however, is essential. Children with postoperative bulbar problems may require prolonged ventilation and go on to require a tracheostomy. Postoperative complications include neurological disability including cranial nerve palsies, worsening of cerebellar dysfunction and new major deficits (40/105[8]) including bulbar problems, cerebellar mutism and apnoeas. Apnoeas are almost always associated with bulbar dysfunction. Postoperative morbidity depends on tumour site, the child's preoperative condition, the operative technique and the extent of tumour removal.

The sitting position in children undergoing posterior fossa surgery potentially facilitates surgical access, improves CSF and venous drainage and lowers ICP. Potential problems include hypotension, venous air embolism (VAE), paradoxical air embolism, pneumocephalus, quadriplegia, and decompressive peripheral neuropathy.[9] The seriousness of potential complications have led to a decline in the use of this position, with most neurosurgeons now choosing the prone or lateral positions for paediatric posterior fossa surgery.

Learning points

- Cerebral tumours are the second most common form of malignancy in children and the most common solid tumour.
- Careful anaesthetic preoperative assessment is vital, including careful parental counselling.

- Adequate invasive intraoperative monitoring is essential because of the risk of blood loss, air embolism and cardiovascular complications.
- A remifentanil infusion is an increasingly useful part of the anaesthetic technique for paediatric neurosurgery because of its extremely short half-life, which allows neurological assessment almost immediately postoperatively.
- All children will require paediatric high dependency or intensive care postoperatively.
- Postoperative complications include respiratory and cardiovascular dysfunction, bulbar dysfunction, vomiting and hydrocephalus.

References

1. Gurney JG, Davis S, Severson RK et al. Trends in cancer incidence among children in the US. *Cancer* 1996; 78: 532–540.
2. Wisoff JH, Boyett JM, Berger MS et al. Current neurosurgical management and the impact of the extent of resection in the treatment of malignant gliomas of childhood: a report of the Children's Cancer Group Trial no. CCG-945. *J Neurosurg* 1998; 89: 52–59.
3. Raimondi AJ. The future perspectives of pediatric neurosurgery. *Child Nerv Sys* 1996; 12: 59–62.
4. Tomita T. Neurosurgical perspectives in pediatric neurooncology. *Child Nerv Sys* 1998; 14: 94–96.
5. Pencalet P, Maixner W, Sainte-Rose C et al. Benign astrocytomas in children. *J Neurosurg* 1999; 90: 265–273.
6. Robertson PL, Zeltzer PM, Boyett JM et al. Survival and prognostic factors following radiotherapy and chemotherapy for ependymomas in children: a report from the Children's Cancer Group. *J Neurosurg* 1998; 88: 695–703.
7. Walker DA, Punt JAG, Sokal M. Clinical management of brain stem gliomas. *Arch Dis Child* 1999; 80: 558–564.
8. Cochrane DD, Gustavsson B, Poskitt KP, Steinbok P, Kestle JRW. The surgical and natural morbidity of aggressive resection for posterior fossa tumours in childhood. *Pediatr Neurosurg* 1994; 20: 19–29.
9. Porter JM, Pidgeon C, Cunningham AJ. The sitting position in neurosurgery: a critical appraisal. *Br J Anaesth* 1999; 82: 117–129.
10. Meridy HW, Creighton RE, Humphreys TRP. Complications during neurosurgery in the prone position in children. *Can Anaesth Soc J* 1974; 21: 450–453.

15

Nephroblastoma (Wilms' tumour)

Peter A Stoddart

Introduction

Despite dramatic improvements in survival rates neoplasia continues to be a major cause of childhood mortality.[1] Nephroblastoma (Wilms' tumour), a common solid tumour of childhood, has an incidence of approximately 7 in one million. Treatment regimens with combinations of surgery and chemotherapy with or without radiotherapy have been developed within international protocols,[2–5] leading to a remarkable improvement in overall survival from $< 10\%$ in 1935 to $> 85\%$ in 1996.[6,7] These children undergo numerous procedures during their treatment, many requiring anaesthesia. The following case depicts the clinical course of a child from presentation.

Case report

A 22-month-old male child was taken to his local casualty department after his mother had noticed a large abdominal mass while bathing him. He had no other significant history. On examination, he weighed 13.6 kg and looked well except for a large right-sided non-tender mass with no signs of jaundice or lymphadenopathy. He was noted to be hypertensive with BP 138/78. Further investigations are shown in Table 15.1

A provisional diagnosis of nephroblastoma was made and he was referred to the regional paediatric surgical centre. His hypertension was treated with nifedipine 7 mg three times daily and atenolol 5 mg three times daily.

A computed tomography (CT) scan of his abdomen and chest was carried out under general anaesthesia. Controlled ventilation was requested by the radiologist to optimize the CT views of the lungs, so following induction of anaesthesia with propofol 50 mg and mivacurium 2.5 mg he was intubated with a 4.5 uncuffed oral endotracheal tube. Anaesthesia was maintained with isoflurane in oxygen-enriched air.

Following the CT scan (see Table 15.2, Figure 15.1) the child now had a provisional diagnosis of bilateral Wilms' tumour or stage V nephroblastoma. This required confirmation before further treatment could be planned so he underwent percutaneous ultrasound-guided trucut biopsy of the left renal pole, open biopsy of the right renal mass and insertion of a Hickman line. The latter was required in view of his poor venous access and because he would have chemotherapy before definitive surgery.

FBC	Hb 9.8 g.dl^{-1}, WCC 6.7 × 10^{9} l^{-1}, Plts 198 × 10^{9} l^{-1}
U & Es	Na 134 mmol.l^{-1}, K 3.9 mmol.l^{-1}, urea 4.2 mmol.l^{-1}
Liver function tests	Normal for age
Urinary VMAs	< 5 mmol.mol^{-1} creatinine
Ultrasound	A large mass arising from right kidney with tumour extension into the renal vein; left kidney appears normal
Chest X-ray	Normal heart and lungs, no sign of metastases

Table 15.1
Initial investigations

His second anaesthetic was induced on his mother's knee with sevoflurane in oxygen-enriched nitrous oxide. Unfortunately the intravenous cannula from his previous anaesthetic had been removed and he had a number of bruises from prior venepunctures. Paracetamol 260 mg had been given an hour earlier for premedication. Intubation was facilitated with rocuronium 8 mg and intraoperative analgesia augmented with fentanyl 50 μg. The procedures took an hour and half during which time he was given a total of 250 ml of Hartmann's solution. He made an uneventful recovery and postoperative analgesia consisted of paracetamol 200 mg 4-hourly for 24 hours with a supplemental dose of oral morphine syrup 5 mg.

The results from the biopsy confirmed bilateral nephroblastoma with favourable histology. Chemotherapy consisting of two doses of dactinomycin (actinomycin D) and doxorubicin plus six doses of weekly vincristine were given prior to definitive surgery with the intention of reducing tumour mass and enabling maximal parenchymal preservation of the left kidney. During this time the boy developed profound bone marrow suppression and alopecia, however his white cell and platelet counts recovered before his major surgery.

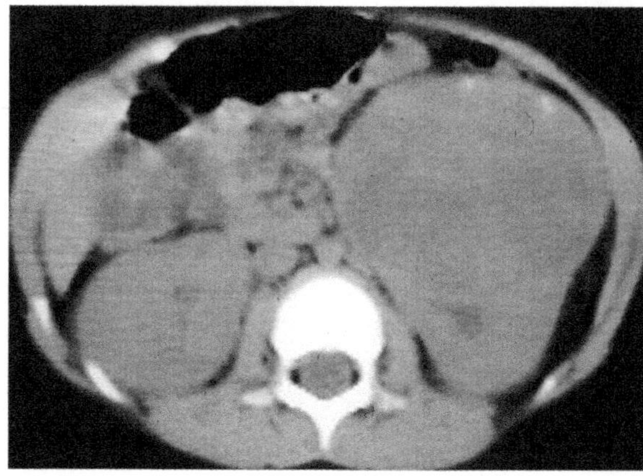

Figure 15.1
Large mass arising from right kidney with presumed tumour/thrombus extension in the renal vein and inferior vena cava to just below the level of the hepatic veins. Left kidney had a small nodule in the upper pole. Para-aortic lymphadenopathy. Normal lung fields.

A repeat abdominal CT scan was performed under general anaesthetic before the surgery to assess the response to chemotherapy (see Table 15.2).

The anaesthetist saw the child and his parents on the oncology ward before surgery. In addition to the routine preoperative assessment, his treatment so far was reviewed and potential venous and arterial access sites were assessed. After discussion of the options for postoperative pain control the parents agreed to a thoracic epidural infusion. They were also taken around the paediatric intensive care and introduced to the nurses and intensive care specialists who initially would be looking after the child following surgery. The boy's antihypertensive treatment was continued preoperatively including the morning of surgery.

Anaesthesia was induced through the Hickman line with propofol 50 mg and fentanyl 75 μg and maintained with isoflurane in oxygen enriched air. Intubation of the

CT scan	Mass arising from right kidney with minimal tumour/thrombus extension in the renal vein; left kidney nodule almost resolved; residual para-aortic lymphadenopathy
Echocardiogram; renal vein Doppler	Normal left ventricular function; renal veins poorly visualized
U & Es	Na 135 $mmol.l^{-1}$, K 4.2 $mmol.l^{-1}$, urea 3.4 $mmol.l^{-1}$
Cross-match	2 units of CMV negative blood
Haematology	Hb 9.8 $g.dl^{-1}$, WCC $5.6 \times 10^9 l^{-1}$, Plts $98 \times 10^9 l^{-1}$, INR 1.1

Table 15.2
Repeat investigations

trachea with a 4.5 uncuffed endotracheal tube was facilitated with rocuronium 10 mg. A size 10FG nasogastric tube was then inserted. The left radial artery was canulated with a 22g cannula and two 18g cannulae inserted into large forearm veins. The Hickman line was transduced to monitor the central venous pressure (CVP). A thoracic epidural catheter was easily inserted at T_{9-10} using an 18G, 5-cm Tuohy needle and a loss of resistance to saline technique. The epidural analgesia was initiated with an incremental dose of 8 ml of 0.25% plain bupivacaine before skin incision. A silastic urinary catheter was inserted to accurately monitor urinary output. Peripheral and nasopharyngeal temperatures were measured. All fluids were warmed with a Hotline™ and the child lay on a warming mattress.

Surgery was performed through a transverse supraumbilical incision. The right-sided tumour had shrunk considerably following the chemotherapy and a nephrectomy with sampling of the local lymph nodes was performed. Once the vena cava had been explored and controlled it was opened and a small amount of residual tumour/thrombus removed but the intima appeared intact. The left renal upper pole had a superficial scar, which was removed with a wedge resection. Estimated blood loss was 350 ml. The CVP was maintained at 8–10 cmH_2O with an infusion of 10 $ml.kg^{-1}.h^{-1}$ of Hartmann's solution, boluses of Gelofusine® and 250 ml of donor blood. A dose of mannitol 0.25 $g.kg^{-1}$ was given prior to mobilizing the right kidney and a second dose as the abdomen was being closed. Some hypertension occurred during dissection of the supranephric structures. This was controlled by increasing the inspired isoflurane and resolved once the dissection was complete.

At the end of surgery, which took 2.5 hours, the child was warm, well perfused, with a base excess of −2 $mmol.l^{-1}$ and a haemoglobin of 9 $g.dl^{-1}$. He was therefore electively extubated and transferred to the paediatric intensive care unit for high dependency care. His urine output which initially had been < 0.5 $ml.kg^{-1}.h^{-1}$ improved overnight with two further fluid challenges of 10 $ml.kg^{-1}$ of normal saline and maintenance of his CVP between 6 and 8 cmH_2O.

Postoperative analgesia was provided with an epidural infusion of 2–4 $ml.h^{-1}$ of 0.125% bupivacaine and 2 $\mu g.ml^{-1}$ fentanyl. A postoperative ileus persisted for 4 days. When he was drinking, the epidural was removed and analgesia continued with regular oral paracetamol. Following surgery the oral antihypertensives were stopped and his blood pressure returned to normal levels for a 2-year-old.

Histology demonstrated some residual tumour, though the thrombus removed from the inferior vena cava had no viable malignant cells. He was discharged home after a week but returned for further chemotherapy. In view of the favourable histology no radiotherapy was planned.

At one year there was no evidence of recurrent disease.

Discussion

A number of syndromes and recognized abnormalities of chromosome 11 are associated with a predisposition to Wilms' tumour especially with bilateral tumours where approximately 25% occur in syndromic children.[2,8] These may present anaesthetic problems in their own right (see Table 15.3).

Presentation in non-syndromic children is usually with an asymptomatic mass, however one-third may have additional symptoms including abdominal pain,

Overgrowth	No overgrowth
Beckwith–Wiedemann syndrome	Aniridia
Hemihypertrophy	Wilms' tumour, aniridia, genitourinary malformations, mental retardation (WAGR syndrome)
Perlman syndrome	Denys–Drash syndrome
Sotos syndrome	Familial Wilms' tumour
Simpson–Golabi–Behmel syndrome	

Table 15.3
Syndromes associated with a predisposition to nephroblastoma, characterized by either overgrowth or no overgrowth

haematuria, a pyrexia of unknown origin, anorexia, vomiting and malaise. Hypertension is not unusual and is secondary to renal ischaemia and raised renin levels. Rarely, erythrocytosis secondary to increased erythropoietin secretion, hypercalcaemia due to high vitamin D levels or acquired von Willebrand disease with bleeding may occur. Differential diagnosis includes neuroblastoma especially if the child has associated hypertension; however, urinary vanillylmandolic acid levels are not raised with Wilms' tumour.

The treatment of Wilms' tumour is a good example of a paediatric tumour where advances in therapy have replaced a previous poor prognosis with an excellent chance of good long-term survival even when initial presentation is with advanced or bilateral tumours. The survival rates for bilateral disease are between 65% and 75% at 5 years.[9,10] Wilms' tumours are bilateral in 5–10% of cases and the aim of therapy is to treat the tumour while preserving as much functioning renal parenchyma as possible and thereby reduce the risk of renal failure or the requirement for renal transplantation in the long term.[9,10] This involves multimodal therapy, as described in this case, associated with the requirement for many anaesthetics especially in young children who tolerate diagnostic procedures poorly. Therefore a good rapport must be established at an early stage with the child and family to improve co-operation and long-term behaviour. The insertion of an indwelling tunnelled central venous catheter, i.e. Hickman line, is especially useful in this age group.

Chemotherapy is associated with significant bone marrow toxicity which may be life-threatening. Platelet counts may fall to $< 10 \times 10^9 l^{-1}$ with a high risk of intracerebral haemorrhage, and profound neutropenia may result in overwhelming sepsis. These effects are normally dose-dependent and recover spontaneously, however the child may need platelet support or growth simulating factor to boost white cell recovery.

Actinomycin D and the anthracyclines such as doxorubicin are known to cause congestive cardiomyopathy and arrhythmias.[11,12] This is associated with high-dose chemotherapy and may occur as a late side effect several years after successful treatment of the initial tumour. Children are routinely screened for this side effect and the child in this case had normal left ventricular function.

Vincristine is associated with neurotoxicity, especially the development of a peripheral neuropathy. This may manifest itself with paraesthesia, reduced sensation and wrist or foot drop. These effects are usually reversible but can cause concern if not appreciated preoperatively. Careful attention to positioning on the table and appropriate padding should be used to protect vulnerable peripheral nerves.

The surgery involves a major retroperitoneal dissection and exploration of the major vessels; furthermore, a partial nephrectomy may be associated with brisk haemorrhage. It is therefore important to have good vascular access and replace any blood loss and fluid shifts with warmed fluids to prevent hypotension and avoid renal hypoperfusion in the face of the reduction in renal parenchyma. Careful attention to the blood pressure, heart rate, temperature gradient and clinical signs of peripheral perfusion must be maintained. A number of drugs, namely dopamine, dopexamine, frusemide (furosemide) and mannitol have been described as renal protective in the potentially poorly perfused kidney. Unfortunately none have been shown to consistently reduce the incidence of renal failure in the ischaemic kidney.[13,18] It is the author's personal preference to use small aliquots of mannitol in an attempt to maintain urine output especially when both kidneys are to be mobilized. However, if there were hypotension or signs of poor cardiac output despite adequate fluid replacement then dopamine is preferable.

Blood transfusion has been associated with many problems ranging from acute transfusion reactions, transmission of infective agents including HIV and hepatitis to potential long-term immunomodulatory effects including increased risk of recurrent tumours and nosocomal infections. Therefore even in the UK where the risk of these adverse outcomes is extremely low, routine postoperative transfusion to maintain a 'normal' haemoglobin level of greater than $10\,g.dl^{-1}$ should no longer occur. Children should only be transfused if clinically indicated and exposure limited to as few donor units as possible.[19,20]

An extensive transverse incision is required to enable dissection of both kidneys; therefore postoperative analgesia must be optimum. A multimodal approach should be utilized. In a child with a normal platelet count a low thoracic epidural using local anaesthesia will block T_{8-10} and can be supplemented with epidural fentanyl.[21,22] This will additionally improve cardiovascular stability by obtunding the hypertensive responses associated with perinephric surgery especially in tumours that secrete vasoactive hormones. Opioids can provide similar effects but may require high doses of fentanyl intraoperatively and a postoperative infusion of morphine. This can increase the risk of postoperative respiratory dysfunction including the need for ventilation. Paracetamol should be added to this regimen but non-steroidal anti-inflammatory drugs (NSAIDs) are contraindicated.

Learning points

- Nephroblastoma is a common solid childhood tumour, treated with combined surgery, chemotherapy and radiotherapy.
- Multiple anaesthetics may be required; therefore the child and family must be treated sympathetically.
- Review the effects of chemotherapy, especially cardiac and haematological.
- Major retroperitoneal laparotomy with potential for significant blood loss; therefore invasive monitoring and avoidance of hypovolaemia required to protect renal function.
- Use multimodal analgesia to provide optimal postoperative pain relief, but avoid NSAIDs.

References

1. Number of deaths by age group. England and Wales, 1998. http://www.statistics.gov.uk/
2. Wiener JS, Coppes MJ, Ritchey ML. Current concepts in the biology and management of Wilms tumor. *J Urol* 1998; 159: 1316–1325.
3. Coppes MJ, Wolff JE, Ritchey ML. Wilms tumour: diagnosis and treatment. *Paediatr Drugs* 1999; 1: 251–262.
4. Haase GM, Ritchey ML. Nephroblastoma. *Semin Pediatr Surg* 1997; 6: 11–16.
5. Farhat W, McLorie G, Capolicchio G. Wilms' tumor. Surgical considerations and controversies. *Urol Clin North Am* 2000; 27: 455–462, viii.
6. Plesko I, Kramarova E, Stiller CA, Coebergh JW, Santaquilani M. EUROCARE Working Group. Survival of children with Wilms' tumour in Europe. *Eur J Cancer* 2001; 37: 736–743.
7. Gatta G, Capocaccia R, Coleman MP, Ries LA, Berrino F. Childhood cancer survival in Europe and the United States. *Cancer* 2002; 95: 1767–1772.
8. Knudson AG Jr, Strong LC. Mutation and cancer: a model for Wilms' tumor of the kidney. *J Natl Cancer Inst* 1972; 48: 313–324.
9. Tomlinson GS, Cole CH, Smith NM. Bilateral Wilms' tumor: a clinicopathologic review. *Pathology* 1999; 31: 12–16.
10. Kumar R, Fitzgerald R, Breatnach F. Conservative surgical management of bilateral Wilms' tumor: results of the United Kingdom Children's Cancer Study Group. *J Urol* 1998; 160: 1450–1453.
11. Burrows FA, Hickey PR, Colan S. Perioperative complications in patients with anthracycline chemotherapeutic agents. *Can Anaesth Soc J* 1985; 32: 149–157.
12. McQuillan PJ, Morgan BA, Ramwell J. Adriamycin cardiomyopathy. Fatal outcome of general anaesthesia in a child with adriamycin cardiomyopathy. *Anaesthesia* 1988; 43: 301–304.
13. Bracco D, Parlow JL. Best evidence in anesthetic practice. Prevention: dopamine does not prevent death, acute renal failure, or need for dialysis. *Can J Anaesth* 2002; 49: 417–419.
14. Galley HF. Can acute renal failure be prevented? *J R Coll Surg Edinb* 2000; 45: 44–50.
15. Ralph CJ, Tanser SJ, Macnaughton PD, Sinclair DG. A randomised controlled trial investigating the effects of dopexamine on gastrointestinal function and organ dysfunction in the critically ill. *Intensive Care Med* 2002; 28: 884–890.
16. Filler G. Acute renal failure in children: aetiology and management. *Paediatr Drugs* 2001; 3: 783–792.
17. Reddy VG. Prevention of postoperative acute renal failure. *J Postgrad Med* 2002: 48: 64–70.
18. O'Leary MJ, Bihari DJ. Preventing renal failure in the critically ill. There are no magic bullets – just high quality intensive care. *BMJ* 2001; 322: 1437–1439.
19. Canadian Medical Association. Guidelines for red blood cell and plasma transfusion for adults and children. *CMAJ* 1997; 156: 1S–23S.
20. American Society of Anaesthesiologists Task Force on Blood Component Therapy. Practice guidelines for blood component therapy. *Anesthesiology* 1996; 84: 732–747.
21. Tobias JD, Lowe S, O'Dell N, Holcomb GW 3rd. Thoracic epidural anaesthesia in infants and children. *Can J Anaesth* 1993; 40: 879–882.
22. Wolf AR, Eyres RL, Laussen PC et al. Effect of extradural analgesia on stress responses to abdominal surgery in infants. *Br J Anaesth* 1993; 70: 654–660.

16

Laser therapy for laryngeal papillomas

Paul Reynolds and Robert Weatherly

Introduction

Recurrent respiratory papillomatosis (RRP) is a relatively rare viral disease of the larynx that often presents in early life with signs and symptoms of airway obstruction. These patients often require multiple, repeated anaesthetics for laryngeal microsurgery. Anaesthetic and surgical management of a child with RRP is presented.

Case presentation

An otherwise healthy 3-year-old 15-kg male presented to the Paediatric Otolaryngologists with a history of increasing hoarseness and stridor. His tolerance to activity had diminished over the past few months and he had complained of increasing dysphagia. Past medical history was positive for removal of a laryngeal papilloma at 1 year of age at an outside hospital. On physical examination he was comfortable at rest, but became hoarse when asked to vocalize. He had a harsh quality to his breathing that was audible even without a stethoscope as he increased his activity. He had no nasal flaring, sternal retractions or other symptoms of respiratory distress.

Awake fibreoptic laryngeal examination demonstrated a 'ballvalving' lesion in the laryngeal airway, directly between the vocal cords. He was scheduled for microscopic laryngoscopy and bronchoscopy for airway stabilization and removal of the lesion using a carbon dioxide laser under general anaesthesia.

The following day, the child arrived in the operating room accompanied by his mother fasted and unpremedicated. An inhalation induction with sevoflurane was performed with no difficulty maintaining airway patency. Standard monitors (EKG, end-tidal CO_2, pulse oximetry, non-invasive blood pressure and temperature) were placed, as was an intravenous line. 20 µg of fentanyl, 150 µg of glycopyrrolate, and 10 mg of dexamethasone were administered intravenously. Once an adequate plane of anaesthesia was obtained, the vocal cords were sprayed with 2 cc of 2% lignocaine. The otolaryngologist performed suspension laryngoscopy. With the patient breathing spontaneously, anaesthesia was maintained with propofol infused at 200–300 $\mu g.kg^{-1}.min^{-1}$ and isoflurane in a 30% O_2 and air mixture insufflated into the hypopharynx via a metal endotracheal tube (Norton tube, A.V. Mueller, Chicago, IL, USA). The patient's eyes were covered with moist eye pads and cloth tape, while moist towels were placed over the patient's face and neck.

Direct laryngoscopy revealed a large, pedunculated papilloma, attached to the left anterior true vocal cord, partially obstructing and 'ballvalving' the laryngeal opening (see Figure 16.1). The mass was fibrous in character and was difficult to remove with the microdebrider (Xomed, Jacksonville, FL, USA). The lesion was then grasped with cupped forceps, and with tension applied, the carbon dioxide laser was used to remove the mass (see Figure 16.2). Great care was taken not to allow the mass to fall into the airway. Upon completion of the procedure, the airway was returned to the anaesthesiologists, and the patient was awakened in the operating room, prior to transfer to the postanaesthesia care unit (PACU). The patient's airway remained patent and unobstructed throughout the postoperative phase and the patient required no additional analgesics. The child was discharged home less than 2 hours after arrival in the PACU.

Following his original presentation 6 months previously, the patient returned to the operating room on two occasions for additional microscopic laryngoscopy and removal of smaller recurrent papillomas using a microdebrider under general anaesthesia. The patient tolerated all subsequent procedures without incident.

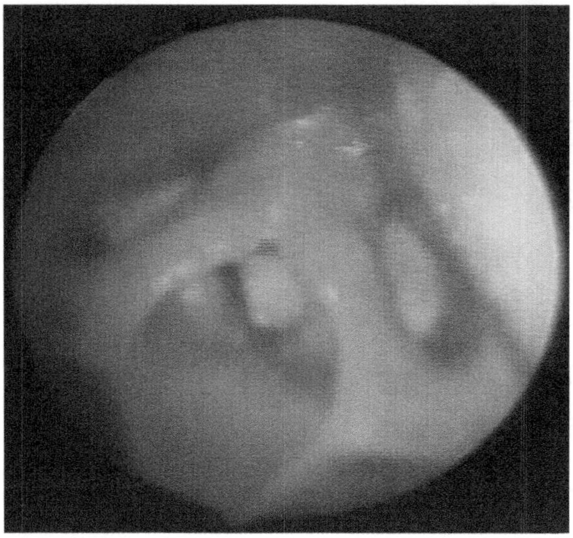

Figure 16.1
Photograph of the larynx with a 'ballvalving' laryngeal papilloma partially obstructing the glottic opening.

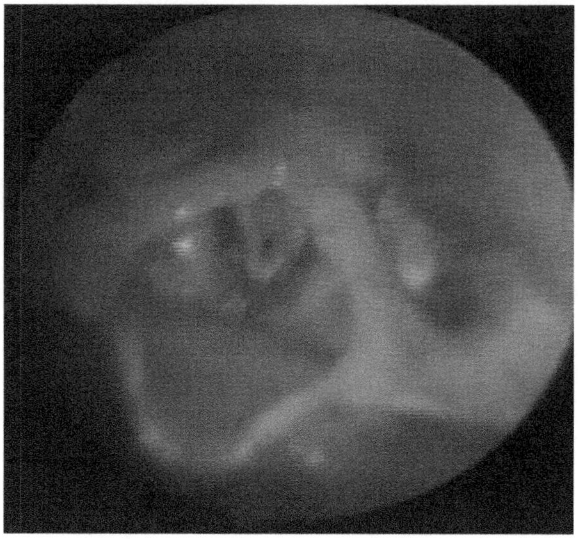

Figure 16.2
Same view as Figure 16.1, during inspiration.

Discussion

RRP is caused by the human papillomavirus (most commonly types 6 and 11), and has the potential for poor if not fatal outcome because of airway involvement and risk of malignant conversion.[1] The course of the disease is variable, with some patients exhibiting mild symptoms with eventual regression after limited interventions, while others require frequent, unremitting procedures to maintain airway patency. The juvenile form of the disease is much more aggressive than the adult form. The lesions occur in the airway where ciliated and squamous epithelium is juxtaposed, such as the laryngeal surface of the epiglottis, the undersurface of the vocal folds, and the carina, and are thought to be secondary to virally induced epithelial changes.[2] Lesions can also occur throughout the respiratory tract and the upper gastrointestinal tracts. Vertical transmission of the disease to infants probably occurs from mothers infected with the human papillomavirus during birth, although the exact mechanism of transmission may differ in selected cases. The incidence of RRP in the United States is relatively rare, with approximately 1500–2500 new cases per year. In most series, RRP is diagnosed between 2 and 3 years of age.[3]

The relative rarity of the disease and the complexity of the management make it prudent to care for children with RRP at major medical centres and children's hospitals. Children with RRP may require dozens of surgical procedures during their lifetime to maintain airway patency, with intervals as short as weekly. This represents a significant burden to the child and family in terms of airway difficulties, voice changes and time away from family, school and work.

Preoperative evaluation should include a careful history of obstructive airway symptoms. Signs of upper airway obstruction can be variable, not all patients who have obstructing lesions present with classic high-pitched inspiratory stridor. Some patients have air hunger, voice changes, dysphagia (usually from the competition required to breathe while swallowing), and exercise intolerance as their primary complaints. A patient who looks comfortable at rest may worsen at times of stress, such as crying or during induction of anaesthesia. Physical examination may reveal signs of respiratory insufficiency or distress such as tachypnoea, nasal flaring, suprasternal retractions, or use of accessory muscles of respiration.

Preoperative investigations are usually limited in RRP. Awake, flexible fibreoptic evaluation of the airway is often helpful in confirming the diagnosis (as in our patient), but is not always performed and is dependent upon the age and compliance of the patient and the skill of the endoscopist. The use of sedatives for airway evaluation outside the operating room can be extremely risky in the absence of skilled personnel and equipment necessary to secure the airway. Chest X-ray may be helpful if pulmonary disease is suspected.

Once the patient is scheduled for surgical intervention, there must be excellent communication between the anaesthesiologist and otolaryngologist preoperatively. Plans regarding airway management should be agreed upon, and equipment made available, including all equipment required for a surgical airway. Because of the potential for loss of airway, sedative premedication should be avoided. Since many of these children present as toddlers, where separation from parents can be stressful and agitating to both parent and child, and crying or agitation can worsen an already compromised airway, parents will often accompany the child to the induction room or operating room at our institution so as to avoid the use of a sedative premedicant. The otolaryngologist must be present during induction of anaesthesia, in case the need for an immediate surgical airway arises. At our institution, inhalational agents (sevoflurane or halothane) are the preferred induction agents. After the patient has been anaesthetized, standard monitors are placed, and an intravenous line is secured. Four different methods have been employed to secure the airway for bronchoscopy/laryngoscopy and microlaryngeal surgical removal of the papilloma.

Spontaneous ventilation[4]

As described in this case report, once an adequate plane of anaesthesia has been obtained, the vocal cords are sprayed with a maximum of $6\,mg.kg^{-1}$ of lignocaine. This topical anaesthetic may reduce the amount of maintenance anaesthetic required by blunting the response to stimuli caused by manipulation of the larynx. The otolaryngologist then performs suspension laryngoscopy. With the patient breathing spontaneously, anaesthesia is maintained by insufflation of volatile anaesthetic, and intravenous propofol, infused at $200–300\,\mu g.kg^{-1}.min^{-1}$. Recently, we have added remifentanil as a separate infusion of $0.05–0.1\,\mu g.kg^{-1}.min^{-1}$ to the maintenance anaesthetic. With careful titration of these infusions, volatile anaesthetic concentrations can be reduced, while preserving a regular pattern of spontaneous respirations. A 30% O_2 and air mixture (to minimize the risk of airway fire with the use of lasers) is insufflated into the hypopharynx via a metal endotracheal tube (Norton tube, A.V. Mueller). The primary advantage of this technique is that it permits the patient to breathe spontaneously thereby facilitating the diagnosis of dynamic airway abnormalities (such as laryngo or tracheomalacia), that would otherwise be masked by positive pressure ventilation. In addition, spontaneous respirations allow for a clear line of sight from which the surgeon may use the laser. This is particularly helpful in patients with subglottic lesions. Furthermore, maintaining spontaneous respirations and avoidance of muscle relaxant can be life saving in the event of acute airway loss. Finally, avoiding positive pressure ventilation can theoretically diminish the potential of distal seeding of papilloma virus due to mechanical spread from endotracheal tube placement or dispersion by jet ventilation. Disadvantages of this technique include the potential for aspiration, hypoventilation and resultant hypoxemia, and conversely, coughing and movement due to inadequate anaesthesia. Therefore intravenous and volatile anaesthetics must be carefully titrated to provide the ideal balance. This technique requires experience and patience.

Intubation with metal or wrapped tube

After induction of anaesthesia, the trachea can be intubated with either a metal tube or an endotracheal tube wrapped in metal tape (3M, St. Paul, MN, USA). This can be accomplished with or without muscle relaxant. Advantages of this technique include the ability to give positive pressure ventilation during laser removal of papilloma while protecting the airway from papilloma debris, smoke, or other material that could be aspirated. Hypoventilation or hypoxaemia can be avoided through controlled ventilation, while higher inspired oxygen concentrations, if required, can be used (if there is no airway leak around the tube). Disadvantages include obstruction of the surgical field by the endotracheal tube, aspiration of accidentally dislodged papilloma upon tube placement, or distortion of the airway by the tube itself. If the wrapped tube has any areas uncovered, the tube may be ignited if contact is made with the laser.

Venturi jet ventilation

This method of ventilating a patient's lungs without the aid of an endotracheal tube has been used in both adults and children with great success in the treatment of laryngeal papillomatosis. A metal catheter is clamped inside a laryngoscope and connected to an adjustable oxygen source at a pressure of 50 psi. With the catheter directed into the laryngeal opening, the operator uses a trigger to inject the jet of oxygen, timing the breaths with the surgeon's actions. Room air is entrained along with the oxygen jet, thus decreasing the FiO_2.[5] Advantages to this technique for laser papilloma removals include the absence of an endotracheal tube and a lower FiO_2, diminishing the risk of airway fires. Total intravenous anaesthesia and a muscle relaxant are required for this technique. Since jet ventilation makes use of a very high-pressure source (50 psi is equivalent to 3500 cm H_2O), it is imperative that the anaesthesiologist be certain the jet is aimed through the laryngeal inlet, and not at mucosa. Initial ventilations should begin at less than 10 psi and should be gradually increased as chest wall movements are observed and breath sounds are auscultated. High pressures applied directly to the distal airways may cause pneumothorax or pneumomediastinum. If the jet is not kept in perfect alignment, gastric dilatation may occur, possibly leading to regurgitation and aspiration through an unprotected airway.

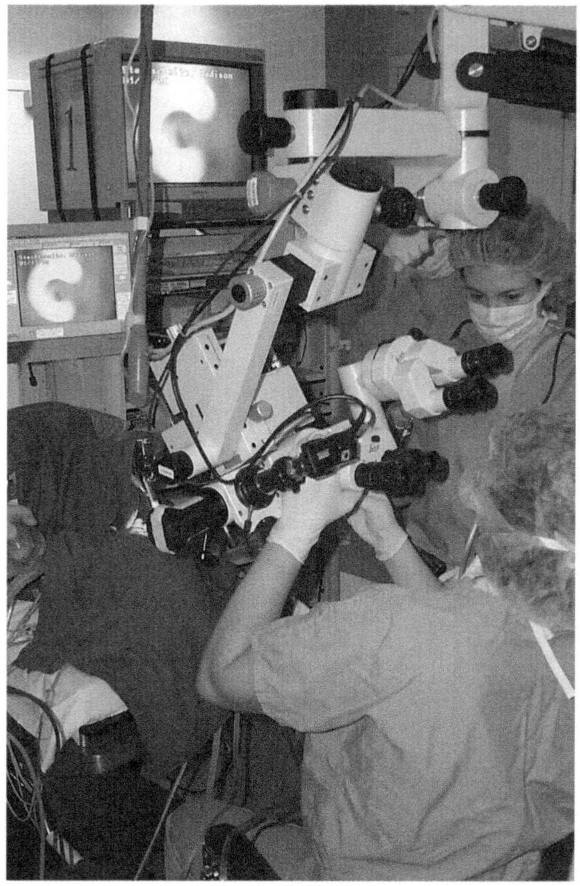

Figure 16.3
The child is covered with moist towels, and the carbon dioxide laser mounted to an operating microscope is used to remove the papilloma.

Apnoeic oxygenation

This form of anaesthesia for laryngeal papilloma surgery involves intermittent intubations of the larynx with standard endotracheal tubes and hyperventilation with 100% oxygen. The endotracheal tube is then removed from the surgical field while the surgeon is directing the laser at the lesion. When the anaesthesiologist determines the patient requires further ventilation, the surgeon will stop the procedure, reinsert the tube, and the patient will be ventilated for a short period of time. The tube is then removed, and surgery resumed. This technique requires a muscle relaxant in combination with either an inhalation agent or intravenous anaesthetic. Advantages include the absence of a combustible tube at the time of laser application, and the ability to intermittently ventilate the patient during the procedure. The major disadvantage to this technique is knowing when to stop operating. Waiting too long between intubations can lead to hypercarbia and/or hypoxaemia. Additionally, repeated intubations to an already traumatized airway can lead to postoperative supra- or subglottic oedema.

Although no one technique is foolproof, each technique has its merits. The anaesthesiologist caring for the child with RRP should be familiar with each technique. If one method fails (e.g. the patient begins coughing during spontaneous ventilation), the anaesthesiologist may have to select another technique to continue with the procedure.

No discussion about RRP is complete without mention of laser safety. Although the microdebrider is being used more frequently in the treatment of RRP,

92% of otolaryngologists still use the CO_2 laser.[2] Laser safety involves protecting the patient and all operating room personnel. Prevention of an airway fire is best accomplished by detailed discussion of the case between the anaesthesiologist and the surgeon. Key points are limiting the availability of the oxidizer (oxygen), controlling the ignition source (laser beam), and trying to eliminate the fuel source (non-flammable endotracheal tube or *no* endotracheal tube). The most commonly employed means of accomplishing this task are using a solid metal or metal-wrapped endotracheal tube, spontaneous respirations with no endotracheal tube, or intermittent apnoea with or without jet ventilation. All patient surfaces exposed to potential laser scatter should be covered with moist towels. All personnel working in the operating room should wear laser resistant eyewear. In addition, operating room personnel should wear laser masks to filter out small-aerosolized particles.

In summary, the anaesthetic and surgical management of recurrent and respiratory papillomatosis poses a unique challenge. Successful management of this condition calls upon the resourcefulness and attention to detail of the anaesthesiologist and requires detailed communication between the anaesthesiologist and surgeon, awareness of the unique anaesthetic and surgical considerations.

Learning points

- RRP is caused by the human papillomavirus, has the potential for poor if not fatal outcome because of airway involvement and risk of malignant conversion.
- Children with RRP may require dozens of surgical procedures during their lifetime to maintain airway patency, with intervals as short as weekly.
- Preoperative evaluation should include a careful history of obstructive airway symptoms, some of which may not be 'classic'.
- Preoperative investigations are usually limited in RRP. Awake, flexible fibreoptic evaluation of the airway is often helpful in confirming the diagnosis.
- Once the patient is scheduled for surgical intervention, there must be excellent communication between the anaesthesiologist and otolaryngologist preoperatively.
- Because of the potential for loss of the airway, sedative premedication should be avoided.
- The otolaryngologist must be present during induction of anaesthesia, in case the need for an immediate surgical airway arises.
- Four different methods have been employed to secure the airway for microlaryngeal surgical removal of the papilloma: spontaneous ventilation, intubation with metal or wrapped tubes, Venturi jet ventilation, and apnoeic oxygenation.
- Laser safety involves protecting the patient and all operating room personnel.
- Key points to avoiding a laser fire are limiting the availability of the oxidizer (oxygen), controlling the ignition source (laser beam), and trying to eliminate the fuel source (non-flammable endotracheal tube or *no* endotracheal tube).

References

1. Armstrong L, Derkay C, Reeves W et al. Initial results from the national registry for juvenile-onset recurrent papillomatosis. *Arch Otolaryngol Head Neck Surg* 1999; 125: 743–748.
2. Derkay C. Task force on recurrent respiratory papillomas. *Arch Otolaryngol Head Neck Surg* 1995; 121: 1386–1391.
3. Derkay C, Malis D, Zalzal G et al. A staging system for assessing severity of disease and response to therapy in recurrent respiratory papillomatosis. *Laryngoscope* 1998; 108: 935–937.
4. Hermen J, Bennett M, Hirshman C. Anaesthesia for laser surgery. *Anesth Analg* 1983; 62: 218–229.
5. Sosis M. Anaesthesia for laser surgery. *Int Anesth Clin* 1990; 28: 119–131.

17

Anaesthesia for a child with Apert syndrome and a congenital abnormality of the hand

Philip M D Cunnington and Robert Bingham

Introduction

There are many congenital anomalies of the hand that require surgical correction. They form a spectrum of disease from simple anomalies, e.g. clinodactyly, that require only a single surgical procedure, to complex anomalies, e.g. radial club hand which may require multiple procedures over a prolonged period of time. These anomalies may occur in isolation or as part of a congenital syndrome.

The perioperative management of these cases presents the anaesthetist with a number of challenges related to the assessment of congenital disease and its anaesthetic implications, the conduct of anaesthesia and postoperative pain management. Effective communication with the family is particularly vital as these children are likely to require multiple anaesthetics as their treatment progresses.

Correction of syndactyly is a frequently performed surgical procedure (incidence 1 : 2000 approximately) and is associated with many congenital syndromes (Table 17.1). Apert syndrome is one of the congenital syndromes associated with syndactyly and the following history describes such a case.

History

A 2-year-old girl presented for division of central complex syndactyly of her left hand. The routine preoperative anaesthetic assessment the evening before surgery revealed a complex past medical history.

She had been born at 38 weeks' gestation via vaginal delivery. She was immediately noted to be dysmorphic with craniofacial and limb abnormalities and suffering from choanal stenosis. She had upper airway obstruction, this was mild at rest and became more pronounced during sleep. During this time she was diagnosed as having Apert syndrome and in addition to the obvious external craniofacial and limb abnormalities she was also found to have a cleft palate and a small ostium secundum atrial septal defect.

She had undergone repair of her cleft palate at 8 months of age, which resulted in a worsening of her obstructive sleep apnoea. The obstruction was improved by insertion of a nasopharyngeal airway, which remained in situ for her return home. Otherwise, anaesthesia had been uneventful; there had been no difficulties in intubation and there was no family history of anaesthetic problems. Anaesthesia for a computed tomography scan (spontaneous ventilation via a laryngeal mask airway) had also been uneventful.

Review of systems revealed that she had been discharged from the cardiology clinic, an echocardiogram demonstrating closure of the atrial septal defect. She had been well for the previous 9 months with no further need for the nasopharyngeal airway but was awaiting a craniofacial assessment with a view to cranial reconstructive surgery. There was no suggestion of raised intracranial pressure. She had no known allergies and was not taking any regular medication.

Physical examination revealed brachycephaly, frontal bossing and a flat occiput. She still exhibited a degree of maxillary retrusion and had flat faces and proptosis with a depressed nasal bridge and copious nasal secretions. She had good mouth opening, no obvious tonsillar hypertrophy, dental crowding but no loose teeth. She also demonstrated a full range of neck movements.

Auscultation of the chest revealed normal heart sounds and vesicular breath sounds with transmitted upper airway noises. She had symmetrical central syndactyly of both hands, thumb and great toe malformations. She weighed 12.2 kg and was on the 50th percentile for height and weight.

Syndrome	*Findings*	*Anaesthetic Implications*
Apert	Craniosynostosis, complex syndactyly, mid-face hypoplasia	Upper airway obstruction, difficult airway, IV access
Pfeiffer	Brachycephaly, craniosynostosis, simple syndactyly, broad thumbs	Occasional choanal atresia, laryngomalacia, tracheomalacia, bronchomalacia
Saethre-Chotzen	Craniosynostosis, maxillary hypoplasia, syndactyly	May have raised intracranial pressure
Carpenter	Acrocephaly, mandibular and maxillary hypoplasia, syndactyly, polydactyly, VSD, ASD, patent ductus arteriosus, tetralogy of Fallot, TOGA	Cardiovascular abnormality in 50%
VATER	Vertebral anomalies, anal atresia, tracheo-oesophageal fistula, radial dysplasia, VSD	VSD in 20–30%
Holt-Oram	Upper limb abnormality, cardiac defect, narrow shoulders	Cardiac defect may be VSD, ASD, patent ductus arteriosus or arrhythmias
TAR	Thrombocytopenia, bilateral radial hypoplasia/aplasia	Abnormal platelet function, associated with tetralogy of Fallot, congenital heart disease in up to 33%
Epidemolysis Bullosa	Blister formation, digital fusion, anaemia, growth retardation, malnutrition	Difficult IV access, careful positioning
Ladd (lacrimo-auricluo-dento-digital)	Radial defects, thumb triphalangy or duplication, clinodactyly, syndactyly, nasolacrimal obstruction/ aplasia, cup shaped ears, hypodontia	
Poland's sequence	Syndactyly, axillary webbing, unilateral defect of pectoralis major	Dextrocardia in left sided Poland sequence
Oculodentodigital	Micropthalmia, small teeth, enamel hypoplasia, syndactyly	
Oro-facial-digital (I)	Cleft tongue, abnormalities of teeth, cleft palate, cleft lip, hypoplasia of alae nasi, digital asymmetry, simple syndactyly	
Oro-facial-digital (II)	Cleft tongue, cleft lip, high arched or cleft palate, mandibular hypoplasia, syndactyly	
Trisomy 13	Defects of eyes, nose, holoprosenchephaly, polydactyly, cardiac defects	VSD, ASD, patent ductus arteriosus, dextrocardia in up to 80%

Table 17.1
Congenital syndromes associated with deformities of the hand and their anaesthetic implications

Following discussion with the parents it was decided to perform a gaseous induction because of difficulties in obtaining intravenous access for her last procedure. At this time the potential methods of postoperative analgesia were discussed including the use of an axillary brachial plexus block and the administration of diclofenac suppositories.

Since she was well with good exercise tolerance and no suggestion of intercurrent disease, no additional investigations were performed.

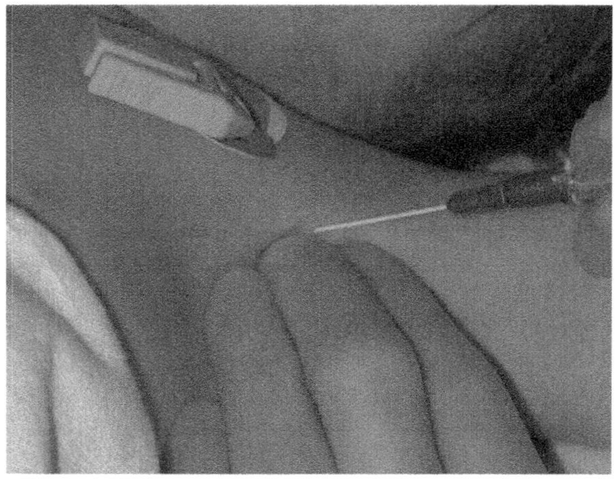

Figure 17.1
Left axillary brachial plexus block, using a 22G parallel-sided intra-venous cannula.

Management

The next morning, following routine checks of the anaesthetic machines and equipment, the patient was transferred into the anaesthetic room accompanied by her father. She was calm and co-operative and a pulse oximeter probe was applied to her left foot. A gaseous induction was then performed using sevoflurane 8% in oxygen and nitrous oxide (F_IO_2 0.5) delivered via a T-piece initially held in the hand and later with a clear plastic facemask. This was well tolerated and she was soon unconscious; the father was then escorted from the room.

Additional monitoring, consisting of ECG and non-invasive blood pressure, was applied and intravenous access secured in the right long saphenous vein using a 22g cannula. During the next minute she developed signs of upper airway obstruction with tracheal tug and paradoxical respiration which were not completely relieved with simple airway manoeuvres and distending pressure. Following insertion of an oropharyngeal airway, however, her respiratory pattern was much improved. A 7-mg dose of atracurium was administered and she was intubated without difficulty with a 5.0-mm tracheal tube. Positive pressure ventilation with a rate of 20 min^{-1} and pressures of 18/4 cmH_2O was commenced. The sevoflurane was then substituted for isoflurane, an oropharyngeal temperature probe was inserted, her eyes were protected with simple eye ointment and she was positioned for a left axillary brachial plexus block (see Figure 17.1).

The patient was placed supine with her left arm pulled straight up so as to lie alongside her head, in such a way that the loose tissues of the axilla were placed under tension, although this resulted in some 'winging' of her scapula. The skin was then prepared with 0.5% chlorhexidine in methylated spirit. The arterial pulse was then palpated and traced to the point of maximum pulsation over the head of the humerus. Using a sterile technique, a 22g parallel-sided intravenous cannula was then introduced through a small skin incision and advanced, at an angle of 45° to the skin, aiming at a point anterior to the artery, until a 'click' was felt corresponding to puncture of the neurovascular sheath. The cannula was then advanced over the needle for a short distance. Some resistance was felt and it was not possible to fully advance the cannula. Following a negative aspiration test, 0.5 $ml.kg^{-1}$ of 0.25% plain bupivacaine was injected. There was no resistance to the injection despite distal compression of the sheath, which was maintained in an attempt to aid the spread of local anaesthetic solution proximally.

The patient was then transferred into the operating theatre, positioned for surgery and a tourniquet applied to her left upper arm and the cuff inflated to 250 mmHg. An intravenous infusion of Hartmann's solution was commenced and a total of 20 $ml.kg^{-1}$ administered in theatre.

There was a small and transient increase in heart rate when the first incision was made but this rapidly settled and heart rate and blood pressure remained constant throughout the procedure. A division of complex syndactyly left hand was performed. A full-thickness skin graft was taken from the left groin following infiltration with a further 4 ml of 0.25% plain bupivacaine. The duration was 75 minutes with virtually no blood loss. Once the dressings had been applied the isoflurane was switched off and 100%

oxygen administered, she was extubated when awake and transferred to the recovery room breathing oxygen.

A full handover was given to the recovery nurse including the details of the axillary brachial plexus block and intravenous fluid administration. Instructions regarding limb care and postoperative analgesia were given verbally and paracetamol (oral $20\,mg.kg^{-1}$, max. $100\,mg.kg^{-1}.24hr^{-1}$), diclofenac (oral $1\,mg.kg^{-1}$, max. $3\,mg.kg^{-1}.24hr^{-1}$) and codeine phosphate (oral $1\,mg.kg^{-1}$, 4-hourly) were prescribed. The intravenous infusion was discontinued but the cannula left in situ until the patient was taking oral fluids.

The patient remained in the recovery room for 20 minutes during which time her observations of arterial saturation, non-invasive blood pressure and pain score remained stable and she required no further analgesia. She was discharged, pain free, to the paediatric ward.

Her recovery on the ward was unremarkable and she was able to take oral fluid within 2 hours. Over the first 24 hours she required one dose of diclofenac which was administered 8 hours after the insertion of the axillary brachial plexus block and two subsequent doses of paracetamol.

Outcome

The patient was discharged home on the second postoperative day and was given an outpatient appointment to see the Clinical Nurse Specialist for review of her dressings 4 days later. The remainder of her recovery was uneventful and she was scheduled for corrective surgery on her right hand 8 months later.

Discussion

There are many congenital syndromes that may confront the anaesthetist when performing anaesthesia for hand surgery. Many other organ systems may be affected and so a knowledge of the nature and extent of these conditions is essential to enable the anaesthetist to identify potential problems during the preoperative assessment and to plan appropriate anaesthesia. Those conditions affecting the airway, respiratory system, cranial vault and cardiovascular system are of particular importance (Table 17.1).

Apert first defined a syndrome of craniosynostosis, midface hypoplasia and retrusion and symmetric syndactyly of the hands and feet (acrocephalosyndactyly) in 1906.[1–3] It is inherited in an autosomal dominant fashion with the majority of cases being sporadic. Mutations of the fibroblast growth factor receptor 2 (FGFR2) cause Apert syndrome and different mutations in the same gene cause Crouzon syndrome and Pfeiffer syndrome.

The features of Apert syndrome are listed in Table 17.2. The features of most importance to the anaesthetist are those involving the airway, cranial vault and cardiovascular system.

The airway problems are as a result of the craniosynostosis. This premature closure of the cranial sutures results in arrested growth of the skull perpendicular to the fused suture and compensatory growth in other directions. In Apert syndrome this involves the coronal sutures leading to brachycephaly (short skull) and involving the calvaria, base and face. The anterior cranial fossa is shortened and therefore limits the area for development of the nasomaxillary complex. The nasal cavity, palate and maxilla are all shortened. The middle cranial fossa is rotated to a more vertical position which also contributes to the reduction in the size of the pharynx.[4] These anatomical changes along with possible choanal stenosis, cleft palate, dental crowding and hypertrophy of lymphoid tissue make for potential airway problems. The narrow nasopharyngeal and pharyngeal spaces are easily obstructed by the posterior movement of the tongue towards the posterior pharyngeal wall which also compresses the soft palate or cleft palatal tags against the posterior pharyngeal wall. Therefore there is a meeting of the tongue, velum and posterior pharyngeal wall in the upper oropharynx as well as movement of the lateral pharyngeal walls medially opposing each other. The tendency for this to happen is reduced but not completely removed by midfacial surgery, e.g. Le Fort III osteotomy. A craniosynostosis release may be required if raised intracranial pressure has occurred as a result of the fusion of cranial sutures. Intracranial hypertension may be exacerbated by chronic carbon dioxide retention.

Airway management of these children should be approached with caution and prior preparation. A thorough assessment is made preoperatively with particular reference to any past anaesthetic records. A full range of airway equipment should also be immediately available including the soft plastic facemasks, which will mold more easily to the child's retruded midface, and a range of oropharyngeal airways as sizing and insertion may be difficult due to the altered nasopharyngeal dimensions and the dental overcrowding.

System	*Findings*
Craniofacial	Craniosynostosis, frontal bossing, flat occiput, midface hypoplasia, flat faces, proptosis, hypertelorism, depressed nasal bridge, cleft palate or bifid uvula, dental crowding, choanal stenosis or atresia
Extremities	Symmetrical syndactyly of fingers and toes, osseous and / or cutaneous thumb and great toe malformations
Cardiovascular	ASD, VSD, overriding aorta, coarctation of the aorta, pulmonary stenosis
Musculoskeletal	Joint aplasia or ankylsosis, synostosis of radius and humerus, cervical spine fusion at C5-6
Pulmonary	Glottic stenosis, anomalous tracheal cartilage
Gastrointestinal	Ectopic anus, oesophageal atresia, pyloric stenosis
Renal	Polycystic kidney, hydronephrosis
Central nervous system	Agenesis of the corpus callusum, limbic malformations, absent septum pellucidum, ventriculomegaly, mental retardation, hearing deficit
Growth and development	Normal birth weight and length, slower growth in childhood

Table 17.2
Features of Apert syndrome

The decision on the mode of induction of anaesthesia depends on the individual patient but intravenous access may be difficult in these patients owing to the congenital limb abnormalities, past attempts at access and lack of patient co-operation.

The decision to intubate must also be carefully considered, but laryngoscopy is not usually difficult in patients with midfacial hypoplasia. A well placed laryngeal mask airway may provide a suitable airway for shorter procedures.

Effective analgesia is of course an essential part of the anaesthetic and axillary brachial plexus blockade is a simple and effective technique for hand surgery, allowing for rapid emergence and good intraoperative analgesia extending into the postoperative period. The avoidance of opioids may be particularly useful in those at risk of upper airway obstruction or obstructive sleep apnoea.

The innervation of the upper limb is from the roots of C5–T1 via the brachial plexus. Several different approaches to blocking this plexus have been described. These include interscalene block,[5] parascalene block,[6] subclavian block,[5] supraclavicular block,[7,8] infraclavicular block[9] and axillary block.

The axillary approach is the commonest brachial plexus block used in children and is associated with a low risk of significant complications and good analgesia of both ulnar and medial nerves, although the radial nerve distribution may not be so complete. It also does not reliably block the musculocutaneous nerve and the medial cutaneous nerve of the arm as they are not as closely related to the axillary artery. It is notable that in Apert syndrome it is occasionally difficult to abduct the arm sufficiently due to relative fixing of the scapula.

The axillary approach to the brachial plexus was first described by Hirschel in 1911[10] and is now used for a number of indications, e.g. analgesia for hand surgery, vascular insufficiency and vascular access procedures. It is easy to perform and has a low incidence of complications.[11] There are two main techniques used for axillary brachial plexus block:

1. Immobile needle technique – two puncture or single injection.
2. Cannulation of the neurovascular sheath.

Cannulation of the neurovascular sheath is commonly used in children. A simple cannula over the needle technique using a 22G cannula allows the cannula to be inserted an appropriate distance into the sheath. This may have advantages in children: once it lies within the neurovascular sheath, further advancement is less likely to cause damage to nerves or to puncture vessels; also the tip is likely to lie more proximally and may produce more effective block of the musculocutaneous nerve and the radial aspect of the forearm; injection of local anaesthetic solution or movement of the arm to aid spread is less likely to cause displacement of the cannula than with an immobile needle; it is also possible to leave the cannula in situ postoperatively or thread a catheter through it, to allow continuation of the analgesia in the postoperative period.[12]

In theory, the use of a peripheral nerve stimulator should aid the accurate placement of the local anaesthetic solution. In practice, however, good results have been achieved using the cannula over the needle alone and false positive results may occur with the use of a peripheral nerve stimulator in small children.

In the study of the cannula technique by Fisher et al, oral codeine phosphate was only required in 38% of 250 patients a mean time of 9 (+ 4.7) hours postoperatively. On average 0.6 doses of codeine, 0.8 doses of diclofenac and 1.5 doses of paracetamol were administered per patient over the first 24 hours after initiation of the block.[12] The complication rate was extremely low with no significant complications, although inadvertent intravenous injection is a potential hazard.

The commonest local anaesthetic solution used for upper limb blocks involving the brachial plexus is the amide agent bupivacaine and it is usually used in a dose of $0.5\,ml.kg^{-1}$ of 0.25%. Only the unbound, unionized fraction is able to penetrate into the cell but the diffusion into the nerve cell membrane seems to be greater, especially in small children, therefore lower concentrations are required to produce a block in comparison with adults.[13] Neonates and infants also have lower levels of alpha 1-acid glycoprotein which is the protein complex to which bupivacaine binds. They are therefore more vulnerable to the development of toxic free plasma levels and the use of lower doses in these age groups has been advocated. Bupivacaine is cardiotoxic as well as neurotoxic and may produce profound cardiovascular depression before any clinical evidence of seizures. This may include impaired contractility, bradycardia, hypotension and ventricular tachyarrhythmias. It has direct effects on the myocardium to facilitate re-entrant arrhythmias and may also have neurogenic effects in increasing the autonomic outflow from the brainstem by blocking GABA receptors.[14] Bupivacaine remains bound more avidly to cardiac tissue than lignocaine or ropivicaine and the treatment of cardiotoxicity may require prolonged advanced life support and the use of antiarrhythmic agents.

Because of the cardiotoxicity of bupivacaine there has been recent interest in ropivicaine, which is the N-n-proplyl homologue of bupivacaine that has had a single S-isomer produced for clinical use. Studies of its use in other regional blocks and a preliminary study in axillary block in children suggests that it has the potential to be as effective as bupivacaine with the addition of greater cardiovascular safety.[15]

Learning points

- Many children who require anaesthesia for correction of congenital hand abnormalities will have important associated disease that may be life threatening.
- Apert syndrome is associated with abnormalities of the airway, cranial vault and cardiovascular system.
- Regional anaesthesia is safe and effective in children and the use of peripheral nerve blocks should be considered where feasible.
- The use of cannula over the needle technique for axillary brachial plexus block is simple, effective and has a low incidence of complications.
- Although complications are rare, there is a risk of cardiotoxicity and monitoring with ECG, non-invasive blood pressure and pulse oximetry should be maintained during the performance of the block and resuscitation equipment and drugs should be immediately available.
- Effective communication is vital, not only with patients and parents but also with other colleagues to co-ordinate the treatment of multiple problems which may require multiple anaesthetics.

References

1. Apert ME. De'lacrocephalosyndactylie. *Bull Mem Soc Med Hop Paris* 1906; 23: 1310–1330.
2. Jones KL. Smiths Recognisable Patterns of Human Malformation, 4th Edn. Philadelphia PA: W.B. Saunders, 1988.
3. Wheaton SW. Two specimens of congenital cranial deformity in infants associated with fusion of the fingers and toes. *Trans Pathol Soc Lond* 1894; 45: 238.
4. Gregory GA. Pediatric Anesthesia, 3rd Edn. New York: Churchill Livingstone, 1994.
5. Winnie AP. Interscalene brachial plexus block. *Anesth Analg* 1970; 49: 455–466.
6. Dalens B. A New Approach to the Brachial Plexus in Children: comparison with the supraclavicular approach. *Anesth Analg* 1987; 6: 1264–1268.
7. Kulenkampff D, Persky MA. Brachial plexus anesthesia: its indications, technique and dangers. *Ann Surg* 1928; 87: 883.
8. More 1981
9. Raj PP, Montgomery SJ, Nettles D, Jenkins MT. Infraclavicular brachial plexus block – a new approach. *Anesth Analg* 1973; 52: 897–904.
10. Hirschel G. Die Anasthesierung des plexus brachialis bei operationen an der oberen extremitat. *Munchener Med Wochenschr* 1911; 58: 1555–1556.
11. Dalens B, Mansoor O. Safe selection and performance of regional anesthetic techniques in children. *Curr Opin Anesthiol* 1994; 7: 257–261.
12. Fisher WJ, Bingham RM, Hall R. Axillary brachial plexus block for perioperative analgesia in 250 children. *Paediatr Anaesth* 1999; 9: 435–438.
13. Warner MA, Kunkel SE, Offord KO et al. The effects of age, epinephrine and operation site on duration of caudal analgesia in pediatric patients. *Anesth Analg* 1987; 66: 995–998.
14. Peutrell JM, Mather SJ. Regional Anaesthesia for Babies and Children. Oxford University Press, 1997.
15. DA Conceicao MJ, Coelho L, Khalil M. Ropivicaine 0.25% compared with bupivacaine 0.25% by the caudal route. *Paediatr Anaesth* 1999; 9: 229–233.

18

Multilevel orthopaedic surgery in a child with cerebral palsy

JA Nolan

Introduction

Cerebral palsy is a non-progressive disorder of movement and posture, which is caused by damage to the developing central nervous system either antenatally or perinatally.

It is the commonest cause of childhood motor disability with an incidence of around 2 per 1000 live births in developed countries.

Children often present to orthopaedic surgeons because of postural disorders and gait abnormalities due to muscle imbalance, and many will require multiple orthopaedic procedures. Operations commonly performed include femoral and tibial osteotomies, and tendon transfers and releases to reduce muscle spasm. These may be performed as separate procedures or together in one stage as a 'multilevel' operation, either involving one limb or bilaterally.

These children often have associated medical problems that influence the anaesthetic technique, and may respond differently to particular drugs used in the perioperative period. They may also be on medication with significant anaesthetic implications.

This chapter highlights some of the challenges these children present to the anaesthetist.

Case history

A 14-year-old girl with dystonic diplegia was scheduled for multilevel orthopaedic surgery. She was born at 26 weeks' gestation and had significant perinatal problems with recurrent apnoeas requiring ventilatory support. The diagnosis of spastic diplegia was made at the age of 2 years when she was still unable to walk, and her main preoperative problems were difficulty with climbing stairs and trouble with balance.

Her speech and hearing were normal, as was her cognitive development, but she had a tendency to temper tantrums and attention seeking. There was a family history of epilepsy but no other neurological abnormalities, and no history of problems with anaesthetics. She had mild asthma but medical history was otherwise unremarkable and her only medication was a salbutamol inhaler on an occasional basis.

On examination she was a happy and co-operative girl weighing 52 kg. She was able to walk unaided although she had poor balance with a fixed flexion deformity of both hips and difficulty with fine finger co-ordination. There was mild dystonia of the upper limbs and more severe dystonia of the lower limbs, but no contractures. Ankle clonus was present. Her mother had been providing daily physiotherapy in the form of stretching exercises, and previous treatment had involved plastercasts. Computed tomography scans revealed bilateral medial femoral torsion and compensatory external tibial torsion. She presented for soft tissue release of psoas, adductor longus and gracilis and release of hamstrings.

Investigations

A full blood count, urea and electrolyte and blood glucose level were normal. Blood was grouped and saved.

Surgery and anaesthesia

In the anaesthetic room she suddenly became frightened and refused to co-operate. Several attempts to calm her failed but cannulation was eventually successful with the help of distraction therapy from her mother. Anaesthesia was induced with fentanyl 100 µg and propofol 120 mg through a 22-gauge cannula in the dorsal left hand and maintained with oxygen, air and isoflurane. Muscle relaxation was provided with rocuronium 30 mg and she was intubated with a size 7.0 endotracheal tube. After induction two 18-gauge cannulae were inserted in the right hand and forearm. Granisetron was administered by slow intravenous injection. A diclofenac suppository was inserted (50 mg) and intravenous cefuroxime 1.5 g was given.

An epidural catheter was then sited under sterile conditions in the L3/4 interspace using an 18-gauge Tuohy needle and the catheter fed 4 cm into the epidural space and secured in position. A urinary catheter was then inserted.

Initial analgesia was provided with 20 ml bupivacaine 0.25% given in 5-ml increments into the epidural space, after which an infusion of bupivacaine 0.125% with clonidine 2.5 $\mu g.ml^{-1}$ was commenced at 10 $ml.h^{-1}$ (range 5–15 $ml.h^{-1}$).

Intravenous fluids were warmed, inspired gases humidified and a hot air blanket placed over the patient.

Standard monitoring was used including a nerve stimulator, and core temperature was monitored with a nasopharyngeal probe. Tape and padding were placed over the eyes and the patient was placed in the prone position taking care to protect pressure points.

The patient was ventilated using a circle system and low flows. Respiratory rate was 12 breaths per minute and tidal volume 450 ml. Peak airway pressure was 14–15 cmH_2O.

Bilateral semitendonosus tendon transfers were performed after proximal division and medial tunnelling. The skin was sutured and a sterile dressing applied. The patient was then turned supine and redraped and bilateral tenotomies of psoas, adductor longus and gracilis performed. Rectus femoris tendon transfers were performed through a midline longitudinal incision above the knee.

The procedure lasted 3 hours and the patient received 1 litre of colloid in addition to Hartmann's solution at a maintenance rate of 90 $ml.h^{-1}$.

At the end of the procedure the patient was extubated awake and transferred to the recovery area. Intravenous maintenance fluid was continued at 90 $ml.h^{-1}$ and the epidural infusion maintained at a rate of 10 $ml.h^{-1}$. Analgesia was supplemented with regular 4-hourly paracetamol (15 $mg.kg^{-1}$) and parenteral diclofenac 100 mg daily. Oral/parenteral diazepam 5–10 mg was prescribed as rescue therapy for muscle spasms.

She was managed on the ward as a 'high dependency' patient with a nurse-to-patient ratio of approximately 1:3, and physiotherapy input was started on day 1 with regular turning and attention to pressure areas.

She remained relatively sedated on the ward after her surgery. The following morning she was reviewed by the acute pain team (on-call anaesthetist and 'acute pain nurse'); she was awake and comfortable and her epidural was continued at 10 $ml.h^{-1}$. Her mother had been with her overnight but, as she was settled, left her that morning. Later in the day she became irritable and distressed and was seen again by the on-call anaesthetist on behalf of the pain team who gave her a 5 ml epidural bolus and diazepam 5 mg intravenously for presumed muscle spasm. She did not settle, however, and became increasingly agitated. When her mother returned to the ward she explained to the nurse that her problem was constipation and she was prescribed laxatives and eventually settled.

She was reviewed by the pain team twice a day and remained generally comfortable for the remainder of her postoperative course. Her epidural remained at 10 $ml.h^{-1}$ for 2 days after which it was reduced to 5 $ml.h^{-1}$ and was stopped on day 4. She had no episodes of nausea.

Discussion

Children with cerebral palsy manifest features attributable to central nervous system damage such as cognitive impairment, behavioural disturbance, hearing and visual defects and seizures. The gastrointestinal and respiratory systems are also commonly involved, usually to a greater extent in those with a greater degree of spasticity.

Aetiology and classification of cerebral palsy

The role of asphyxia and perinatal complications in the aetiology has been overemphasized in the past. It is now thought that events occurring in the early antenatal period predispose to complications that are only manifest at the time of delivery and may be misdiagnosed as perinatal asphyxia.[1] Aetiologies differ according to gestational age. The clinical picture evolves over time and the degree and type of disability depend on the extent and site of cerebral pathology. The Swedish classification below is the most commonly used:

Spastic (70%):
- Quadriplegia (27% of all cases of cerebral palsy)
- Diplegia (21%)
- Hemiplegia (21%)

Dyskinetic (10%):
- Dystonia
- Athetosis
- Chorea

Ataxic (10%)
Mixed (10%).

Spastic cerebral palsy results in the development of contractures and may be associated with intellectual disability and epilepsy. Bulbar muscle involvement may lead to feeding difficulties and increased risk of aspiration. Dyskinetic cerebral palsy is associated with deafness, dysarthria and drooling but often no intellectual impairment. In ataxic cerebral palsy balance and speech disorders occur and intellectual disability and epilepsy are often associated.

Preoperative considerations/ management

Communication

Preoperative management poses a challenge because of the difficulty communicating with many of these children. The majority of the communication problems occur in children with severe cerebral palsy associated with quadriplegia. Behavioural problems and attention deficit disorders are particularly common in children who do not have intellectual impairment.

Gastrointestinal tract

Gastro-oesophageal reflux and oesophagitis are common and may be difficult to detect, but night time waking may be a manifestation. If the child is on antireflux therapy this should be continued. Many other children will demonstrate reflux on pH studies or upper gastrointestinal endoscopy but will not be on medication and these children may not require reflux prophylaxis prior to surgery.

Some children may be fed by nasogastric tube or gastrostomy because of pseudobulbar palsy and impaired swallowing, and in severe cases may suffer from malnutrition with electrolyte imbalance and anaemia requiring correction.

Constipation can be a problem because of gut dysmotility and may be worsened by inadequate fluid intake. Children may be on regular laxative treatment and this may result in electrolyte imbalance, which should be corrected before surgery.

Respiratory

Poor bulbar control and a weak cough contribute to common problems such as pulmonary aspiration, recurrent chest infections and chronic lung disease with retained secretions. Spinal deformity may result in a restrictive lung defect and preoperative physiotherapy and antibiotics may be needed. The airway should be assessed for ease of intubation because of the increased incidence of malocclusion (see Figure 18.1).

Central nervous system

Epilepsy occurs in about 30% of children with cerebral palsy, tonic–clonic and complex partial seizures being the most common. Anticonvulsant medication should be continued up to and including the day of surgery. It may be possible to give drugs rectally or intravenously throughout the perioperative period if they cannot be tolerated orally or via nasogastric tube. Many anticonvulsants, however, have long half-lives and a 24-hour period may elapse without levels becoming subtherapeutic.

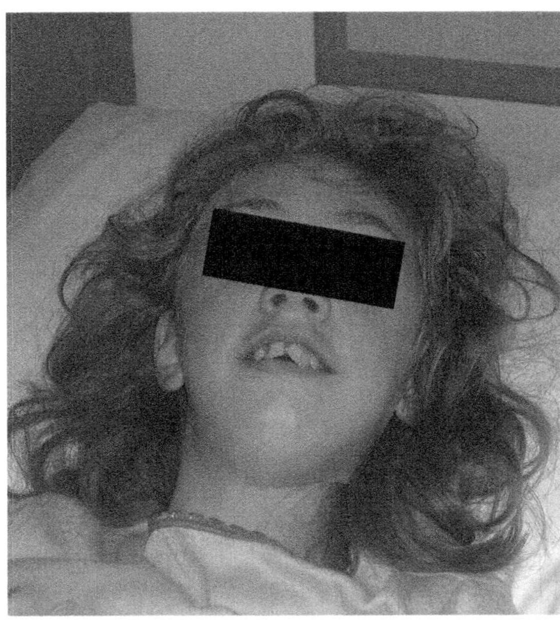

Figure 18.1
'Overbite' in a child with cerebral palsy.

Drug interactions

When taking the drug history it is important to be aware of certain drugs and their anaesthetic interactions, most of which are well described. Baclofen, benzodiazepines and dantrolene are not uncommonly used to treat pain from muscle spasm. Baclofen may be given orally or intrathecally. Intrathecal baclofen reduces spasticity at lower doses than are needed orally and is usually given via a subcutaneous pump connected to an intrathecal catheter.[2] Sudden withdrawal may result in seizures and hallucinations requiring intravenous diazepam. Baclofen has also been implicated in delayed arousal and hypotension in the perioperative period[3,4] but treatment should not be stopped perioperatively. If an intrathecal catheter must be removed prior to surgery baclofen should be given at an appropriate oral dose and started prior to catheter removal.

Other commonly prescribed drugs include antireflux agents, antacids and laxatives. Carbamazepine may be prescribed to treat dystonia and levodopa can be used for the treatment of athetosis.

Allergy to latex is particularly common in cerebral palsy[5] and seems to be associated with multiple previous exposures to latex, particularly involving mucous membranes. Any such history must be established at the preoperative visit.

Anaesthesia

Sedative premedication may reduce anxiety and muscle spasm but should be used with caution in those with respiratory impairment. Antireflux premedication should be given if the child has symptomatic reflux or is on regular prophylaxis. Topical local anaesthetic (EMLA® or topical/amethocaine) for cannulation is routine for intravenous induction, although some may require a gas induction because of difficult venous access. These children are often frequent hospital attenders and their parents or carers usually have a good deal of insight into their behaviour and will know how they have coped with previous anaesthetics.

It is often helpful to have carers in the anaesthetic room until the child is asleep. If the child has symptoms of reflux a rapid sequence induction should be performed, but vascular access is sometimes difficult owing to spasticity or dystonia and an inhalational induction in the sitting position in the child 'at risk' may be more practical. Required doses of induction agents may well be reduced by about 20%. Intravenous fluids should be considered in the anaesthetic room once a cannula is in place if there has been prolonged preoperative fasting. These children are often underweight for their age and it is tempting to downsize endotracheal tubes; however, sizing is better related to age than weight.

A lumbar epidural should ideally be sited in the anaesthetic room for children undergoing lower limb surgery, as postoperative pain and spasm may otherwise be very difficult to control.

Children with cerebral palsy seem to have a greater incidence of opioid-induced nausea and vomiting, and prophylactic antiemetics should be considered.

There are few drugs that should be avoided in cerebral palsy. Sensitivity to suxamethonium probably does not occur[6] but resistance to non-depolarizing neuromuscular blocking agents has been reported,[7] although this is probably not clinically relevant. MAC (minimum alveolar concentration) may be reduced in cerebral palsy. Drug responses are otherwise no different unless the child has associated organ dysfunction such as renal failure, in which case drugs such as pethidine with epileptogenic metabolites should be given with caution. 'Proconvulsant' anaesthetic agents should be avoided, although most of these actually raise the seizure threshold in normal patients while lowering it in those 'at risk'.

Children must be positioned with care on the operating table because of the presence of contractures, and with appropriate padding of pressure areas.

Temperature regulation is often abnormal in cerebral palsy due to hypothalamic dysfunction. Devices available to minimize intraoperative hypothermia include warming mattresses, hot air warming blankets such as the Bair Hugger® device and warmed fluids. Intraoperative hypothermia may contribute to a delayed time to awakening.

Postoperative problems (immediate)

Pain

Pain in the recovery area may be magnified if the child is disorientated, as is often the case with intellectual disability, deafness or visual impairment. Perioperative analgesia in multilevel surgery is particularly important because of the nature of the procedure and the incidence of muscle spasms. Regional analgesia with local anaesthetics (bupivacaine 0.125%) has an important role to play, and is mentioned in more detail later.

Irritability
Several factors may contribute to irritability on emergence from anaesthesia, including pain, disorientation and poor communication as a result of sensory deficits and intellectual impairment. Involvement of carers again early in the recovery phase reduces anxiety and may speed recovery.

Hypothermia
If not managed appropriately in theatre and continued in the recovery area this will result in prolonged recovery.

Postoperative nausea and vomiting
This is a particular problem when opiates have been used and prophylactic antiemetics should be considered in theatre.

Postoperative problems (delayed)

Spasms
Muscle spasms are a particular problem in children undergoing multilevel surgery, and many will have a history of chronic spasms. Children may require regular oral or intravenous diazepam in addition to epidural analgesia. If spasms remain a problem oral baclofen may also be needed. Clonidine, when added to bupivacaine epidurally, reduces muscle spasms with a reduction in the requirement for diazepam. Avoidance of epidural opiates also reduces the incidence of postoperative nausea and vomiting.[8]

A commonly used epidural technique would be bupivacaine 0.125% with clonidine 2–2.5 $\mu g.ml^{-1}$ run at 0.1–0.4 $ml.kg^{-1}.h^{-1}$. The level of insertion should take into account the dermatomal levels of skin incision, which may extend from L1 to S1 resulting in inadequate analgesia if inserted too high or too low. This dose of clonidine should not result in any haemodynamic compromise but may cause sedation.

Diazepam 0.3–0.5 $mg.kg^{-1}$ orally, or 0.1–0.2 $mg.kg^{-1}$ intravenously should, however, be prescribed at least on an as needed basis for all children who have had lower limb surgery.

Pain and muscle spasms may be a problem for several days after major orthopaedic surgery and epidural infusions are usually continued for 2–4 days, by which time simple analgesics such as paracetamol, non-steroidal anti-inflammatory drugs and codeine phosphate should be sufficient (Figure 18.2). Diazepam on a regular or as needed basis may be needed for several days after discontinuing the epidural.

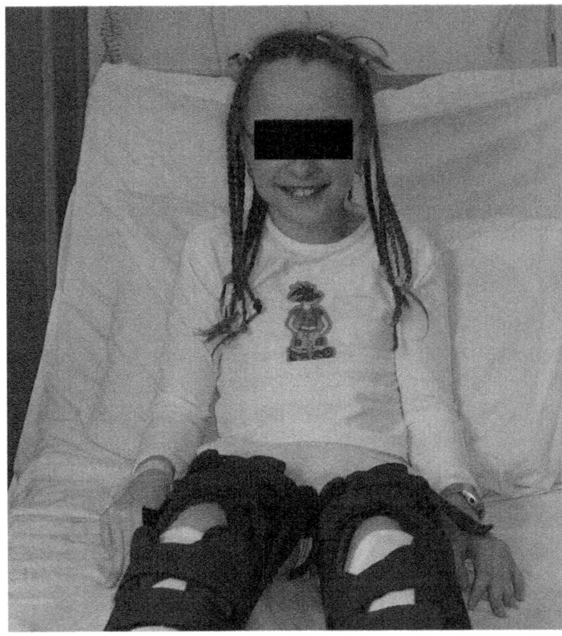

Figure 18.2
48 hours after multilevel surgery, epidural catheter removed.

Assessment of pain
Pain assessment in children with cerebral palsy can be challenging due to intellectual disability or poor communication. Behavioural indicators such as facial grimacing, moaning and altered sleep patterns are often unreliable due to the diversity of patient responses.[9,10] Pain scales may also lack sensitivity due to elevated pain thresholds in children with developmental disability.[11] However, there is evidence that the pain experience may be blunted in these children due to an altered neurological system and ability to communicate pain, without this actually reflecting true pain insensitivity.[12]

The 'non-communicating children's pain checklist' which uses social behaviour, facial gestures, body movements and physiological signs, has been validated and shown to be reliable and reproducible for these children in the postoperative period without the need for familiarity with the individual.[13] It is important also to remember other medical problems that may be causing discomfort, such as gastro-oesophageal reflux and urinary retention.

The parent or guardian, however, is usually the best at recognizing pain in these children.

Learning points

- Cerebral palsy is a non-progressive disorder although clinical manifestations may change with time.
- Children with cerebral palsy will have other disorders attributable to central nervous system damage.
- Communication is a common problem, particularly in the more severely affected.
- Respiratory and gastrointestinal systems are commonly involved.
- A history of latex allergy should be sought during the preoperative visit.
- MAC may be reduced and opioid-induced nausea is common.
- Disturbances of temperature regulation may lead to hypothermia and delayed recovery.
- Epidural analgesia is recommended for postoperative pain and muscle spasm.

References

1. Truwit CL, Barkovich AJ, Koch TK, Ferriero DM. Cerebral palsy: MR findings in 40 patients. *Am J Neuroradiol* 1992; 13: 67–78.
2. Albright AL. Intrathecal baclofen in cerebral palsy movement disorders. *J Child Neurol* 1996; 11 (Suppl 1): S29–35.
3. Gomar C, Carrero EJ. Delayed arousal after general anaesthesia associated with baclofen. *Anesthesiology* 1994; 81: 1306–1307.
4. Still JC, Schumacher K, Southorn A et al. Bradycardia and hypotension associated with baclofen used during general anaesthesia. *Anesthesiology* 1986; 64: 255–258.
5. Delfico AJ, Dormans JP, Craythorne CB, Templeton JJ. Intraoperative anaphylaxis due to allergy to latex in children who have cerebral palsy: a report of six cases. *Dev Med Child Neurol* 1996; 39: 194–197.
6. Dierdorf SF, McNiece WL, Rao CC et al. Effect of succinylcholine on plasma potassium in children with cerebral palsy. *Anesthesiology* 1985; 62: 88–90.
7. Moorthy SS, Krishna G, Dierdorf SF. Resistance to vecuronium in patients with cerebral palsy. *Anesth Analges* 1991; 73: 275–277.
8. Nolan J, Chalkiadis GA, Low J et al. Anaesthesia and pain management in cerebral palsy. *Anaesthesia* 2000; 55: 32–41.
9. Giusiano B, Jimeno MT, Collignon P, Chau Y. Utilization of a neural network in the elaboration of an evaluation scale for pain in cerebral palsy. *Meth Inform Med* 1995; 34: 498–502.
10. McGrath PJ, Rosmus C, Canfield C et al. Behaviours caregivers use to determine pain in non-verbal, cognitively impaired individuals. *Dev Med Child Neurol* 1998; 40: 340–343.
11. Biersdorff KK. Incidence of significantly altered pain experience among individuals with developmental disabilities. *Am J Ment Retard* 1994; 98: 619–631.
12. Oberlander TF, O'Donnell ME, Montgomery CJ. Pain in children with significant neurological impairment. *Dev Behav Pediatr* 1999; 20: 235–243.
13. Breau LM, Allen Finley G, McGrath PJ, Camfield CS. Validation of the non-communicating Children's Pain Checklist – Postoperative Version. *Anesthesiology* 2002; 96: 528–535.

19

Scoliosis repair in a child with Rett syndrome

Gillian R Lauder

Introduction

Scoliosis is derived from the Greek word meaning curvature or crooked. Scoliosis is a coronal plane deformity of the spine that is greater than 10% and has structural rotation at the apical segment. The incidence of scoliosis is 1.8 per 1000 of school age children in the United Kingdom. Rett syndrome is a progressive neurological disorder. It is an inherited condition, prevalent in 1 in 10,000 females,[1] the gene is carried on the X chromosome and only affects girls. The incidence of scoliosis in Rett syndrome increases with age affecting 80% of those who reach puberty.[2] Scoliosis correction is contemplated in these patients to prevent deterioration of respiratory function or to improve seating position. The anaesthetic challenges of scoliosis correction in a child with Rett syndrome include recognition of the potential problems associated with the syndrome and delivery of an appropriate anaesthetic that takes into consideration the important issues of minimizing homologous blood transfusion and preservation of spinal cord function.

Case history

A 15-year-old girl with Rett syndrome and a rapidly progressive scoliosis presented for scoliosis correction.

Preoperative assessment revealed the findings noted in Table 19.1. Liaison between the orthopaedic surgeon, paediatrician and the anaesthetist concluded that the benefit of surgery outweighed the potential risks in this case. Prior to surgery baseline somatosensory evoked potentials (SSEPs) were recorded. On the day of surgery the patient was premedicated with oral diazepam 1 hour prior to transfer to theatre. In the anaesthetic room the patient was fully monitored. An in situ cannula was flushed and then used for intravenous induction of anaesthesia with propofol 4 mg.kg^{-1}, fentanyl 3 µg.kg^{-1} and vecuronium 0.1 mg.kg^{-1}. Following tracheal intubation with a reinforced cuffed endotracheal tube the lungs were ventilated with 40% oxygen in air. The endotracheal tube was secured, tincture of benzoin was applied to the face to ensure the tape securing the endotracheal tube was adherent. A nasogastric tube was inserted and placed on free drainage. Total intravenous anaesthesia (TIVA) was maintained with infusions of propofol 9–15 mg.kg^{-1}.hr^{-1} and alfentanil 20–50 µg.kg^{-1}.hr^{-1}. Neuromuscular blockade was continued with an infusion of vecuronium 0.1–0.2 mg.kg^{-1}.hr^{-1}. Two large-bore intravenous cannulae were inserted. Prophylactic antibiotics (cefuroxime 30 mg.kg^{-1}) were administered. Right radial artery cannulation and right internal jugular triple lumen catheterization were performed under sterile conditions. An oesophageal temperature probe was inserted. The eyes were lubricated, taped and padded. A urinary catheter was inserted and the patient transferred into the operating theatre.

The patient was positioned for the first stage of the procedure in the right thoracotomy position. All invasive and non-invasive monitoring was re-established. Neurophysiology technicians instituted SSEP monitoring. Mean arterial pressure was maintained at 55–60 mmHg with TIVA. No further agent was required to manipulate the blood pressure. Neuromuscular blockade was monitored to maintain one twitch using a train-of-four monitor. A bolus dose of 400,000 KIU of aprotonin was infused over 30 minutes followed by an infusion of 200,000 KIU.hr^{-1} until the end of the procedure. Ventilation was manipulated to maintain good oxygenation and normocapnia. Maintenance fluids were connected via a peripheral cannula and bolus fluids were set up via a fluid warmer

Past medical history	Rett syndrome; no seizures	
ASA Grade	III	
Social history	Permanently resident in a school for children with special needs	
Regular medications	Lactulose 15 ml TDS Baclofen 10 mg TDS	
Allergies	None known	
Examination	Alert but uncommunicative Scoliosis Normal airway Chest clear, SaO_2 97% in air Normal heart sounds, pulse 110 min^{-1}, BP 90/60 mmHg, mean arterial pressure 70 mmHg	
Investigations	*Weight*	22.2 kg
	FBC	Hb 12.2 $g.dl^{-1}$, Plat $203 \times 10^9 l^{-1}$, WBC $6.1 \times 10^9 l^{-1}$
	Clotting	PT 14.4 s, INR 1.1, APPT 25.9 s, fibrinogen 3.21 $g.l^{-1}$
	U+Es	Na^+ 140 $mmol.l^{-1}$, K^+ 4.3 $mmol.l^{-1}$, urea 4.4 $mmol.l^{-1}$, creatinine 49 $\mu mol.l^{-1}$
	ECG	NAD, normal QTc interval
	Chest X-ray	Lung fields clear
	Spine X-ray	Right thoracolumbar curve, the angle between T9 and L3 measures 70 degrees
	Lung function	Patient unable to perform lung function tests
	ABGs	pH 7.35, pO_2 11.7 kPa, pCO_2 4.9 kPa, HCO_3^- 23.4 $mmol.l^{-1}$, BE –1.6
	Crossmatch	Six units

Table 19.1
Initial investigations

to the other peripheral cannula. A warm air device was used to maintain core temperature. A right lateral thoracotomy along the 9th rib and five anterior discectomies were performed uneventfully with minimal blood loss.

The patient was transferred to the prone position for the second stage of the procedure. Bilateral air entry was confirmed and the patient ventilated to achieve normocarbia. Positioning was checked to ensure that there was no pressure on the abdomen, no change in airway pressure, no pressure on the eyes, no stretch of the brachial plexi and that all pressure points were padded. All invasive and non-invasive monitoring was again re-established. Neurophysiology technicians reinstituted SSEP monitoring. Later in the procedure SSEPs were recorded via a bipolar epidural electrode placed by the surgeon. Mean arterial pressure was maintained at 55–60 mmHg with TIVA. The aprotonin infusion continued. A posterior spinal fusion with a double rod system, hooks, screws and titanium cables was performed from T2 to the pelvis to achieve a good correction without significant change to the

SSEP latency and amplitude. The procedure took 9 hours. 3100 ml of blood (1.85 blood volumes) was lost. The patient received three units of homologous donated blood, 1130 ml of cell-saved blood, platelets and fresh frozen plasma. Haematocrit, electrolyte, coagulation, glucose and gases were serially monitored. Normothermia was achieved with a warm air device. An epidural catheter was placed under direct vision by the surgeon at T8.

The patient was transferred intubated, ventilated, sedated and fully monitored to the paediatric intensive care unit. On admission the patient was stable, warm and well perfused. The patient was initially ventilated then weaned to synchronized intermittent mandatory ventilation and pressure support. Baseline bloods and gases were stable with slightly deranged clotting which resolved with further fresh frozen plasma (FFP). A chest X-ray revealed a right pneumothorax that was drained. Sedation was achieved with morphine and propofol infusions. A 0.125% solution of plain bupivacaine was infused at 8 $ml.kg^{-1}$ through the epidural. The patient was extubated 28 hours postoperatively. The chest drain was removed 36 hours postoperatively. Physiotherapy was instituted during her stay on the intensive care unit and continued until her discharge from hospital. The patient was transferred to the ward on the second day after her scoliosis correction. Analgesia on the ward was maintained with regular paracetamol, diclofenac and the epidural infusion. The epidural was stopped 3 days postoperatively. The patient's stay on the ward was prolonged by difficulties with feeding and constipation. The patient was discharged 21 days postoperatively.

Discussion

This patient presented a number of problems for anaesthesia which are summarized in Table19.2 below.

Preoperative	Problems associated with Rett syndrome Problems associated with severe scoliosis; restrictive lung defect

Peroperative	Haemorrhage and massive blood transfusion
	Large intravenous fluid requirements
	Oliguria
	Hypothermia
	Air embolism
	Pneumothorax/haemothorax
	Need for spinal cord function monitoring
	Aim to extubate at end of procedure
	Periorbital/airway oedema
	Positioning:
	    Retinal thrombosis
	    Brachial plexus injury
	    Peripheral nerve injury
	    Minimize intra-abdominal pressure

Postoperative	Possible elective postoperative ventilation Potentially difficult pain relief Haemorrhage, hypovolaemia Oedema Ileus Syndrome of inappropriate antidiuretic hormone Root pain may occur due to one of the pedicle screws

Table 19.2
Problem list

Rett syndrome was first described by Andreas Rett in 1996. The aetiology of Rett syndrome is unknown. The gene for Rett syndrome has been isolated to the X chromosome; mutation of this gene results in excessive amounts of methyl cytosine binding protein. Central nervous system changes in neurons and neurotransmitters have been described by Naidu.[3] Deceleration of head growth between 2 and 4 months of age is the first sign that is often unrecognized. Patients usually present after the first year of age with a delay in reaching their milestones; they then lose milestones already gained. The anomalies seen in Rett syndrome include seizures in 30–50% of patients,[3] an abnormal EEG, autistic behaviour, microcephaly, gait ataxia, axial hypotonia, spasticity, loss of purposeful hand movements and stereotypic hand movements. Rett syndrome patients display respiratory anomalies in the awake state only.[1] Young Rett syndrome patients demonstrate prolonged inspiration. Older Rett syndrome patients demonstrate prolonged breath holds, which are terminated by a Valsalva manoeuvre. Blood pressure and heart rate swings occur during these breathing abnormalities.[1] Rett syndrome patients may have a long QTc interval[4] and/or low cardiac vagal tone with low baroreflex sensitivity. Sudden and unexpected death occurs in 26% of patients.[4] High pain threshold due to raised cerebrospinal fluid β-endorphin levels has been reported as have oropharyngeal dysfunction, gastro-oesophageal dysmobility[5] and severe constipation.[3]

The neurodevelopmental delay of these patients presents communication problems for anaesthesia and postoperative recovery. The respiratory anomalies and prolonged QTc interval require careful investigation. Assessment of respiratory status of the case described proved impossible so a baseline blood gas analysis was performed to help predict outcome. She was electively ventilated postoperatively to minimize the potential respiratory complications, whereas a non-syndromic child undergoing scoliosis correction should be extubated at the end of the procedure to enable clinical assessment of cord function. Postoperative feeding difficulties and constipation significantly delayed our patient's discharge home.

Minimizing homologous blood transfusion

The risks associated with homologous blood transfusion include viral infections, bacterial infections, alloimmunization, immunomodulation, graft versus host disease, metabolic imbalance and transfusion mismatch due to human error.[6–8] Growing medical and parental concern about these potential hazards necessitates the need to avoid or at least minimize homologous blood transfusion. This can be achieved by one or more of the following measures: predonation of blood if the patient is greater than 30 kg,[9,10] supplemented with oral iron and possibly subcutaneous erythropoietin,[7,11] acute normovolaemic haemodilution,[12] good surgical technique and haemostasis, correct positioning of the patient when prone, hypotensive anaesthesia (only with adequate cord monitoring), cell saver, aprotonin,[6,13–15] transenamic acid,[15] intrathecal opiates,[16] and monitored use of coagulation products. Lower postoperative haemoglobin levels should be accepted (in patients with no respiratory or cardiac disease) to reduce the need for postoperative transfusions.

There is insufficient good quality evidence of the safety or effectiveness of these techniques in the paediatric population. Hence, the cost effectiveness, the logistics and the risks involved for each one of these blood salvage techniques needs to be carefully considered for each individual case.

Hypotensive anaesthesia for scoliosis correction

There are studies to support the use of controlled hypotension during paediatric scoliosis correction.[17–19] A number of agents have been used including β-adrenergic antagonists, calcium channel blockers, directly acting vasodilators and inhalational agents. However, Bridwell et al[20] recommend normotensive anaesthesia for those patients undergoing anterior and posterior surgery on the same day as these patients pose a greater risk for neurological deficit due to hypoperfusion of a vascular aetiology.

Anaesthesia

There are multiple anaesthetic plans that would be appropriate for this patient. The one presented above is an example of one approach. Whatever plan is adopted a meticulous approach, as usual, is essential and includes liaison with the surgeon, cell-saver technician and the neurophysiology technician.

Once the endotracheal tube is secured, ensure that there is bilateral air entry then check baseline gases to confirm good oxygenation and normocarbia. Hypocarbia reduces blood flow to the spinal cord and should be avoided. Whenever the patient is moved these checks need to be repeated to ensure that the endotracheal tube has not been dislodged. A nasogastric tube left on free drainage prevents gastic secretions from loosening the tapes on the endotracheal tube and decreases intra-abdominal pressure.

Invasive monitoring (central venous pressure, arterial line) is essential to evaluate the enormous fluid shifts and losses, especially as urine output is an unreliable sign of adequate hydration during this procedure.[21] The arterial trace monitors the beat-to-beat blood pressure and allows for serial assessment of blood gases, acid-base status, electrolytes, glucose and haematocrit. As the fluid requirements are enormous all administered fluid should be warmed. The urine should be collected in a urometer to document hourly urine output.

Prophylactic antibiotics need to be administered at the beginning of the procedure. When TIVA is used for anaesthesia the site of infusion must be visible to the anaesthetist.

Positioning the patient in the prone position needs to be carefully coordinated to prevent trauma to the patient and accidental removal of monitoring lines and/or cannulae. Once in the prone position scrupulous attention to detail is required. The lubricated, padded and taped eyes should be set into the well of a head ring to ensure that there is no pressure on the eyes. This will help to prevent retinal thrombosis. The thorax should not be compressed. The abdomen should hang freely to minimize intra-abdominal pressure to encourage venous return through the inferior vena cava and reduce venous return via the vertebral venous plexus. This will reduce perioperative blood loss from venous ooze. All pressure points need to be checked and padded to prevent peripheral nerve injury. To safeguard against brachial plexus injury the axillae should not be stretched. All these checks need to be repeated every time the patient position is changed.

The coagulation status needs to be monitored; it is likely that clotting factors and/or platelets will be required once the patient has lost one blood volume. The ionized calcium may fall with infusions of FFP and should be replaced centrally.

Scoliosis correction can take a number of hours and once the patient is prone there is a large area of exposed skin. The patient may cool rapidly. Hypothermia needs to be avoided to prevent deleterious effects on coagulation, changes in the latency of SSEP signals and maximize conditions for extubation at the end of the procedure. Maintenance of normothermia can be achieved with warm air devices.

Surgery

With regard to the surgical correction of scoliosis in the syndromic child, as in this case, after exposure of the full length of the spine (Figure 19.1) instrumentation commences distally with insertion of multiple pedicle screws to provide secure distal foundation. The proximal foundation is usually achieved through the use of hooks in a claw construct. The intermediate vertebrae may be secured with screws, hooks, or in this case sublaminar cables correcting the translation of the apex vertebra to the contour of the rods (Figure 19.2). Third-generation implants are cross-linked and after thorough decortication bone graft is applied over the instrumented vertebrae before wound closure.

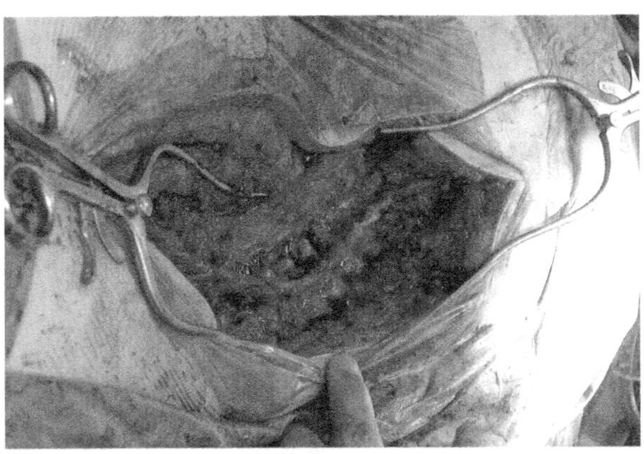

Figure 19.1
Full exposure of scoliosis of the spine.

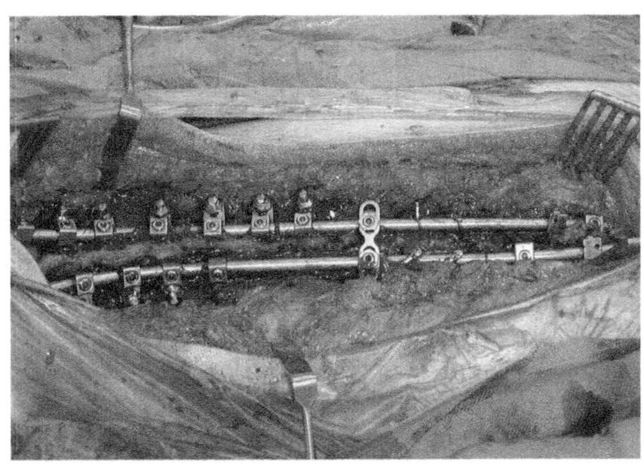

Figure 19.1
The same spine after instrumentation.

Cord function

The overall incidence of major neurological deficit caused by correction of spinal deformity in paediatric and adult patients is 0.37%. The risk is increased if the patient has hyperkyphosis or is undergoing a combined anterior and posterior repair on the same day.[20] The use of spinal cord monitoring with SSEP has been found to correlate with neurosurgical outcome.[22] Monitoring of cord function signals the need for early intervention by the surgeon and/or anaesthetist. Intraoperative cord function can be monitored with SSEPs. Other methods used include motor-evoked potentials (MEPs) and/or a wake-up test. Nuwer has recently reviewed the techniques and literature.[23]

SSEPs are a measurement of the electrical potentials evoked by stimulation of the sensory system. The response of constant current stimulation of the median, tibial and rarely the sural nerve is recorded at the cortex or from a bipolar electrode placed epidurally by the surgeon. Baseline SSEPs are recorded in order to exclude neurological dysfunction and also to determine the feasibility of operative monitoring. Neurophysiology technicians monitor the latency and amplitude of the recordings continuously during anaesthesia and surgery. An SSEP amplitude drop of greater than 50% is deemed significant. SSEP responses are sensitive to various anaesthetic agents.[24] It is important to be cognizant of the effects of anaesthetic agents on SSEP monitoring and provide suitable anaesthesia. Responses recorded from the cerebral cortex are more sensitive to the effects of anaesthetic agents than the epidurally recorded responses. Neuromuscular blockade reduces muscle artifact on the recorded SSEPs. SSEP monitoring is pathway specific; an injury to the cord not involving the sensory pathway will not be detected. Global cord monitoring may be possible with combined SSEPs and MEPs.[25]

MEPs assess function of the motor cortex and the descending motor pathways. MEPs are recorded peripherally in response to stimulation of the motor cortex or spinal cord. The peripheral response is recorded by measuring compound muscle action potentials through fine wire electrodes within muscles. MEP monitoring is technically difficult and presently more of a research tool than a clinical monitoring device. Neuromuscular blocking agents would obliterate the MEP response.

Both SSEPs and MEPs are suppressed by volatile agents, cold, hypoxia, hypercarbia and spinal ischaemia. If SSEPs or MEPs change then it may be necessary to do a wake-up test. During a wake-up test the patient is allowed to wake in the middle of scoliosis surgery to demonstrate motor power. This can only be done if the patient is intellectually competent and has been warned/consented preoperatively. The hazards are accidental extubation, air embolism on deep inspiration and dislodgement of fixators. The wake-up test gives a false sense of security as it only tests motor power at one time point.

Prevention of neurological compromise requires careful preoperative assessment of the patient, delicate surgical exposure and instrumentation, avoidance of excessive traction forces, accurate cord monitoring, awareness that hypotension reduces cord blood flow and an understanding that all these factors are additive.[26]

Postoperative analgesia

The lack of communication with a Rett syndrome patient prevents adequate pain assessment so demands effective postoperative pain relief. The respiratory impairment associated with Rett syndrome also dictates that the analgesic techniques adopted have minimal respiratory side effects. A multimodal approach to prevention of pain needs to be adopted. Regular paracetamol, regular diclofenac (only after coagulation status has been normalized) and epidural analgesia sometimes in combination with intravenous opiates (patient-controlled, nurse-controlled or infusions) may be required. Postoperative epidural analgesia significantly decreases the incidence of pulmonary morbidity compared with other analgesic therapies.[27] Epidural analgesia, with a correctly sited epidural catheter, is reported as safe and efficacious in children undergoing spine fusion surgery[28–30] and has been reported in a child with Rett syndrome.[31] Tobias et al have reported a dual epidural catheter technique in a series of 14 patients.[30] However, there are concerns regarding the use of epidural analgesia for scoliosis correction, i.e. the possibility of increased risk of infection from the epidural catheter and the masking of the signs of neurological injury.[32]

Dearlove and Walker[33] have reported the combined use of a morphine infusion and interpleural bupivacaine as postoperative analgesia for Rett syndrome patients following scoliosis correction. Goodarzi has reported that intrathecal opioids provide continuous postoperative pain relief for 14.5 hours (range 0–38 hours) without additional analgesic drugs following spinal fusion in children.[16] Whatever mode of analgesia is adopted for Rett syndrome patients the parental input into the adequacy of the analgesia is essential.

Learning points

- Careful preoperative evaluation of patients is required to assess the risk–benefit ratio of performing corrective scoliosis surgery.
- All attempts should be made to avoid homologous blood transfusion during and following corrective scoliosis surgery.
- Neurological deficit can be minimized by careful attention to preoperative assessment, good surgical technique, good haemodynamic control using invasive cardiovascular monitoring and continuous monitoring of spinal cord function.
- Anaesthetic management requires a meticulous approach to ventilation and patient position, with maintenance of normothermia and normovolaemia despite the large peroperative exposure and enormous fluid shifts.
- Most patients should be extubated at the end of the procedure to allow immediate and continuous postoperative assessment of cord function.
- Postoperative analgesia can be difficult; a multimodal approach may be the best regimen for these patients.

Acknowledgement

My thanks to Mr Ian Nelson, Consultant Orthopaedic Surgeon, for describing the surgical procedure.

References

1. Kerr AM, Julu POO. Recent insights into hyperventilation from the study of Rett syndrome. *Arch Dis Child* 1999; 80: 384–387.
2. Banta JV, Drummond DS, Ferguson RL. The treatment of neuromuscular scoliosis. *AAOS Instructional Course Lectures* 1999; 48: 551–562.
3. Naidu S. Rett syndrome: natural history and underlying disease mechanisms. *Eur Child Adolesc Psychiatr* 1997; 6 Suppl 1: 14–17.
4. Ellaway CJ, Scholler G, Leonard H et al. Prolonged QT interval in Rett Syndrome. *Arch Dis Child* 1999; 80: 470–472.
5. Motil KJ, Schultz RJ, Browning K et al. Oropharyngeal dysfunction and gastroesophageal dysmotility are present in girls and women with Rett syndrome. *J Pediatr Gastroenterol Nutr* 1999; 29: 31–37.
6. De Ville A. Blood saving in paediatric anaesthesia. *Paediatr Anaesth* 1997; 7: 181–182.
7. De Ville A, Govaerts MJM. 4th European Congress of Paediatric Anaesthesia. Paris 1997.
8. Williamson LM, Lowe S, Love EM et al. Serious hazards of transfusion (SHOT) initiative: analysis of the first two annual reports. *BMJ* 1999; 319: 16–19.
9. Vanderlinde ES. Clinical review; autologous transfusion. *BMJ* 2002; 324: 772–775.
10. Moran MM, Kroon D, Tredwell SJ, Wadsworth LD. The role of autologous blood transfusion in adolescents undergoing spinal surgery. *Spine* 1995; 20: 532–536.
11. Sonzogni V, Crupi G, Poma R et al. Erythropoietin therapy and preoperative autologous blood donation in children undergoing open heart surgery. *Br J Anaesth* 2001; 87: 429–434.
12. Brustowicz RM. Cotrel-Dubousset Instrumentation for Scoliosis. In: *Common Problems in Paediatric Anaesthesia*. Linda Stehling (ed.). Mosby Year Book,
13. Rochette A, Canaud N, Gariglio A et al. Aprotonin decreases transfusion requirements by 50% in posterior spinal fusion. *Anesthesiology* 1997; 87(Suppl 3): A1068.
14. Capdevila X, Calvet Y, Biboulet P et al. Aprotonin decreases blood loss and homologous transfusions in patients undergoing major orthopedic surgery. *Anesthesiology* 1998; 88: 50–57.
15. Fremes SE, Wong BI, Lee E et al. Meta-analysis of prophylactic drug treatment in the prevention of postoperative bleeding. *Ann Thorac Surg* 1994; 58: 1580–1588.
16. Goodarzi M. The advantages of intrathecal opioids for spinal fusion in children. *Paediatr Anaesth* 1998; 8: 131–134.
17. Tobias JD. Fenoldopam for controlled hypotension during spinal fusion in children and adolescents. *Paediatr Anaesth* 2000; 10: 261–266.
18. Tobias JD. Sevoflurane for controlled hypotension during spinal surgery: preliminary experience in five adolescents. *Paediatr Anaesth* 1998; 8: 167–170.
19. Tobias JD, Lowe S, Deshpande JK. Nicardipine perioperative applications in children. *Paediatr Anaesth* 1995; 5: 171–176.
20. Bridwell KH, Lenke LG, Baldus C, Blanke K. Major intraoperative neurological deficits in pediatric and adult spinal deformity patients. Incidence and etiology at one institution. *Spine* 1998; 23: 324–331.
21. Cregg N, Mannion D, Casey W. Oliguria during corrective spinal surgery idiopathic scoliosis: the role of antidiuretic hormone. *Paediatr Anaesth* 1999; 9: 505–514.
22. Nuwer MR, Dawson EG, Carlson LG et al. Somatosensory evoked potential spinal cord monitoring reduces neurologic deficits after scoliosis surgery: results of a large multicenter survey. *Electroencephalogr Clin Neurophysiol* 1995; 96: 6–11.
23. Nuwer MR. Spinal cord monitoring. *Muscle Nerve* 1999; 22: 1620–1630.
24. Kumar A, Bhattacharya A, Makhija N. Evoked potential monitoring in anaesthesia and analgesia. *Anaesthesia* 2000; 55: 225–241.

25. Owen JH, Sponseller PD, Szymanski J, Hurdle M. Efficacy of multimodality spinal cord monitoring during surgery for neuromuscular scoliosis. *Spine* 1995; 20: 1480–1488.
26. Winter RB. Neurologic safety in spinal deformity surgery. *Spine* 1997; 22: 1527–1533.
27. Ballantyne JC, Carr DB, de Ferranti S et al. The comparative effects of postoperative analgesic therapies on pulmonary outcome: cumulative meta-analysis of randomized, controlled trials. *Anesth Analg* 1998; 86: 598–612.
28. Turner A, Lee J, Mitchell R et al. The efficacy of surgically placed epidural catheters for analgesia after posterior spinal surgery. *Anaesthesia* 2000; 55: 370–373.
29. Watcha MF, Smith R, Safavi F, Hackney G. Postoperative analgesia with epidural hydromorphone after spine fusion surgery in children. *Anesth Analg* 1996; 82: S478 [Abstract].
30. Tobias JD, Gaines RW, Lowry KJ et al. A dual epidural catheter technique to provide analgesia following posterior spinal fusion for scoliosis in children and adolescents. *Paediatr Anaesth* 2001; 11: 199–203.
31. Konen AA, Girish PJ, Kelly CK. Epidural analgesia for pain relief after scoliosis surgery in a patient with Rett's syndrome. *Anesth Analg* 1999; 89: 451–452.
32. Purnell RJ. Scoliosis correction and epidural analgesia. Prolonged block following Harrington rod insertion. *Anaesthesia* 1982; 37: 1115–1117.
33. Dearlove OR, Walker RWM. Anaesthesia for Rett Syndrome. *Paediatr Anaesth* 1996; 6: 155–158.

20

Magnetic resonance imaging in an infant with a cystic hygroma

MRJ Sury

Introduction

Modern imaging techniques frequently require the patient to remain still for prolonged periods of time. This can be impossible to achieve without general anaesthesia especially in a small infant with an airway that may be compromised. The challenge of providing safe anaesthesia for a baby with a congenital neck swelling is described.

History

A 3.5-kg term new-born presented with a soft fluctuant mass in the left side of the neck. The mass was the size of a small orange and extended from the base of the neck to the mandible; the tongue was obviously large. There were no signs of airway obstruction but because the baby did not suckle effectively nasogastric tube feeding was commenced. The most likely diagnosis was a cystic hygroma and this was supported by the cystic appearance seen on the ultrasound scan. A chest X-ray suggested that there was no extension into the thorax but magnetic resonance imaging (MRI) was requested to determine the true limits of the hygroma.

Overnight, while awaiting the scan, the swelling enlarged and become less fluctuant. Also, the baby developed inspiratory stridor although the oxygen saturation was 95% in air. The haemoglobin concentration decreased from 17.5 $g.dl^{-1}$ to 14.0 $g.dl^{-1}$ and haemorrhage into the hygroma was suspected. Urgent surgery was proposed following the MRI scan.

Assessment for anaesthesia established that the large tongue restricted access to the mouth but probably there was room for insertion of a laryngoscope. The nostrils were patent. The parents were advised that maintaining a clear airway during anaesthesia would be hazardous and that urgent tracheostomy might be necessary. A unit of blood was cross-matched for surgery and an intravenous cannula was inserted. Intramuscular premedication with 70 μg atropine was administered 60 minutes before induction of anaesthesia. The MRI department was not a suitable environment for either technically demanding aspects of anaesthesia or for tracheostomy and the case was therefore managed in the operating theatre until the airway was secure.

The difficult intubation equipment was made ready and the ENT team were prepared for possible urgent tracheostomy. When the patient arrived in the anaesthetic room it was obvious that the stridor was louder and that sternal recession had developed since the assessment in the ward a few hours previously. The surgeons were consulted and it was agreed that whatever the MRI findings and whether or not surgery was performed, it would be safer if the patient had a tracheostomy.

The intravenous line was flushed and the nasogastric tube was aspirated. Anaesthesia was induced with oxygen and halothane and facemask anaesthesia was deepened gradually with the intention of maintaining spontaneous ventilation until the larynx was visualized and, if possible, the trachea intubated. Gas exchanged was improved by the application of continuous positive airway pressure via the breathing system. When the baby had central and small pupils and regular quiet respirations the airway was examined with a Miller laryngoscope. By sliding the laryngoscope blade to the right of the enlarged tongue and by pressing the anterior neck only the epiglottis could be seen; tracheal intubation was not attempted. A laryngeal mask size 1 was inserted which provided a clear airway and it was possible to assist ventilation gently.

The tracheostomy proceeded uneventfully and once the trachea was intubated, atracurium 2 mg was given and anaesthesia was maintained with isoflurane. The temperature of the baby was maintained by the use of a warm air mattress during surgery and by insulation with plastic bubble wrapper for the transfer to MRI. For the transfer the intravenous sedative drugs midazolam and fentanyl were administered and portable monitors were attached (ECG, pulse oximeter, non-invasive blood pressure, and capnography). Manual pulmonary ventilation with oxygen was used via an Ayres T-piece.

During MRI, atracurium paralysis was maintained, and the baby was mechanically ventilated with 1% isoflurane in 33% oxygen and 66% nitrous oxide via a T-piece connected to a pressure generator ventilator. Monitors were situated in an observation room next to the scanner and were connected to the patient by long cables. Twenty minutes into the scan the blood pressure measurement equipment failed and although all pulses were easily palpable, the saturation pickup (which registered 99%) became intermittent. The saturation signal improved after the isoflurane was discontinued and after 70 ml of Hartmann's solution was administered. Further blood pressure recording was unsuccessful for the remaining 20 minutes of scanning although the blood pressure recording outside the scanner was normal immediately afterwards.

The patient was transferred to the intensive care to await a decision on the surgical management. The MRI scans confirmed that the neck mass was cystic and extended into both the tongue and into the apex region of the right thorax. There was no evidence of a haematoma. The surgeons revised their decision and advised the parents that complete surgical excision was not possible and that conservative management should be tried with injections of the streptococcal derivative 'OK432'.

Discussion

Cystic hygroma

Lymphangiomas are tumour-like masses caused by congenital malformations of lymphatic tissue. They contain abnormal lymphatic channels of varying size and a cystic hygroma is a lymphangioma with macroscopic cysts that can be as large as several centimetres in diameter. Typically there is no clear demarcation of the 'tumour' and although benign, the hygroma appears to infiltrate into surrounding tissue and this makes complete surgical excision difficult and recurrence rates are high.

The natural history of the disease is unpredictable; the hygroma may shrink either spontaneously or with aspiration of the cysts and injection of a streptococcal derivative 'OK432'. Often however, lymph accumulates slowly and occasionally there is an acute increase in size due to haemorrhage or infection in the cysts and in these circumstances urgent surgical excision is warranted.

Magnetic resonance imaging

MRI requires the patient to lie still and supine for 20–60 minutes in a noisy and enclosed space: in infants and small children this can be achieved only if they are asleep. A small infant without airway compromise may sleep naturally and lie still enough after a feed, and if possible, this should be tried first. However, if there is any likelihood of hypoxia, the patient must have a secure airway and be anaesthetized.[1,2]

The scanner generates an image from electromagnetic signals created by a strong and fluctuating magnetic field and while clinical MRI has no proven harmful effects, the scanner has three major restrictions on equipment.[3–5]

1. The magnetic field of a superconducting magnet scanner is 1.5 Tesla and has the power to pull even very heavy magnetic equipment into the core of the field; for example, a molybdenum steel oxygen cylinder is particularly dangerous.
2. Electrical equipment can emit electromagnetic noise that disrupts the image. Even if the apparatus is outside the scanner, any conducting cable entering the scanning room must pass through a filter to remove troublesome signals.
3. The fluctuating magnetic field can induce electric current in any conductor and this can both interfere with electrical equipment and also cause heating of wires that can burn skin if they are in contact.

There are two broad approaches to the problem of the magnetic restrictions on equipment for anaesthesia and monitoring, and one must consider where induction and recovery and resuscitation (if necessary) could take place in safety. The options are as follows.

A 'magnetic-safe' area exists

Ideally, if there is a 'magnetic-safe' area next to the scanner this could be used to allow the use of conventional equipment certainly during induction and recovery, and perhaps for the entire procedure. During scanning itself, conventional monitors placed outside the scanning room can connect to the patient by long cables and this may be a distance of approximately 10 m. Non-invasive blood pressure and gas analysis equipment uses non-conducting cables and is easy to arrange but unfortunately, the extra length of tubing causes significant damping on the blood pressure signal of small infants because of their high heart rate and low pulse pressure – blood pressure recordings may be intermittent in small infants. Only the ECG and the pulse oximeter must be modified to be MRI compatible; the pulse oximeter is connected to the patient via a long fibreoptic cable and is less sensitive than conventional monitors; the ECG electrodes and cables have to be non-magnetic and the signals passed through a filter to remove electromagnetic noise (this is usually installed by the manufacturer of the scanner). For unstable patients such as those transferred from intensive care, invasive monitoring can be achieved[6] but long manometer lines will be needed to connect to monitors outside the scanning room. Alternatively, expensive MRI-compatible monitors are available that have integral filters and electrical circuits protected from magnetic flux and can be used next to the scanner.

Any anaesthesia equipment in the scanning room can be either non-magnetic or secured to prevent accidents. Medical gases should be piped because steel gas cylinders are too dangerous and non-magnetic aluminium oxygen cylinders are expensive and have a low capacity. The length of anaesthesia breathing circuits can be extended without increasing resistance appreciably for small infants.[7] 'As a rule' in an emergency, equipment such as laryngoscopes should not be taken into the scanner but rather the baby should be carried out to the safe area.

There is no 'magnetic-safe' area

If there is no 'magnetic-safe' area, all equipment must be compatible with the magnetic field. Care must be taken even with small items such as scissors and laryngoscopes. Whereas this may seem the simplest solution, it brings with it the problem of maintaining a sufficient stock or reserve of special equipment to cater for all reasonable eventualities. There may be circumstances where incompatible equipment is required and the management of a patient may be compromised by the lack of a safe area. If such a circumstance can be foreseen, both induction of anaesthesia and recovery may need to take place in a safe area even if this means transferring the patient some distance to and from the scanner.

Anaesthesia in an infant with a difficult airway

A large cystic hygroma may obstruct the airway and make identification of the laryngeal inlet very difficult. The normal resting oxygen consumption in a new-born is 6.6 ml.kg.$^{-1}$min^{-1} and because this is approximately twice that of an adult, failure to ventilate the lungs will result in more rapid oxygen desaturation than in an adult.

Assessment

Partial airway obstruction in an infant is marked by an increasing respiratory and heart rate, sternal and costal recession, and nasal flaring. Obstruction outside the thorax is worse during inspiration and inspiratory stridor or snoring may be heard. Signs of hypercarbia and hypoxia may develop and are followed shortly by 'collapse' and hypoxic cardiac arrest. A baby with unpredictable airway obstruction may deteriorate during scanning and it is wise to make the airway safe first. In deciding how to manage the airway the following should be examined:

1. Face. Can a mask be applied on the face to effect manual chest expansion? A mask with a soft seal should be effective.
2. Access via the mouth. Can a laryngoscope or airway be inserted? This may be difficult if the tongue is large.
3. Access via the nose. Are the nostrils patent to allow insertion of a nasal airway? This may be vital to maintain oxygenation during fibreoptic laryngoscopy or tracheostomy.
4. Stridor. Stridor indicates tracheal, laryngeal or pharyngeal obstruction. The true site of obstruction may not be apparent until laryngoscopy.
5. Access to the neck. Can a tracheostomy be performed? If the hygroma is large this may be very difficult.
6. Are there mobile structures that could obstruct the larynx during positive pressure mask ventilation? This is possible in lymphangiomas and haemangiomas and will make it important to maintain spontaneous ventilation until the airway can be examined with a laryngoscope.
7. Is neck movement restricted? This is unlikely in this baby but should be checked for because an immobile or short neck will add to difficulty with laryngoscopy.

Anaesthesia plan

Clearly, anaesthesia and airway management in this patient is potentially difficult and unsuitable for a remote and technically restrictive environment such as an MRI scanner. Attempts to maintain a clear airway may fail during anaesthesia and therefore it is wise to maximize safety by ensuring that a tracheostomy can be performed promptly; the parents must be warned of this possibility. Anaesthesia should therefore start in an operating theatre so that necessary skills and equipment are at hand. Later, with the airway secured, the baby can be transferred to the scanner and then returned either to the operating theatre for surgery or to a suitable recovery area.

Induction

A weak neonate in extremis should be laryngoscoped and intubated without anaesthesia. However, laryngoscopy in an awake and lusty infant is both distressing to the patient and associated with hypoxia and therefore not recommended. The safest course of action is to perform a gentle and unhurried inhalational induction with either halothane or sevoflurane in oxygen. Atropine premedication is preferred for drying secretions and preventing bradycardia. If the nostrils are not patent the mouth must be held open. Under sufficient anaesthesia, an oral airway should be inserted and if this fails a laryngeal mask or nasal airway can be tried. The application of continuous positive pressure via the breathing system is often helpful to increase the patency of the airway.

Laryngoscopy

With deeper levels of anaesthesia the airway can be examined with a laryngoscope. If the glottis is seen easily and there are no reasons to believe that positive pressure mask ventilation will be difficult, muscle relaxation with suxamethonium will allow smooth tracheal intubation. The short action of suxamethonium may allow return to spontaneous respiration in time to prevent catastrophe if either intubation or assisted ventilation fails. With less confidence the trachea may be intubated without muscle relaxation, but if anaesthesia is too deep there is the possibility of cardiorespiratory depression and if it is not deep enough, laryngospasm can occur.

A straight-bladed laryngoscope such as a Miller is preferred in infants because the normal epiglottis is long and needs to be lifted away from the glottis. The straight blade can also be passed to the side of the tongue and even underneath it. If this manoeuvre fails to visualize the glottis, other methods are available but are time-consuming and have variable success according to the skills and experience of the anaesthetist. A tracheostomy can be performed without prior tracheal intubation and if the surgeons have already decided that a tracheostomy is required this could be performed before the MRI scan. Alternatively the following methods of tracheal intubation or laryngoscopy are available.

1. Blind, via the nose. This is unlikely to be successful in a neonate and the hygroma or pharynx or larynx may be traumatized.
2. Light wand assisted. In a darkened room the light of a wand will reveal its position and can be guided into the trachea. A tracheal tube, previously loaded on the wand, can then be pushed off into the trachea.
3. Flexible fibreoptic. Either via a nostril or the mouth a fibrescope can assist the placement of a tracheal tube.[8] If the scope is inserted into the trachea it will obstruct breathing and cause hypoxia and a safer technique involves first passing a guide-wire via the suction port of the fibrescope into the trachea. The fibrescope is then removed but if a tracheal tube is railroaded over the wire it will usually kink because it is too flexible. It is better to use a respiratory exchange catheter first because it does not kink easily and a tracheal tube can be inserted over it smoothly.[9] Also, respiratory exchange catheters are hollow and allow both capnography monitoring to check on the position of the tip and the delivery of oxygen. While the glottis is being sought by the fibrescope there must be two patent airway orifices: one for breathing and one for the scope itself. Unfortunately the size 1 laryngeal mask is too small for a fibrescope that has a suction port.
4. Bullard Laryngoscope®. This is a robust rigid fibreoptic tool with a blade shaped like a hook that slides over and behind the tongue. A good view of the glottis is usually achieved without the manipulation of the airway structures that sometimes is necessary with conventional blades. There is a suction port through which a respiratory exchange catheter can be passed. If successful, this method is quicker than the flexible fibreoptic method.

Complete airway obstruction

Great care must be taken to avoid this situation by gathering together the best skills available. If airway obstruction cannot be overcome, the following possibilities must be considered.

1. Can anaesthesia be reversed to allow the baby to recover its own airway? This is unlikely because the obstruction is likely to happen when the anaesthesia is 'committed'.
2. Is laryngoscopy and intubation possible? If artificial airways have proved ineffective laryngoscopy must be attempted. The stimulation of laryngoscopy should cause increased respiratory effort and movement and may even bring the glottis into view.
3. If there is laryngospasm it can usually be overcome with suction and application of continuous positive pressure: muscle relaxation at this stage is hazardous and not recommended.

If obstruction persists the surgeon must perform a prompt tracheostomy.

Learning points

- A cystic hygroma can obstruct the airway and make anaesthesia hazardous.
- Anaesthesia management of an infant with a difficult airway is safest if spontaneous ventilation is maintained until either the larynx has been identified easily or the trachea has been intubated.
- Difficult airway procedures should take place in an operating theatre with the necessary equipment and staff available, including the facility for tracheostomy.
- During transport, small infants must be kept warm and monitored if they are anaesthetized or sedated.
- There are restrictions and limitations on equipment in MRI scanners. Special equipment is necessary and ideally there should be an adjacent area 'safe' from the magnetic field.

References

1. Egelhoff JC, Ball WS Jr, Koch BL, Parks TD. Safety and efficacy of sedation in children using a structured sedation program. *Am J Roentgenol* 1994; 168: 1259–1262.
2. Sury MRJ, Hatch DJ, Deeley T et al. Development of a nurse-led sedation service for paediatric magnetic resonance imaging. *Lancet* 1999; 353: 1667–1671.
3. Peden CJ, Menon DK, Hall AS et al. Magnetic resonance for the anaesthetist. Part II: Anaesthesia and monitoring in MR units. *Anaesthesia* 1992; 47: 508–517.
4. Sury MRJ, Johnstone G, Bingham RM. Anaesthesia for magnetic resonance imaging of children. *Paediatr Anaesth* 1992; 2: 61–68.
5. Hall S. Paediatric anaesthesia outside the operating room. *Can J Anaesth* 1995; 42: R68–R72.
6. Tobin JR, Spurrier EA, Wetzel RC. Anaesthesia for critically ill children during magnetic resonance imaging. *Br J Anaesth* 1992; 69: 482–486.
7. Jackson E, Tan S, Yarwood G, Sury MRJ. Increasing the length of the expiratory limb of the Ayres T-piece: implications for remote mechanical ventilation in infants and young children. *Br J Anaesth* 1994; 73: 154–156.
8. Chadd GD, Crane DL, Phillips RM, Tunell WP. Extubation and reintubation guided by the laryngeal mask airway in a child with the Pierre–Robin syndrome. *Anesthesiology* 1992; 76: 640.
9. Hasan MA, Black AE. A new technique for fibreoptic intubation in children. *Anaesthesia* 1994; 49: 1031–1033.
10. Borland LM, Casselbrant M. The Bullard laryngoscope. A new indirect oral laryngoscope (pediatric version). *Anesth Analges* 1990; 70: 103–104.

21

Empyema in a 4-year-old boy

Peter A Stoddart

Introduction

The incidence of complicated pneumonia including empyema is increasing.[1–4] The management of parapneumonic empyema is controversial but depends on the successful drainage of the pleural fluid.[5–9] The natural history of the disease is well described and should be staged prior to treatment.[10–12] The child may require repeated surgical interventions and have significant respiratory impairment. The following case illustrates some of the anaesthetic challenges.

Case history

A 4-year-old boy was admitted to his local hospital with a short history of poor appetite, malaise and a fever of 39 °C. He had previously been well, attained all his milestones at the correct time and was up to date with his immunizations. He had missed 3 days of nursery school 2 weeks previously due to an acute upper respiratory tract infection but appeared to have recovered with his cough and coryza resolving. However, in the last 2 days he had developed a nocturnal cough. On examination he looked tired and was pale. He weighed 15.8 kg. His respiratory rate was 28 bpm and pulse oximetry demonstrated that his saturations were between 92% and 95% in air. On auscultation the breath sounds were markedly reduced on the left with a dull percussion note. For further investigations see Table 21.1.

A diagnosis of postpneumonic pleural effusion was made and the local paediatricians asked the on call surgical registrar to aspirate the effusion and send a sample for culture. Anaesthesia was induced uneventfully with propofol 60 mg and fentanyl 15 mg. He was allowed to spontaneously breath isoflurane in an air/oxygen mixture through a size 2 laryngeal mask airway. 100 ml of turbid pleural fluid was easily aspirated and sent for culture and analysis. A 20G chest drain was inserted and connected to an underwater seal. He made an uneventful recovery from his anaesthetic and was returned to the ward.

He was started on intravenous cefuroxime 500 mg 6-hourly, with paracetamol 240 mg 4-hourly as needed for analgesia and as an antipyretic. Unfortunately he only drained a further 40 ml of fluid through his chest drain over the next 24 hours and so it was removed. His fever did not settle and a repeat chest X-ray at 48 hours showed the effusion was unresolved. After discussion with the regional paediatric unit he was transferred for further treatment.

On arrival an ultrasound scan of the chest was performed which demonstrated a large left-sided effusion with multiple loculations, pleural thickening and atelectasis especially of the left lower lobe. In view

FBC	Hb 10.3 g.dl^{-1}, WCC 14.6 × 10^{9} l^{-1}, platelets 356 × 10^{9} l^{-1}
U&Es	Na 134 mmol.l^{-1}, U 7.6 mmol.l^{-1}, K 4.7 mmol.l^{-1}, Cr 76 mmol.l^{-1}
Blood cultures	–ve
Chest X-ray (see Figure 21.1)	A large left-sided pleural effusion without significant mediastinal shift

Table 21.1
Investigations from district general hospital

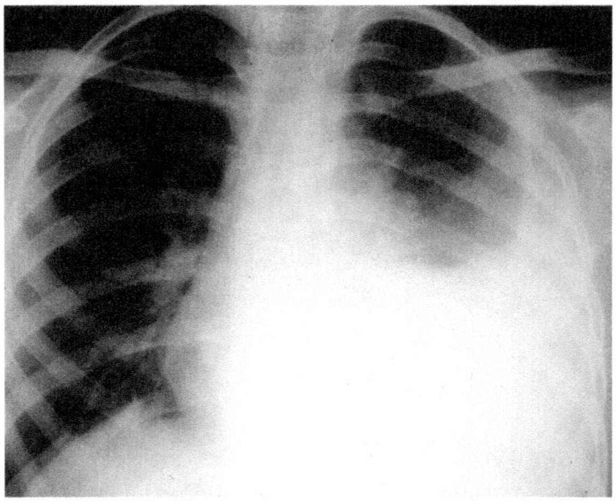

Figure 21.1
Left-sided empyema

Biochemistry	Protein 4.2 g.dl^{-1}, glucose 3.1 mmol.l^{-1}, pH 7.10, LDH > 1000 IU.dl^{-1}
Microscopy and culture	WCC > 500 cells.ml^{-1}, no growth

Table 21.2
Pleural fluid biochemistry and microbiology results

of the continuing fever and the ultrasound findings the child was taken to theatre the same evening for a thoracotomy and open decortication of empyema.

Definitive management

The boy still had saturations in the low 90s despite nasal oxygen 2 l.min^{-1}, a respiratory rate of 34 bpm and a temperature of 39.5 °C. He was cross-matched for 2 units of blood. At the preoperative visit postoperative analgesia was discussed and verbal consent for epidural analgesia and the use of rectal diclofenac was obtained. With his mother present, he tolerated preoxygenation and monitoring of his saturations and ECG prior to induction of anaesthesia. Anaesthesia was induced with propofol 55 mg, fentanyl 50 µg and atracurium 10 mg. An uncut non-cuffed 5.5-mm endotrachial tube was easily inserted into the right main bronchus and withdrawn to the trachea to ventilate both lungs. An additional 18G cannula was inserted into the brachiocephalic vein in the left forearm and a 22G cannula into the left radial artery. A thoracic epidural catheter was inserted at T5/6 using a 5 cm 18G Tuohy needle and a loss of resistance to saline technique. An initial dose of 8 ml plain 0.25% racemic bupivacaine was given slowly prior to skin incision. A urinary catheter was inserted to monitor urine output interoperatively and because of the small risk of postoperative urinary retention with epidural analgesia.

A left mini-thoracotomy at T4/5 revealed a thick coat of gelatinous empyema that was adherent to the underlying lung. The small amount of free fluid was aspirated and sent for further microbiological investigation. The empyema was evacuated and the adherent component carefully peeled from the underlying lung. This resulted in a blood loss of approximately 130 ml but enabled the left lung to be fully inflated. Air leaks were searched for by applying gentle positive end-expiratory pressure (PEEP) with the chest cavity containing warmed saline. Two 20G chest drains were inserted before the chest was closed. During the procedure the child's temperature rose to 40 °C and his heart rate climbed initially to 124 bpm but with no change in blood pressure. Over an hour he was given 330 ml of Hartmann's solution plus 200 ml of Gelofusine® and the heart rate settled to 100 bpm with a temperature of 38.5°C. At the end of surgery a 12.5 mg suppository of diclofenac was inserted per rectum. He was extubated uneventfully on the operating table and transferred to the recovery unit.

Postoperative analgesia was maintained with an epidural infusion of bupivacaine 0.125% with 2 µg.ml^{-1} of fentanyl at a rate of 3–4 ml.h^{-1}. This was supplemented with paracetamol 240 mg 4-hourly, and ibuprofen 80 mg 6-hourly, both of which also acted as antipyretics. Over the following 48 hours his fever resolved, he was able to co-operate with physiotherapy and when the volume of fluid drained reduced the chest drains were removed. Culture of the pleural fluid was negative. He was discharged home on the fourth postoperative day. At follow-up 3 months later he had started infant school and had no residual respiratory symptoms.

Discussion

Empyema in children has a number of causes but usually follows a previous community acquired pneumonic illness in an otherwise well child.[13,14] Rarely it may follow a neglected aspiration of foreign body with the development of parenchymal lung abscess. If a foreign body is suspected a bronchoscopy should also be performed under general anaesthesia.

The treatment is controversial especially since the introduction of fibrinolytics to aid the drainage of loculated pus and the increased use of video-assisted thoracoscopy (VAT). Management depends on staging of the disease process.[7,15] A skilled ultrasonographer can usually assess the size of the effusion, the presence of loculations, the thickness of any adherent peel and the extent of the underlying atelectasis.[16,17] The treatment options include simple aspiration of the effusion with microbiological examination of the fluid, chest tube drainage with or without additional fibrinolysis using streptokinase or urokinase,[18–21] VAT with decortication[7,14,22,23] or open thoracotomy with decortication.[6,24–26] Even simple drainage with a chest tube as in this case often requires general anaesthesia.

Community acquired infections may be sterile by the time the child presents in hospital, but because of the range of infectious agents that can potentially cause empyema broad-spectrum antibiotics are usually prescribed and given for 2–3 weeks.[8,10]

The type of anaesthesia required depends on the surgical intervention.[27] Thoracoscopy invariably requires one-lung ventilation of the contralateral lung.[28] In a small child selective endobronchial intubation or endobronchial blockers can be used since suitably small double-lumen tubes are rarely available. Single lung anaesthesia can lead to hypoxaemia especially if there continues to be an underlying pneumonic process. The low saturations usually respond to a combination of increases in FiO_2 and the application of PEEP to the ventilated lung. Once the affected lung has been decorticated it is essential to ensure it can be expanded by applying periods of gentle but sustained PEEP. This also allows identification of air leaks from the lung which if large may need to be repaired. With open thoracotomy we find that simple tracheal intubation with a correctly sized tube is usually satisfactory unless there is a significant lung abscess or a large bronchopleural fistula.

Thoracotomy is extremely painful and effective analgesia is important for recovery. Good analgesia simplifies management of the chest tubes and enables the physiotherapists to maintain lung expansion. A multimodal approach improves the efficacy of the analgesia and reduces the potential side effects. In this case a thoracic epidural was inserted[29] which we find produces excellent analgesia. The use of an epidural catheter is controversial if the child is pyrexial because of concerns about systemic sepsis but in our unit we feel that the benefit of high quality analgesia outweighs the theoretical risks of infection especially when the empyema is sterile and broad-spectrum systemic antibiotics have been administered. Other centres have used continuous paravertebral block with a catheter either inserted by the surgeon under direct vision[30] or the anaesthetist using a loss of resistance technique.[31] Alternatively a morphine infusion or in an older child patient-controlled analgesia can provide good pain relief but usually with increased sedation. Regular non-steroidal anti-inflammatory drugs and paracetamol are opioid sparing and are useful antipyretics.[32]

Decortication can be associated with considerable blood loss so donor blood should be available. Evacuation of the empyema often results in an initial systemic septic episode presumably due to the absorption of a range of cytokines. Hypotension may occasionally require ionotropic support though it is usually short-lived and self-limiting. The fever usually resolves rapidly and the child becomes less systemically unwell over the first 24 hours. The epidural infusion or intravenous morphine infusion should be continued until the chest tubes are removed but following this the child can rapidly progress to simple analgesics.

Complete recovery over the subsequent months is usually the norm though occasionally restrictive type defects may be demonstrated.[8,33]

Learning points

- . Treatment of a parapneumonic empyema requires a multidisciplinary approach.
- All children should be staged with ultrasonography before planning definitive treatment.
- Open thoracotomy usually results in rapid recovery though other methods are often initially tried.
- Single lung anaesthesia may be required but is not essential except to prevent soiling of the contralateral lung with either blood or pus, to control a large bronchopleural fistula, or for thoracoscopic procedures.
- Excellent postoperative analgesia is essential to allow the physiotherapists to keep the affected lung fully expanded.

References

1. Tan TQ, Mason EO Jr, Wald ER et al. Clinical characteristics of children with complicated pneumonia caused by Streptococcus pneumoniae. *Pediatrics* 2002; 110(1 Pt 1): 1–6.
2. Byington CL, Spencer LY, Johnson TA et al. An epidemiological investigation of a sustained high rate of pediatric parapneumonic empyema: risk factors and microbiological associations. *Clin Infect Dis* 2002; 34: 434–440.
3. Playfor SD, Smyth AR, Stewart RJ. Increase in incidence of childhood empyema. *Thorax* 1997; 52: 932.
4. Thompson A, Reid A, Shields M et al. Increased incidence in childhood empyema thoracis in Northern Ireland. *Ir Med J* 1999; 92: 438.
5. Angelillo Mackinlay TA, Lyons GA, Chimondeguy DJ et al. VATS debridement versus thoracotomy in the treatment of loculated postpneumonia empyema. *Ann Thorac Surg* 1996; 61: 1626–1630.
6. Carey JA, Hamilton JR, Spencer DA et al. Empyema thoracis: a role for open thoracotomy and decortication. *Arch Dis Child* 1998; 79: 510–513.
7. Cassina PC, Hauser M, Hillejan L et al. Video-assisted thoracoscopy in the treatment of pleural empyema: stage-based management and outcome. *J Thorac Cardiovasc Surg* 1999; 117: 234–238.
8. Chan PW, Crawford O, Wallis C, Dinwiddie R. Treatment of pleural empyema. *J Paediatr Child Health* 2000; 36: 375–377.
9. Waller DA. Thoracoscopy in management of postpneumonic pleural infections. *Curr Opin Pulmon Med* 2002; 8: 323–326.
10. Teixeira LR, Villarino MA. Antibiotic treatment of patients with pneumonia and pleural effusion. *Curr Opin Pulmon Med* 1998; 4: 230–234.
11. Bryant RE, Salmon CJ. Pleural empyema. *Clin Infect Dis* 1996; 22: 747–762; quiz 763–764.
12. Light RW. A new classification of parapneumonic effusions and empyema. *Chest* 1995; 108: 299–301.
13. Givan DC, Eigen H. Common pleural effusions in children. *Clin Chest Med* 1998; 19: 363–371.
14. Doski JJ, Lou D, Hicks BA et al. Management of parapneumonic collections in infants and children. *J Pediatr Surg* 2000; 35: 265–268; discussion 269–270.
15. Chan W, Keyser-Gauvin E, Davis GM et al. Empyema thoracis in children: a 26-year review of the Montreal Children's Hospital experience. *J Pediatr Surg* 1997; 32: 870–872.
16. Shankar S, Gulati M, Kang M et al. Image-guided percutaneous drainage of thoracic empyema: can sonography predict the outcome? *Eur Radiol* 2000; 10: 495–499.
17. Khakoo GA, Goldstraw P, Hansell DM, Bush A. Surgical treatment of parapneumonic empyema. *Pediatr Pulmon* 1996; 22: 348–356.
18. Kilic N, Celebi S, Gurpinar A et al. Management of thoracic empyema in children. *Pediatr Surg Int* 2002; 18: 21–23.
19. Meier AH, Smith B, Raghavan A et al. Rational treatment of empyema in children. *Arch Surg* 2000; 135: 907–912.
20. Robinson LA, Moulton AL, Fleming WH et al. Intrapleural fibrinolytic treatment of multiloculated thoracic empyemas. *Ann Thorac Surg* 1994; 57: 803–813; discussion 813–814.
21. Thomson AH, Hull J, Kumar MR et al. Randomised trial of intrapleural urokinase in the treatment of childhood empyema. *Thorax* 2002; 57: 343–347.
22. Angelillo-Mackinlay T, Lyons GA, Piedras MB, Angelillo-Mackinlay D. Surgical treatment of postpneumonic empyema. *World J Surg* 1999; 23: 1110–1113.
23. Chen LE, Langer JC, Dillon PA et al. Management of late-stage parapneumonic empyema. *J Pediatr Surg* 2002; 37: 371–374.
24. Galea JL, De Souza A, Beggs D, Spyt T. The surgical management of empyema thoracis. *J R Coll Surg Edinb* 1997; 42: 15–18.
25. Shankar KR, Kenny SE, Okoye BO et al. Evolving experience in the management of empyema thoracis. *Acta Paediatr* 2000; 89: 417–420.
26. Gofrit ON, Engelhard D, Abu-Dalu K. Post-pneumonic thoracic empyema in children: a continued surgical challenge. *Eur J Pediatr Surg* 1999; 9: 4–7.
27. Haynes SR, Bonner S. Review article: anaesthesia for thoracic surgery in children. *Paediatr Anaesth* 2000; 10: 237–251.
28. Tobias JD. Anaesthetic implications of thoracoscopic surgery in children. *Paediatr Anaesth* 1999; 9: 103–110.
29. Tobias JD, Lowe S, O'Dell N, Holcomb GW 3rd. Thoracic epidural anaesthesia in infants and children. *Can J Anaesth* 1993; 40: 879–882.
30. Karmakar MK, Booker PD, Franks R, Pozzi M. Continuous extrapleural paravertebral infusion of bupivacaine for post-thoracotomy analgesia in young infants. *Br J Anaesth* 1996; 76: 811–815.
31. Lonnqvist PA, Olsson GL. Paravertebral vs epidural block in children. Effects on postoperative morphine requirement after renal surgery. *Acta Anaesthesiol Scand* 1994; 38: 346–349.
32. Pickering AE, Bridge HS, Nolan J, Stoddart PA. Double-blind, placebo-controlled analgesic study of ibuprofen or rofecoxib in combination with paracetamol for tonsillectomy in children. *Br J Anaesth* 2002; 88: 72–77.
33. McLaughlin FJ, Goldmann DA, Rosenbaum DM et al. Empyema in children: clinical course and long-term follow-up. *Pediatrics* 1984; 73: 587–593.

22

Day case anaesthesia for orchidopexy (including the snotty child)

Liam J Brennan

Introduction

Day case management is appropriate for a wide range of the commoner paediatric surgical procedures (including orchidopexy). Children make excellent candidates for day surgery as they are usually fit, healthy and free of chronic disease. However, a common problem is the child presenting on the day of surgery with a snotty nose. Do you cancel the case or do you proceed? What are the potential risks? A discussion of this dilemma and other aspects of paediatric day case management are included in the case that follows.

Case history

George, a 3-year-old Caucasian boy, weight 16 kg, presented to the Day Surgery Unit via the surgical outpatient clinic with a left undescended testis requiring orchidopexy. His suitability for day case management was assessed with his mother (a single parent with one other child) by an experienced paediatric nurse utilizing a screening questionnaire. It was noted that George suffered from recurrent upper respiratory tract infections requiring frequent antibiotic therapy and that he was awaiting an ENT outpatient appointment. However, at the time of the screening visit his mother regarded George as being well and reported no other significant medical history. The day unit nurse booked George's operation for 3 weeks' time, explained the day of admission procedures and emphasized the Unit's starvation policy (6 hours for milk and solid food; 3 hours for clear fluids). She also provided George's mother with an information leaflet.

On the day of surgery George was admitted to the Day Unit but was noted to have purulent nasal secretions by the nursing staff. Prior to the arrival of medical staff EMLA® cream was applied to prominent veins on the dorsum of both hands according to the Unit's standing instructions. George was then introduced to the play therapist who engaged him in structured play to prepare him for anaesthetic induction (Figure 22.1).

On arrival of the consultant anaesthetist the admitting nurse reported her concern about George's 'snotty nose' and the history of recurrent respiratory infection. When assessed by the anaesthetist George was playful, very active and had no cough. His mother explained that George's snotty nose was always present and had not worsened since the screening visit to the Day Unit. She considered her son to be well and had not deemed it necessary to consult her GP about his condition. On examination George appeared well and very settled in his new environment. Although purulent secretions were noted the nasal airway was unobstructed. He was apyrex-

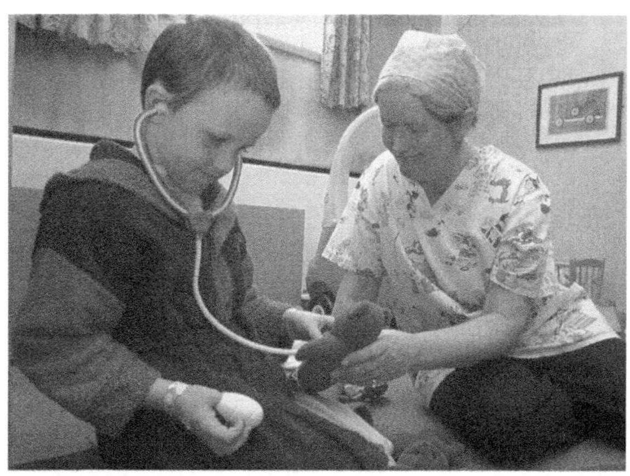

Figure 22.1
Play therapist working with a child prior to anaesthetic induction.

ial and ENT examination revealed enlarged but noninflamed tonsils. Chest examination was unremarkable.

The anaesthetist decided that it was safe to proceed with the operation that day. He explained that he planned to use an intravenous induction and obtained verbal consent for an ilioinguinal block and rectal dicloflenac for perioperative analgesia. As George was not unduly anxious no sedative premedication was prescribed.

George arrived in the anaesthetic room accompanied by his mother. Venous cannulation was performed without difficulty aided by appropriate distraction by the play therapist. After instituting routine monitoring intravenous induction proceeded with propofol ($4\,mg.kg^{-1}$) and alfentanil ($10\,\mu g.kg^{-1}$). A size 2 laryngeal mask airway was inserted without difficulty and anaesthesia was maintained with nitrous oxide, oxygen and isoflurane via a T-piece breathing system. Prior to the start of surgery a left ilioinguinal block was performed (6 ml 0.25% bupivacaine) and 2 ml of the same local anaesthetic was infiltrated subcutaneously in the left hemi-scrotum.

A diclofenac rectal suppository (12.5 mg) was inserted. During the procedure, 150 ml of Hartmann's solution was infused and ondansetron (1.5 mg) was administered as antiemetic prophylaxis.

At the completion of surgery George was transferred to the recovery room and after regaining consciousness he was reunited with his mother on the day unit ward. Two hours later, George was fully awake and in no apparent pain. He had taken a drink, eaten some breakfast cereal and had passed urine. The surgeon and the anaesthetist reviewed George and deemed him fit for discharge. His mother was provided with a postoperative information sheet (including contact telephone numbers) and was supplied with paracetamol and ibuprofen elixirs. She was instructed to give George paracetamol 250 mg and ibuprofen 75 mg four times daily regularly for the next 3 days. On telephone follow up by the day unit nursing staff 2 days later George was very well with minimal pain and no other postoperative problems.

Discussion

Paediatric day surgery is becoming increasingly popular in Europe, Australasia and North America. In the USA 60% of all paediatric surgery is performed on an ambulatory basis. The spur for this development has primarily been economic as transferring suitable procedures to day surgery attracts large cost savings. For example, in Cambridge the costs for day case circumcision are 46% of the inpatient equivalent.[1] Besides these financial considerations, avoiding inpatient admission is highly beneficial for children and their families. Behavioural problems, disrupted sleep patterns and regression of developmental milestones are all sequelae of inpatient admission avoided by day care. In our case history, George's mother was a single parent with another child for whom an overnight stay in hospital is best avoided at all costs.

A well developed screening programme is essential for consistently successful day-stay management. Preventable cancellation on the day of surgery is decreased so avoiding waste of operating time and resources. In addition by completing many of the admission formalities, stress for the child and parents on the day of surgery is minimized. Nurse-led assessment by experienced personnel using a preoperative questionnaire works particularly well in day case practice and has been validated for adults and children. Written information should also be supplied to parents, emphasizing important issues such as preoperative fasting times.

Preoperative investigation of children prior to day surgery is hardly ever justified. Routine full blood count estimation is not required as even in the presence of mild anaemia there is no evidence that this affects morbidity or influences perioperative management for day case procedures.[2] The possible exception to this embargo is sickle cell screening for those children from racially susceptible groups.

Careful psychological preparation of the child for day surgery is essential. This is because on the day of surgery there is little time between admission and anaesthetic induction to orientate the child and parents to the day's events and so develop a rapport. In addition, sedative premedication is not routinely used for day cases making careful preparation of the child of added importance. At the screening visit or on the day of surgery, play specialists, through the medium of structured play can provide a relaxed atmosphere which helps to allay the anxieties of the child and parents (Figure 22.1). In particular they are able to explain the process of anaesthetic induction and to recognize the unduly anxious child who might benefit from sedative premedication.

Sedative premedication may occasionally be required for children coming for repeated procedures or those who have previously had a bad perioperative experience. It may also benefit some children with special needs with whom it may be difficult to gain a rapport. Traditional sedative premedicants are unsuitable as they are associated with excessive postoperative sedation and delayed discharge. Increasingly, interest has focused on the use of midazolam.[3] The standard intravenous formulation is given orally (0.5–0.75 $mg.kg^{-1}$) producing useful sedation within 15–30 minutes but without delaying postoperative recovery time. As the intravenous formulation is bitter, it is best administered mixed with a suitably flavoured vehicle such as a small volume of fruit squash, lemonade or paracetamol elixir. Intranasal midazolam can also be used but is associated with nasal stinging making it a less acceptable alternative.

Deciding on the appropriate management for day surgery of a child with a respiratory infection is controversial. The problem is commonplace as it is estimated that 20–30% of children have a 'runny nose' for most of the year.[4] Cancelling all of these children is inappropriate as the majority of them have a benign, non-infectious rhinitis or their symptoms are attributable to adenoidal hypertrophy. Deferring surgery in these cases confers no clinical benefit. However, a proportion of these children may have the early stages of a more severe upper or lower respiratory infection, childhood exanthema or even a life-threatening condition such as bacterial meningitis. Anaesthesia in these circumstances can be hazardous with increased incidence of perioperative respiratory complications such as laryngospasm, bronchospasm and atelectasis. The incidence of these problems is increased 11-fold if the trachea is intubated and are more common in infancy.[5]

Clearly there is no one correct approach to this problem except that each child should be assessed on an individual basis by an experienced anaesthetist.[6,7] All children with moderate or severe respiratory infection should be postponed. Clinical indicators of severity should be sought to assist in the decision-making process (Table 22.1).The threshold for cancellation should be lower in infancy or in the presence of a history of asthma. If the case is cancelled most authorities recommend a 2-week deferral for upper respiratory infection but 4 weeks if there is lower respiratory tract involvement.

- Malaise and irritable behaviour
- Fever (>37.5 °C)
- Productive cough
- Purulent nasal secretions
- Abnormal auscultatory sounds

Table 22.1
Indicators of moderate/severe respiratory infection

In George's case, his symptoms of snotty nose are long-standing and it is likely that adenoidal hypertrophy will be the likely diagnosis at his forthcoming ENT appointment. His mother and the anaesthetist agree that George is constitutionally well. On examination, George is apyrexial, has no cough and his chest is normal to auscultation. In deciding to proceed that day, the anaesthetist has judged George's symptoms to be long-standing and not complicated by an infective exacerbation. He has also been mindful that cancellation of the case would be extremely disruptive for a single parent.

Careful attention to postoperative symptom control is crucial for consistently successful paediatric day surgery. Uncontrolled pain and intractable postoperative nausea and vomiting (PONV) are the commonest causes of unexpected admission after day surgery.[8] As long-acting opioids are associated with excessive sedation and PONV they should be avoided in day surgery and analgesia instead should hinge on liberal use of local anaesthesia and non-steroidal anti-inflammatory drugs (NSAIDs).

In our case study, local anaesthesia was provided by an ilioinguinal block supplemented by subcutaneous infiltration of more bupivacaine in the scrotum. This is necessary because although the ilioinguinal block provides excellent analgesia for the groin incision it does not cover the scrotal incision since the scrotum is innervated by the pudendal nerves.[9] Caudal anaesthesia would have been a suitable alternative but it is a neuroaxial block associated with concurrent lower limb weakness and the potential (albeit rare) for serious complications such as intrathecal injection, intravascular injection and epidural abscess formation. Many paediatric anaesthetists believe that peripheral nerve blocks should be used whenever possible reserving central blocks for situations where they are the only suitable option.

A NSAID, in this case rectal diclofenac (approx.1 $mg.kg^{-1}$), was utilized perioperatively having obtained parental consent for its use. These drugs are particularly useful in day surgery because they are effective in relieving mild to moderate pain, are non-sedating and lack emetic side effects. They are not licensed for use in infancy. Paracetamol can be used as an alternative or in conjunction with NSAIDs. If given

- Vital signs and consciousness level normal for age and preoperative condition of child
- Protective airway reflexes fully regained
- No respiratory distress or stridor
- No unexpected intraoperative anaesthetic events
- No bleeding or surgical complications
- Pain and PONV absent or mild
- Appropriate ambulation for age of child
- Written/verbal instructions issued and lines of contact emphasized
- Escort home by responsible adult in private car or taxi

Table 22.2
Discharge criteria (reproduced with permission from Brennan[7])

Infants (< 1 year)	Paracetamol 15 $mg.kg^{-1}$ 6-hourly
Children (> 1 year)	Paracetamol 15 $mg.kg^{-1}$ 6-hourly ± ibuprofen 5 $mg.kg^{-1}$ 6-hourly or codeine elixir 0.5 $mg.kg^{-1}$ 6-hourly
Older children (> 12 years)	Compound paracetamol/ codeine preparation e.g. co-codamol ± ibuprofen 200–400 mg qds

NB Analgesia prescribed regularly not as required

Table 22.3
Postdischarge analgesia regimens

orally before surgery a loading dose of 20 $mg.kg^{-1}$ is appropriate but when administered rectally the loading dose should be increased to 30 $mg.kg^{-1}$ as absorption via the rectal mucosa is erratic.

PONV can be a major problem after orchidopexy. Minimizing the impact of the problem includes avoiding excessive preoperative fasting, maintaining adequate perioperative hydration, avoiding too early postoperative oral intake and the use of antiemetic prophylaxis.[10] In George's case, his mother was given clear instructions to maintain oral fluids until 3 hours before admission, a bolus of intravenous fluid was given peroperatively and ondansetron (0.1 $mg.kg^{-1}$) was administered at the start of surgery. Ondansetron, a 5HT-3 antagonist, was chosen as it produces minimal sedation and is devoid of extrapyramidal side effects.

Once reunited with his mother, George was allowed home once he had met the Unit's discharge criteria (Table 22.2). Adequate oral analgesia was provided on departure and his mother was instructed to administer the pain relief regularly for 3 days (Table 22.3). The importance of educating parents to give postdischarge analgesia on a regular rather than on an as required basis cannot be overemphasized. In a study of 551 children in Finland, only 78% of all children reported to have postoperative pain on the day of surgery received analgesia and this decreased to 60% by the next day. This study also demonstrated that inadequate pain relief after discharge was associated with behavioural problems for up to 4 weeks postoperatively, whereas children with little or no pain did not experience such problems.[11]

Telephone follow-up by day unit staff provides reassurance for parents and allows simple problems to be discussed and resolved thus decreasing pressure on primary care services. It also fulfills a useful audit function as data regarding postoperative pain, PONV and surgical morbidity can be collected and so contribute to improving the service.[1]

Learning points

- Day case management confers major benefits for children and families.
- A multidisciplinary team of experienced personnel is required to provide high quality day care.
- Children with respiratory infections should be assessed on an individual basis by an experienced anaesthetist; mild or perennial symptoms may not preclude day case anaesthesia.
- Scrupulous attention to perioperative symptom control, especially pain and PONV is essential for successful children's day surgery.
- Postdischarge analgesia should be prescribed on a regular basis rather than as required.

References

1. Brennan LJ. Modern day case anaesthesia for children. *B J Anaesth* 1999; 83: 91–103.
2. Meneghini L, Zandra N, Zannette G et al. The usefulness of routine preoperative laboratory investigations for one day surgery in healthy children. *Paediatr Anaesth* 1998; 8: 11–15.
3. Parnis SJ, Foale JA, Van der Walt JH et al. Oral midazolam is an effective premedication for children having day case anaesthesia. *Anaesth Intens Care* 1997; 20: 9–14.
4. Hannalah RS. Anaesthetic considerations for paediatric ambulatory surgery. *Ambul Surg* 1997; 5: 52–59.
5. Cohen MM, Cameron CB. Should you cancel the operation when a child has an upper respiratory tract infection? *Anesth Analges* 1991; 72: 282–288.
6. Arthur DS, Morton NS, Fyfe AH. Patient selection, assessment and preoperative preparation. In: Morton NS, Raine PA (eds). *Paediatric Day Case Surgery.* Oxford: Oxford University Press, 1994: 10–20.
7. Brennan LJ. Day stay surgery. In: Sumner E, Hatch DJ (eds). *Paediatric Anaesthesia.* London: Arnold, 1999: 509–533.
8. Patel, RI, Hannallah RS. Complications following paediatric ambulatory surgery. *Ambul Surg* 1995; 3: 83–86.
9. McNicol LR. Peripheral nerve blocks. In: Morton NS, Raine PA (eds). *Paediatric Day Case Surgery.* Oxford: Oxford University Press, 1994: 38–53.
10. Baines D. Postoperative nausea and vomiting in children. *Paediatr Anaesth* 1996; 6: 7–14.
11. Kotiniemi LH, Ryhanen PT, Valanne J et al. Postoperative symptoms at home following day case surgery in children: a multicentre study of 551 children. *Anaesthesia* 1997; 52: 963–969.

23

Problems in recovery (postanaesthesia care unit)

Michelle White and Gillian R Lauder

Introduction

The problems arising during recovery have a quoted incidence ranging from 5% to 40%.[1–4] Common problems in recovery are respiratory complications, pain and postoperative nausea and vomiting (PONV). Errors of judgement, communication failure and inadequate preoperative assessment are contributing factors while previous experience, skilled personnel and detection by monitoring help minimize problems when they occur.[4] The development of the recovery room or postanaesthesia care unit (PACU) resulted from the recognition that there are many common and potentially life-threatening complications that may occur during emergence and recovery from general anaesthesia.[3] For this reason the anaesthetist remains responsible for the patient during their recovery room stay.[5]

The recovery of paediatric patients requires specific paediatric equipment and a suitable environment. The management of a child in recovery is based on an 'ABC' (**A**irway, **B**reathing, **C**irculation) approach. This case report highlights a recovery problem. The subsequent discussion describes a paediatric recovery set up, the 'ABC' approach, and reviews the more common recovery problems that recovery staff and paediatric anaesthetists may need to prevent and/or manage.

Case history

A 3-year-old girl with cerebral palsy was admitted for an arthrogram of her hips. She had spastic quadriplegia, cortical blindness and epilepsy. Her epilepsy manifested as generalized tonic–clonic seizures but was well controlled on clonazepam. Her last fit was over 6 months ago and she had received her morning dose of clonazepam. Further medication consisted of ranitidine (which controlled her symptoms of gastro-oesophageal reflux) and lactulose. She had no known allergies and previous general anaesthesia had been uneventful.

On examination, she weighed 11.6 kg, was lying in bed and unable to communicate. Cardiovascular and respiratory examinations were unremarkable. No further special investigations were considered necessary. She was premedicated with topical local anaesthetic cream to both hands and consent obtained for general anaesthesia and administration of rectal drugs.

Anaesthesia was induced via a 22G cannula (Venflon®) with 1 $\mu g.kg^{-1}$ fentanyl and 2 $mg.kg^{-1}$ propofol. A size 2.0 laryngeal mask airway (LMA) was inserted and anaesthesia maintained with spontaneous ventilation of oxygen, nitrous oxide and isoflurane via an Ayres T-piece with Jackson Rees modification. Prophylactic antibiotics and a loading dose of rectal paracetamol were administered. A warming device was not used because the procedure was anticipated to be quick. The arthrogram proceeded uneventfully and she was transferred to the recovery room 30 minutes later.

On arrival in recovery she was unconscious and required manual support of her airway. Her respiratory rate was 25 breaths per minute, with saturations of 100% in 5 $l.min^{-1}$ oxygen via a Hudson® mask. Her pulse was 95 beats per minute and blood pressure 88/27 mmHg (Figure 23.1). Twenty minutes later she was rousable and able to maintain her own airway but still requiring 4 $l.min^{-1}$ of oxygen. Therefore she was kept in recovery for observation and 20 minutes later she had a prolonged apnoea. This resulted in a desaturation to 80%, which resolved with stimulation. She remained in recovery for further observations and appeared intermittently rousable, but given her premorbid state, her level of consciousness was difficult to assess accurately. Over the next hour her airway was maintained but her oxygen saturations fell to 91%, her

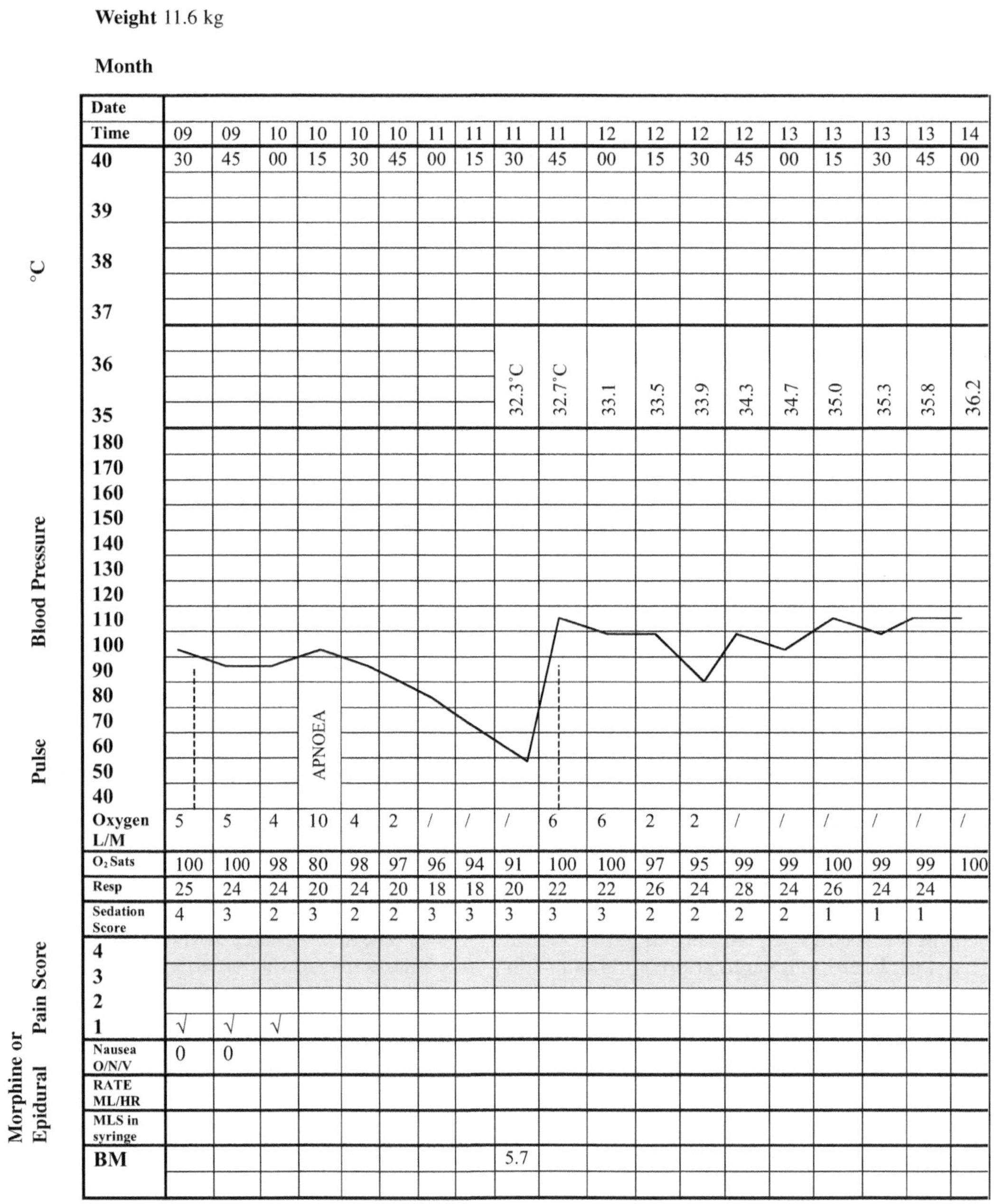

Figure 23.1
Recovery room chart.

heart rate decreased steadily to 50, and she became unrousable. Glucose stix was normal and her temperature found to be 32.3 °C. Oxygen was administered and active external warming measures commenced. Her saturations, heart rate and level of consciousness rapidly improved and over the next few hours her temperature normalized and she was discharged back to the ward.

Discussion

Paediatric recovery room (PACU) set up

The recovery room should be a specially designated, warm and child-friendly area.[5] Protocols covering handover (theatre staff to recovery staff, recovery staff to ward staff), recovery practitioner duties and patient discharge criteria should be available and ideally posted on the wall. Other wall posters include normal age-related values for respiratory and cardiac observations, weight and resuscitation drug doses.

Because detection by monitoring can help minimize problems,[4] the full range of paediatric monitoring including non-invasive blood pressure cuffs, small pulse oximeter probes, and ECG electrodes should be available, as should the full range of sizes of paediatric equipment, including facemasks, airways, breathing systems, nasal prongs, tracheal tubes and laryngoscopes.[5] All these items should also be readily available in latex-free form and stored in a clearly labelled 'latex-free' trolley. A fully equipped resuscitation trolley including a cardiac defibrillator equipped with paediatric paddles must be available and checked daily.

Children require one-to-one supervision throughout their recovery room stay because they are more than twice as likely as an adult to have a complication during recovery from general anaesthesia.[1] Thus staffing levels must reflect this and the staff must be specifically trained in recovery of children because skilled assistance is known to help minimize incidents when they occur.[4,5]

The role of parental presence is controversial but it is recommended that some provision is made for a parent or carer to rejoin their child in recovery as soon as is safely possible. Conclusions from interview data revealed that 100% of parents wanted to be with their child in recovery and that 86% of those allowed to be present felt better as a result of this experience.[6] Parental presence is particularly beneficial if the child is blind, deaf, has behavioural problems, has mental handicap or language or cultural limitations to effective communication. Parents must be willing to comply with nursing requests at all times including being asked to leave PACU if staff deem it necessary.[3,5]

Management

This is based on good communication and an 'ABC' approach.[5,7–11]

Communication

The patient arrives in recovery with an anaesthetist and a theatre practitioner and management begins with a handover which should be listened to carefully and include the following details:

1. Disabilities or previous medical problems explained, including allergies and medications
2. Premedication given
3. State of child and parent on induction of anaesthesia
4. Operation performed
5. Anaesthetic given (including size of endotracheal tube/LMA)
6. Amount of fluid given in theatre and details of blood loss and urine output if appropriate
7. Pain relief given
8. Any problems during the procedure
9. Postoperative fluid and analgesia instructions
10. Any dummies, blankets, comforters, hearing aids or glasses brought with the child.

'ABC' approach

Airway
- If not maintained spontaneously, use manual support or airway adjuncts
- Administer supplemental oxygen and record amount

Breathing
- Record respiratory rate and oxygen saturations every 15 minutes
- Ex-premature infants and term neonates require an apnoea monitor
- Peripheral nerve stimulator and capnography must be immediately available

Circulation
- Record heart rate (and blood pressure for specific cases or at the doctor's request)
- Check surgical wound for bleeding
- ECG monitoring should be immediately available
- Observe intravenous cannulae, wound sites and plaster of Paris casts (POPs) and record every 15 minutes

Disability
- Record level of consciousness on AVPU-type scale (alert, responds to voice, responds to pain, unresponsive)
- Check pupillary light responses and glucose stix if in any doubt or patient at high risk

Environment
- Check temperature in neonates and during lengthy operations

Drugs, drips, drains

- Assess need for analgesia or antiemetics and give as per prescription
- Check intravenous infusions in progress
- Check surgical drains and urinary catheter losses

Documentation and discharge

- Record all the above on the anaesthetic chart or a specifically designed recovery chart
- Do not discharge until discharge criteria are fulfilled

Discharge criteria

The patient may be discharged from recovery when they have met the following criteria:

1. Airway maintained and oxygen saturation levels stable and satisfactory without oxygen
2. Cardiovascularly stable with no bleeding from wound sites
3. Responds to stimuli – eyes open, obeying commands, talking (or other age-appropriate response)
4. Pain free, POP cast comfortable and analgesic regime working satisfactorily
5. Intravenous infusions running freely
6. Drains and catheters working well

Complications

The case above demonstrated two problems which occur in the paediatric recovery room, i.e. apnoea and hypothermia. Apnoea is a common complication and in the case above could have been due to any one of a number of causes including drugs, fits, and/or reflux. Hypothermia in patients with cerebral palsy is common and associated with altered hypothalamic control. There are a multitude of other complications that can occur. Tiret et al reported 27 major complications, including one recovery room death, in a review of 40,240 anaesthetics in children.[12] The incidence of postoperative complications in children range from 0.13% to 40% but the incidence of serious postoperative problems following outpatient surgery in healthy paediatric patients is less than 1%.[1,3] The profile of problems in children differs from adults with respiratory complications and PONV being the commonest while cardiovascular complications are actually very rare. Children are also more likely to experience emergence phenomena and hypothermia. The highest rate of complications occurs in neonates and the lowest rate in the 1–12-month age group.[1,5]

Respiratory complications

Airway and breathing complications are some of the commonest presenting problems in recovery. These include laryngospasm or bronchospasm (up to 40%), prolonged desaturation (19%) and airway obstruction (7–14%). In addition, postextubation stridor, aspiration and pneumothorax all occur with a quoted incidence of between 1% and 5%.[2,4,13] Children at particularly high risk for airway obstruction in the recovery room are those with congenital anomalies (Pierre–Robin, Treacher–Collins or Goldenhar syndromes), those with a history of obstructive sleep apnoea and infants following cleft palate repair.[14] Children with a concurrent respiratory tract infection have up to seven times the likelihood of a respiratory complication and this rises to 11 times if the child's trachea is intubated.[15] Significant medical history such as chronic respiratory disease, neurological impairment and a procedure involving the airway should also be considered predictive of postoperative respiratory complications.[13]

Ex-premature infants are particularly at risk of life-threatening apnoeas and require monitoring for 12–24 hours postoperatively.[7,8] The age at which the ex-premature baby 'outgrows' possible apnoeas is controversial and ranges from 44 to 60 weeks' postconceptual age.[8,9] Term infants less than 44 weeks' postconceptual age are also at risk.[10] Anaemia compounds the problem for the ex-premature infant increasing the incidence of life-threatening apnoeas to 80%.[16] The risk of apnoeas occurs regardless of surgical procedure or anaesthetic technique but regional anaesthesia is associated with a lesser risk although apnoea monitoring remains mandatory.[17,18]

Furthermore, inadequate reversal of neuromuscular blockade causes 7% of cases of inadequate oxygenation/ventilation and is easily overlooked.[4] Partial paralysis with vecuronium causes a decrease in the hypoxic ventilatory response and causes pharyngeal dysfunction, increasing the risk of aspiration.[19,20] Consequently a peripheral nerve stimulator should be readily available, as should capnography, and recovery staff should record respiratory rate, amount of oxygen administered and pulse oximetry as a minimum.[5]

Postoperative nausea and vomiting

PONV is the most frequent side effect of general anaesthesia and the commonest reason for delayed discharge from recovery.[13,21] It is also the commonest cause of unanticipated hospitalization after day case surgery.[22] Although not life-threatening it is a major source of unpleasant experience and recollection for children.[3] The incidence in children ranges from 5% to 80%, although is often quoted as 18–42% it varies depending on patient age, history of car sickness, sex, type of surgery and form of anaesthesia.[1,13,23,24]

Prophylactic administration of antiemetic therapy is not routine because the majority of children do not need it and the commonly used agents have significant adverse effects including sedation, headache and dysphoria.[25] Protocols for management of PONV have been shown to reduce the incidence of moderate to severe postoperative nausea[22,24,25] and in day case surgery prompt curative treatment can be rapidly effective.[25,26] Thus despite PONV being one of the commonest problems occurring in recovery it has been suggested that treatment is more appropriate for selected high-risk patients rather than administering prophylactic antiemetics to all patients.[25,26]

Pain

Untreated postoperative pain causes increased morbidity and mortality, delayed mobilization, prolonged recovery and delayed return to school or playful activities.[27] Pain may also be a contributing factor in postoperative agitation and restlessness.[28]

Historically, pain relief in children has been suboptimal,[29,30] probably due to the misconception that neonates and children do not feel pain. In addition, fears regarding side effects of analgesic drugs (including concerns over addiction) and lack of validated pain assessment tools have confounded the problem. Since the early 1980s these beliefs have gradually been dispelled and there is now an improved understanding and management of pain in children.[31–33]

However, there remains room for improvement. Pain in the recovery phase has been reported by Kokinsky et al to be 75% for mild pain, 20% for moderate pain and 5% for severe pain.[34] Another study by Kotiniemi et al revealed incidences of pain during recovery following day case surgery in hospital as 44% with no pain, 49% with mild pain and 7% with severe pain.[35] In our institution an audit of postoperative pain in 227 consecutive day cases revealed no pain in the recovery room in 95% of children, mild pain in 3%, moderate pain in 1.2% and severe pain in 0.4%.[36]

Pain management begins in the preoperative period with explanation and information given to the family. All types of analgesia appropriate to the planned surgery should be discussed allowing the child and parent some influence in the choice of technique.

Prevention of postoperative pain is the ideal and is more likely if considered pre-emptively. Multimodal therapy involving pharmacological (analgesic drugs and local anaesthetic techniques) and non-pharmacological modes is the basis for this approach. Analgesia must be appropriate to the level of postoperative pain expected. For mild pain, simple analgesics such as paracetamol and/or non-steroidal anti-inflammatory drugs (NSAIDs) usually suffice. For moderate pain, simple analgesics with weak oral opioids are recommended. For severe pain parenteral opioids or regional techniques should be considered.[32] Oral analgesia at the appropriate dose must be given regularly. Parenteral opioid analgesia, if used, must be administered to maintain continuous effective analgesia using either patient-controlled analgesia (PCA) or a continuous infusion.[32] PCA devices can be used for children aged over 5 years. Younger patients or those with learning difficulties will require a continuous infusion or nurse-controlled analgesia (NCA). For certain types of surgery local anaesthetic techniques (for example epidural/caudal, spinal, peripheral nerve blocks) are an alternative. Local anaesthetic infiltration of the surgical incision site at the end of surgery can be effective where appropriate.

Assessment may be difficult especially in the preverbal child but suitable techniques now exist and should be available in the recovery area. For children under 5 years of age, observations of behavioural and physiological changes can be used. Children over 5 years of age can report pain using colour scales, graded pictures of facial expression or visual analogue scales.[27,29] Parental presence in recovery may help to relieve anxiety and fear.[29]

If a child unexpectedly wakes with pain this should be managed immediately using short-acting opioids by the intravenous route until more definitive pain management can be established. Pain that is greater than expected may be of diagnostic significance. The surgical site should be checked and if appropriate reviewed by the surgeon.

All patients in recovery receiving either parenteral opioid infusions or continuous local anaesthetic blockade should be notified to the acute pain team for follow-up. No patient should leave recovery until analgesia is effective.

Emergence phenomena

Occasionally a child will emerge from anaesthesia crying, restless, disorientated and combative. In this situation life-threatening causes such as hypoxia, hypercarbia, hypotension, raised intracranial pressure and metabolic disturbances need to be excluded.[37,38] Other causes include postoperative pain, PONV, sensory deprivation (eye or ear bandages), parental separation, residual central nervous system effects of drugs, fear and anxiety, hunger and thirst.[27,28] In one study in recovery, 58% of distressed children had an attributable cause, which in 25% was due to pain.[28] However, agitation can occur in pain-free children and those not undergoing surgery and seems more common in children under six to 8 years of age.[39]

When other causes are excluded, then disorientation, irritability and restlessness occurs in 10–50% of children during emergence from anaesthesia.[38] Furthermore, emergence may be accompanied by transient symmetric neurological changes such as hyperreflexia, clonus, the Babinski reflex and decerebrate posturing which would otherwise be considered pathological.[27] These symmetrical reflexes can be detected within minutes of discontinuing general anaesthesia and may persist for hours but any focal signs are always abnormal.[27] Inadequate reversal of neuromuscular blockade can also cause abnormal movements and should be excluded. This is another reason to have a peripheral nerve stimulator available.[5]

Disorientation, hallucinations and uncontrolled physical activity may also occur. This hyperactive state commonly occurs after inhalation of volatile anaesthetics and seems to be worst with sevoflurane and desflurane.[27,38,39] There is some suggestion that it may be reduced by the use of preoperative midazolam or intraoperative fentanyl.[40,41]

These emergence phenomena tend to occur during the first 10 minutes of recovery but children who arrive asleep may experience agitation later in their recovery stay.[37] Distress at induction predisposes to distress at arousal.[28]

Gentle reassurance while stroking the child's head or holding their hand are important distractors.

Hypothermia

The incidence of hypothermia in neonates is quoted as 6% compared with 1% for children of all ages.[1] The lower the temperature on admission to recovery then the longer the length of stay.[2]

During surgery heat loss tends to exceed production so body temperature decreases. General anaesthesia typically results in a temperature reduction of 1–3 °C depending on the duration and type of surgery. The main mechanism for cutaneous heat loss is radiation. Convection and conduction from exposed tissues is less important and evaporative losses may become important depending on the type of surgery.[42,43]

Children have a higher surface area to body mass ratio than adults so are more vulnerable to heat loss. Infants maintain normothermia by a combination of vasoconstriction and brown fat thermogenesis but cannot increase their metabolic rate in response to mild intraoperative hypothermia. Over about 1 year of age, non-shivering thermogenesis is replaced by shivering, so hypothermic children tend to shiver postoperatively.[42] Shivering is more effective than non-shivering thermogenesis, increasing heat production by sixfold as opposed to threefold.[43] In addition premature infants and term neonates have little subcutaneous fat and are particularly vulnerable to hypothermia.

Hypothermic neonates are more prone to apnoea, bradycardia, hypoglycaemia, hypotension and acidosis.[3] In adults mild intraoperative hypothermia has been shown to cause prolongation of spontaneous recovery from neuromuscular blockade, thermal discomfort, vasoconstriction, shivering and if below 34 °C, altered platelet function, an increase in bleeding, increased incidence of wound infections, prolonged hospitalization and increased mortality. However, these findings have not been demonstrated in the paediatric population undergoing minor procedures but Booker suggests that ill children and those undergoing major surgery are likely to experience similar problems to adults. Thus he suggests maintaining perioperative normothermia is a prudent strategy.[42]

Hyperthermia

Postoperative fever may result from sepsis or infection, overheating of the patient in the operating room or a metabolic disturbance such as thyroid storm or malignant hyperpyrexia.[3]

Cardiovascular complications

Cardiovascular complications are rarely seen (less than 0.5%) except in those with congenital heart defects.[1] Hypotension is rare but when it occurs may be due to lack of volume replacement, tension pneumothorax or inferior vena cava compression. Hypertension is almost always due to pain but may be due to hypercarbia or emergence delirium. Sinus bradycardia is usually due to hypoxia but may be due to vagal stimulation from a urinary catheter, nasogastric tube or raised intracranial pressure.[3,44,45]

General anaesthetic agents cause a depression of the autonomic nervous system and thus a lack of rapid fluctuations in heart rate and blood pressure.

Conversely recovery is associated with changes in heart rate and blood pressure control as the autonomic inhibition wears off. Children in recovery show an increase in cardiovascular sympathetic drive after major surgery and an overall increase in heart rate and blood pressure variability. But pain, anaemia, blood volume and temperature changes may all also manifest as alterations in autonomic activity and need prompt appropriate treatment.[45]

Drug errors

Drug errors account for 11% of recovery room incidents but the exact causes of these errors are not stated.[4] While human error will never be eliminated entirely, care should be taken to clearly and legibly prescribe on the patient's drug chart any postoperative analgesia, antiemetics, fluids and oxygen that may be needed. An accurate handover will include the patient's usual drug therapy and known allergies as well as the drugs administered in theatre and operative fluid losses and replacement.

Communication failure

All the above management must be recorded in the patient notes either on the anaesthetic record or specifically designed recovery chart.[5] Communication failure contributes to 14% of recovery room incidents and also reflects a lack of preoperative preparation.[4] It should be remembered that the anaesthetist is responsible for the patient until care has been adequately handed over to the recovery staff and an adequate handover includes good, clear, verbal and written communication. This information must also be passed on to ward staff when the patient is discharged from recovery. Given the incidence of drug errors listed above, and communication failure there remains room for improvement in the transmission of information.[4]

When recovery room incidents do occur these should be documented using locally produced 'incident forms'. Properly funded and conducted audit should be undertaken to compare recovery events against national standards. When appropriate, guidelines should be instituted and the audit cycle closed to demonstrate improvement in quality of care.

Learning points

- Problems in recovery are common in children, and include respiratory complications, PONV, pain and emergence phenomena.
- Recovery management necessitates an 'ABC' approach.
- Children require monitoring with appropriately sized equipment and one-to-one nursing care.
- All relevant information must be communicated effectively between healthcare professionals.
- Significant medical history such as chronic respiratory disease, neurological impairment, ex-prematurity and a procedure involving the airway are predictive of postoperative respiratory complications.
- Perioperative hypothermia occurs especially in infants and after long procedures; a high index of suspicion is required for prevention, detection and treatment.
- Recovery room (PACU) practice should be audited to prove or improve quality of care to children.

References

1. Cohen MM, Cameron CB, Duncan PG. Pediatric anesthesia morbidity and mortality in the perioperative period. *Anesth Analg* 1990; 70: 160–167.
2. Hines R, Barash PG, Watrous G, O'Connor T. Complications occurring in the post-anesthesia care unit. *Anesth Analg* 1992; 74: 503–509.
3. Lee B, Wheeler T. Emergence and recovery from anaesthesia for paediatric patients in the post-anaesthesia care unit. *Pediatric Ann* 1997; 26: 461–469.
4. Kluger MT, Bullock MFM. Recovery room incidents: a review of 419 reports from the Anaesthetic Monitoring Study (AIMS). *Anaesthesia* 2002; 57: 1060–1066.
5. Immediate postanaesthetic recovery. Association of Anaesthetists of Great Britain and Northern Ireland, 2002.
6. Graves SA, Berman LS. Caring for children in a general postanesthesia care unit. *Am J Anesthesiol* 1996; 23: 176–181.
7. Ferrari LR. Do children need a preoperative assessment that is different from adults? *Int Anesthesiol Clin* 2002; 40: 167–186.
8. Kurth CD, Spizter AR, Broennie AM, Downes JJ. Postoperative apnea in preterm infants. *Anesthesiology* 1987; 66: 483–488.
9. Welborn LG, Ramirez N, Tae Hee Oh et al. Postanesthetic apnea and periodic breathing in infants. *Anesthesiology* 1986; 65: 658–661.
10. Noseworthy J, Duran C, Khine HH. Postoperative apnea in a full term infant. *Anesthesiology* 1989; 70: 879–880.
11. Recovery Protocol (related best practice standards). 09/21, 09/22 and 09/23. Bristol Royal Hospital for Children.

12. Tiret L, Nivoche Y, Hatton F et al. Complications related to anesthesia in infants and children: a prospective study of 40240 anesthetics. *Br J Anaesth* 1988; 61: 263–269.
13. D'Errico C, Veopel-Lewis TD, Siewert M, Malviya S. Prolonged recovery stay and unplanned admission of the pediatric surgical outpatient: an observational study. *J Clin Anesth* 1998; 10: 482–487.
14. Cauldwell CB. Induction, maintenance and emergence. In: Gregory GA (ed.). *Pediatric Anesthesia*, 3rd Edn. New York, NY: Churchill Livingstone, Inc; 1994: 227–792.
15. Parnis SJ, Barker DS, Van Der Walt JH. Clinical predictors of anaesthetic complications in children with respiratory tract infections. *Paediatr Anaesth* 2001; 11: 29–40.
16. Welborn LG, Hannallah RS, Luban NLC et al. Anemia and postoperative apnea in former preterm infants. *Anesthesiology* 1991; 74: 1003–1006.
17. Lui LMP, Cote CJ, Goudsouzian NG et al. Life-threatening apnea in infants recovering from anesthesia. *Anesthesiology* 1983; 59: 506–510.
18. Williams JM, Stoddart PA, Williams SAR, Wolf AR. Post-operative recovery after inguinal herniotomy in ex-premature infants: comparison between sevoflurane and spinal anaesthesia. *Br J Anaesth* 2001; 86: 366–371.
19. Eriksson LI, Sato M, Severinghaus JW. Effect of a vecuronium-induced partial neuromuscular block on hypoxic ventilatory response. *Anesthesiology* 1993; 78: 693–699.
20. Eriksson LI, Sundman E, Olsson R et al. Functional assessment of the pharynx at rest and during swallowing in partially paralysed humans. *Anesthesiology* 1997; 87: 1035–1043.
21. Patel RI, Hannallah RS. Anesthetic complications following pediatric ambulatory surgery: a three year study. *Anesthesiology* 1988; 69: 1009–1012.
22. Watch MF, White PF. Postoperative nausea and vomiting: its etiology, treatment and prevention. *Anesthesiology* 1992; 77: 162–184.
23. Baines D. Postoperative nausea and vomiting in children. *Paediatr Anaesth* 1996; 6: 7–14.
24. Drake R, Anderson BJ, Persson MA, Thompson JMD. Impact of an antiemetic protocol on postoperative nausea and vomiting in children. *Paediatr Anaesth* 2001; 11: 85–91.
25. Rose JB, Watch MF. Postoperative nausea and vomiting in paediatric patients. *Br J Anaesth* 1999; 83: 104–117.
26. Villeret I, Laffon M, Duchalais A et al. Incidence of postoperative nausea and vomiting in paediatric ambulatory surgery. *Paediatr Anaesth* 2002; 12: 712–717.
27. Yaster M, Sola JE, Pegoli W, Paidas CN. Postoperative management of the pediatric outpatient – surgical and anesthetic aspects. *Pediatr Clin North Am* 1994; 41: 199–219.
28. Holm-Knudsen RJ, Carlin JB, McKenzie IM. Distress at induction of anaesthesia in children. A survey of incidence, associated factors and recovery characteristics. *Paediatr Anaesth* 1998; 8: 383–392.
29. No authors listed. Managing acute pain in children. *Drug Ther Bull* 1995: 33: 41–44.
30. Lichtor JL. Clinical challenges in paediatric ambulatory patients. *Ambulat Surg* 1998: 6; 57–60.
31. Taddido A, Katz J, Ileresich AL, Koren G. Effect of neonatal circumcision on pain response during subsequent routine vaccination. *Lancet* 1997; 349: 599–603.
32. Tobias JD. Postoperative pain management. *Pediatr Ann* 1997; 26: 490–500.
33. Mather L, Mackie J. The incidence of postoperative pain in children. *Pain* 1983; 15: 271–282.
34. Kokinsky E, Thornberg E, Ostlund AL, Larsson LE. Postoperative comfort in paediatric outpatient surgery. *Paediatr Anaesth* 1999; 9: 243–251.
35. Kotiniemi LH, Ryhanen PT, Valanne J et al. Postoperative symptoms at home following day-case surgery in children: a multicentre survey of 551 children. *Anaesthesia* 1997; 52: 963–969.
36. Waterhouse P, Lauder G. There are a few tears at bedtime: results of a paediatric daycase postoperative pain and nausea and vomiting audit. *Paediatr Anaesth* 2001; 11: 753–772.
37. Cole JW, Murray DJ, McAllister D, Hirshberg GE. Emergence behavior in children: defining the incidence of excitement and agitation following anaesthesia. *Paediatr Anaesth* 2002; 12: 442–447.
38. Welborn LG, Hannallah RS, Norden JM et al. Comparison of emergence and recovery characteristics of sevoflurane, desflurane and halothane in pediatric ambulatory patients. *Anesth Analg* 1996; 83: 917–920.
39. Johr M. Postanaesthesia excitation. *Paediatr Anaesth* 2002; 12: 293–295.
40. Hallen J, Rawal N, Gupta A. Postoperative recovery following outpatient pediatric myringotomy: a comparison between sevoflurane and halothane. *J Clin Anesth* 2001; 13: 161–166.
41. Cohen IT, Hannallah RS, Hummer KA. The incidence of emergence agitation associated with desflurane anesthesia in children is reduced by fentanyl. *Anesth Analg* 2001; 93: 88–91.
42. Booker PD. Equipment and monitoring in paediatric anaesthesia. *Br J Anaesth* 1999; 83: 78–90.
43. Kirkbridge DA, Buggy DJ. Thermoregulation and mild peri-operative hypothermia. *Br J Anaesth CEPD Review* 2003; 3: 24–28.
44. Westman HR. Postoperative complications and unanticipated hospital admissions. *Semin Pediatr Surg* 1999; 8: 23–29.
45. Constant I, Laude D, Elghozi JL, Murat I. Assessment of autonomic cardiovascular changes associated with recovery from anaesthesia in children: a study using spectral analysis of blood pressure and heart rate variability. *Paediatr Anaesth* 2000; 10: 653–660.

24

The screaming child

Andy Tatman

Introduction

Anaesthetizing a large screaming child may be very difficult. Besides the practical considerations of anaesthetizing an uncooperative, physically big patient, the issues of competence and the right to refuse treatment become relevant. This chapter will explore such a case.

Case history

A 10-year-old boy presented to the accident and emergency department with an open eye injury which occurred 1 hour prior to admission. He and his brother had been sword fighting with bamboo sticks. He tripped and sustained an eye injury from one of the sticks. On arrival the child was crying and his mother was clearly very upset. The child was very uncooperative and tearful; he complained that his eye hurt. He was given paracetamol 1 g and codeine 35 mg, orally. Despite this the ophthalmic surgeon was unable to assess the degree of injury to the eye and therefore requested an urgent examination under anaesthetic. The child was seen by a trainee anaesthetist who explained the planned procedure and the importance of establishing intravenous access prior to surgery. The findings of the history and examination are summarized in Table 24.1.

Amethocaine 4% gel was applied to the two most promising veins with some reluctance from the child. He was then transferred to the paediatric ward. One hour later, the operating theatre staff were ready to proceed but the child refused to leave the ward. The anaesthetist was called to the ward to find the child shouting and screaming that he did not want to have it done. His mother was visibly upset, his father seemed calmer. The student nurse was unable to reason with him. It become apparent that he was terrified of needles as a result of numerous unsuccessful attempts at venous cannulation during his admission for appendicectomy. A senior anaesthetist was asked for advice.

The eye was at risk from his distress and any further attempts to coerce him were likely to make matters worse, particularly in view of his size. The senior nurse on the ward was asked to help and it was decided to offer the child premedication in the form of midazolam 20 mg (approximately 0.5 mg.kg^{-1}) mixed with neat

Past medical history	Appendicectomy aged 8, otherwise fit and healthy
Anaesthetic history	No problems with previous anaesthesia, apparently difficult venous access
Starvation status	The child ate a full meal 30 minutes prior to his accident
Medications	None
ASA grade	I
Allergies	None known
Examination	Obese, actual weight 50 kg (lean weight estimated to be 35 kg) Normal airway Chest clear, SaO_2 97% in air Normal heart sounds Pulse 100 bpm, BP 110/50 mmHg No other injuries

Table 24.1
History and examination findings

blackcurrant squash (his favourite flavoured drink). This was discussed with the child. He was reassured that the venous cannulation would not hurt with the amethocaine cream but he replied 'that is what they said last time'. He was offered the premedication but refused it, despite some cajoling by his mother, the nursing staff and the anaesthetist.

It was decided that a different approach was needed. His parents were taken on a tour of the ward and the planned procedure was again explained to them. They were given an information booklet about the ward and the operating theatre procedure. The necessity of venous access was reiterated. The mother asked questions and seemed calmer after the tour of the ward.

After discussion and agreement from the ophthalmic surgeon it was decided to use 50% nitrous oxide in oxygen (Entonox®) to facilitate the cannulation. This was explained to the parents.

During the discussions with the parents, the senior sister on the ward established more of a rapport with the child and learnt that he played a lot of computer games. Further enquiry established which were his favourite games. The child was still very anxious, not letting anybody touch him. The purpose of the Entonox® was explained to the child. The senior sister managed to calm him down by encouraging him to breathe slowly and practise with a flavoured facemask. This was attached to an Entonox® apparatus and the child was encouraged to breathe through the mask and to focus on the sound of the valve each time he breathed. It was again explained to the child that a cannula had to be inserted and that it would not hurt. The child was given some control of the situation by being allowed to say when the attempted cannulation could be performed. The cannula was successfully inserted without distress or pain to the child, secured in place and flushed to confirm its patency. His mother was still upset and agreed to stay on the ward, while he was transferred to the anaesthetic room accompanied by his father and the senior sister. His father was asked to support the child in a calm and reassuring manner. The child was permitted to use the Entonox® if necessary.

The theatre staff were prewarned and asked to remain quiet while the number of staff in the anaesthetic room were kept to a minimum. It was agreed beforehand that only the anaesthetist and the father would talk to the child. Once in theatre, the child was preoxygenated with 100% oxygen, via a Mapleson C circuit. The patient was encouraged to focus on the inflation and deflation of the reservoir bag. A pulse oximeter was attached and alfentanil $20\,\mu g.kg^{-1}$ was given intravenously. After 30 seconds, propofol 120 mg, containing 20 mg of lignocaine, was given. Cricoid pressure was applied on loss of the eyelash reflex. The senior sister escorted the father out of the anaesthetic room back to the ward. The cannula was flushed with normal saline and immediately followed with rocuronium 45 mg. The cannula was flushed with normal saline again. A peripheral nerve stimulator was attached and he was intubated with a 6.0 cuffed tracheal tube, once neuromuscular paralysis was complete. The position of the tube was confirmed by auscultation and anaesthesia was maintained with isoflurane in air and oxygen. Prior to the end of surgery, which lasted 90 minutes, he was given ondansetron 4 mg intravenously and codeine 30 mg intramuscularly. On completion of surgery, a wide-bore nasogastric tube was inserted and the stomach emptied. He was extubated awake, in the left lateral position.

The child made an uneventful recovery and displayed no further behavioural problems prior to his discharge 24 hours later.

Discussion

This case is one of those nightmare scenarios. The child has an open eye injury, is not starved, is obese, screaming and uncooperative. It doesn't get much worse. However, the pivotal issue is the full stomach, with the risk of pulmonary aspiration of gastric contents. While discussing the other issues, one must not lose sight of this central issue.

It is not uncommon to be faced with a screaming child, who either refuses to leave the ward or, more commonly, starts screaming once in the anaesthetic room. In many of these situations, there are clues from the initial history that suggest that the child will be upset. If these go unheeded, as in this case, by the time the child is ready to be brought to the anaesthetic room, the situation may be much more difficult to control. Indeed, most children who are very anxious on the ward will come to the operating theatre very anxious, unless there is some preoperative intervention, such as premedication or play therapy.[1] The majority of children are genuinely frightened, whether it is fear of separation in small children or fear of not waking up in older children. However, for a minority of children, there are behavioural problems or complex child–parent power struggles. With these cases, one cannot hope to deal with these problems, which have been reinforced over many years, in the few minutes

Box 1 Predictors of perioperative anxiety
Parental anxiety
Previous bad medical experience
Shy or inhibited children (low self-esteem)
Poor adaptive behaviour
Children with behavioural problems
Low IQ

before surgery. However, an ability to recognize those children with whom problems are likely and the early involvement of senior medical and nursing staff, together with an understanding of the legal issues surrounding a dissenting child, makes their management considerably less complex (Box 1).[2]

This child has a number of risk factors for being very anxious. Obese children, particularly in non-obese communities, commonly have behavioural problems, associated with altered body image, teasing at school and poor self-esteem.[3–5] The previous admission for appendicitis was clearly traumatic for him. It increased his anxiety of medical procedures, in particular venepuncture, which is well known to generate significant anxiety anyway, and he is now highly suspicious of medical staff.[6–9] However, it did tell us that we could probably intubate him successfully. His mother was very anxious and parental anxiety has repeatedly been shown to a strong predictor of whether a child will be distressed.[8,10–13] This is particularly true for smaller children who use social referencing to assess a stranger or new situation. A smiling, happy parent means the stranger is probably okay. A crying parent who is stroking and kissing the child, saying don't worry, mummy loves you, is sending the child very mixed messages.[14]

In order to reduce preoperative anxiety, three aspects need to be tackled.[11] Firstly, the environment must be conducive to minimizing what is already an anxiety provoking experience. Secondly, the anxiety of the parents needs to be addressed by discussion, reading information leaflets and a tour of the ward.[15] Thirdly, the child's anxiety needs to be addressed. Failing to deal with any one of these three aspects can easily undo an attempt to reduce a child's anxiety. Much of the research available refers to planned admissions for elective surgery. However, the principles still apply in the emergency situation; one just has less time to implement them. Dealing with the parents' anxiety was helpful, as was allowing the calmer of the two into the anaesthetic room. Anxious parents in the anaesthetic room make matters worse.[16,17] Setting the environment in the operating theatre beforehand avoided any sudden interruptions that might have tipped the child over the edge again. In the elective situation, problems such as severe anxiety or needle phobia can be tackled before admission, with the help of the departments of clinical psychology and play therapy. Once admitted, the lack of urgency lends itself to a variety of anxiety reducing techniques (Box 2).[18] In this case, we did not have the luxury of time and the operation was 'out of hours'. The techniques available in the emergency situation should be easily learnt and be able to be implemented in a matter of minutes; these are relaxation, focusing/distraction, imagery and positive reinforcement. Before using the techniques, one has to find a 'way in' and get the child's attention. This may be by talking about something unrelated to his medical problem, such as school, films or the latest craze, or in this case, computer games. Once you have the child's attention, try to reduce the overall level of anxiety by getting the child to focus on something, usually breathing. By using imagery, such as getting the child to imagine blowing a feather or that he or she is a balloon and is slowly letting the air out, the breathing is slowed. This produces both relaxation and distraction, thereby lowering the level of anxiety. This allows a more coherent conversation and the development of a rapport. Now one can reassure the child that he or she will be kept informed of what is going to happen, will be involved in the decisions and will not lose control. Positive reinforcement, such as bravery stickers, rarely works in the severely anxious child. Once the child is calmer, it does have a valuable role and is quick and easy to implement. Modelling, again, once the child is calmer can be useful. Modelling shows a similar child,

Box 2 Behavioural and cognitive strategies for preoperative anxiety
Relaxation
Distraction
Modelling
Positive reinforcement
Imagery
Thought stopping
Hypnosis
Memory change
Desensitization

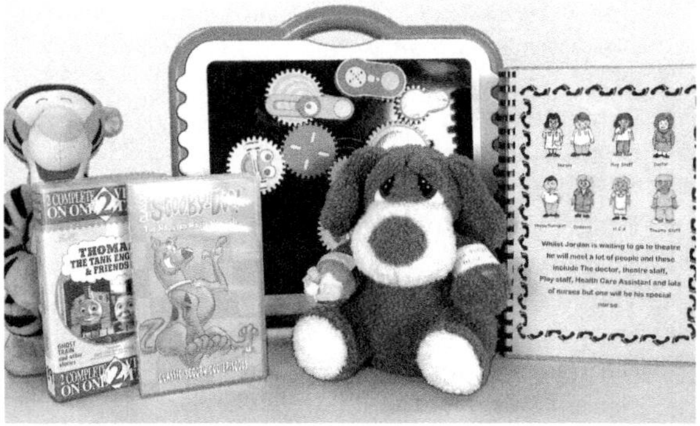

Figure 24.1
Simple devices for distraction and modelling. The toys make a noise and move, adding further to their usefulness for distraction. For smaller children, the bear is a useful modelling tool, with a cannula and an identity bracelet. For older children, the information booklet shows photographs of a child going through the stages of admission, preparation for theatre, transfer to the operating theatre, recovery and discharge.

who is anxious, about to undergo a procedure, but who copes successfully. With older children, this is often best achieved with a video, while with a younger child, a doll or toy with a cannula in situ can be used. Figure 24.1 shows simple devices for distraction and modelling. Some children are self-modellers. They can relate their current experience to a previous one and see that they coped before. Memory change, thought stopping, desensitization and hypnosis all require specialist training and the first three require considerable time to implement, making them unsuitable in the emergency situation.[19]

These techniques will often calm a child sufficiently so that the child will take some form of premedication. However, this may be a particular problem in obese children, as the dose may be difficult to predict. Not enough and the child may be more disturbed. Too much and there is the risk that excessive sedation, in an unstarved patient, will increase the risk of aspiration. Oral or sublingual midazolam, in a dose of $0.5\,mg.kg^{-1}$, is effective in reducing anxiety in many children.[1,20–24] However, it requires the compliance of the child, otherwise it will be rejected. The nasal and rectal routes are alternatives but would be unsuitable in this case. The nasal route is effective but 50% of children cry and many describe it as horrible.[25,26] Rectal administration is unlikely to be achieved without a struggle, particularly in a child of this size. Other orally administered anxiolytics include diazepam, ketamine, oral transmucosal fentanyl citrate and clonidine.[24,27,28] As with oral midazolam, these all require the compliance of the child. Although less popular, the intramuscular route will achieve drug administration if other routes are not available. In this case, intramuscular ketamine would probably have been the next approach, had the Entonox® not worked. Ketamine does increase intraocular pressure, as would restraining the patient while the injection is given. The risk to the eye from the injection must be weighed against the risk from a more uncooperative child at the time of induction. Other intramuscular anxiolytics would include an opioid, either alone or in combination with a phenothiazine or hyoscine, and midazolam. In this case, nitrous oxide/oxygen was used as sedation to achieve venous access. Although amethocaine cream was used to anaesthetize the skin, this does not necessarily improve patient cooperation. 50% N_2O in oxygen abolishes anxiety and pain in nearly 60% of children undergoing venepuncture.[29] Its safety and effectiveness, in the presence of a full stomach, is proven with its routine use in obstetrics. Higher concentrations of N_2O confer no additional benefit but produce excitation and a reduced level of consciousness, with the concomitant loss of protective airway reflexes. In addition to the drug effect, the child was able to focus on his breathing and the sound of the valve, providing both relaxation and distraction, while the cannula was inserted.

The issue of consent in this case is fairly straightforward. The child is a minor and is incompetent. He is under 16 years of age and has an understandable fear of needles but this fear has clouded his understanding of the purpose and nature of the procedure, as well as the consequences of not having the procedure done, i.e. losing the eye. The child's parents and his doctors have a responsibility to ensure that his best interests are served. In this case, he has an open eye injury and without treatment, he will very likely lose the eye. The parents can therefore authorize the treatment of their son, even if he dissents. The law supports parents and doctors who override a dissenting child for urgent or essential treatment. The amount of force or coercion used in achieving this end is an individual decision, but must take into account the consequences of such action, including injuries to staff, the patient, in this case loss of the contents of the eye from struggling, and longer term psychological problems with the child.[30]

The anaesthetic management of the open eye injury largely comprises three elements, the control of intraocular pressure (IOP), the rapid control of the airway and the management of associated injuries, if present.

A sudden rise in IOP may cause a choroidal haemorrhage and expulsion of the contents of the globe. Ketamine and suxamethonium both increase IOP, while thiopentone and propofol both cause a fall in IOP. Non-depolarizing neuromuscular blocking agents either have no effect or produce a fall in IOP. Laryngoscopy with an inadequate depth of anaesthesia or Valsalva manoeuvres, such as crying, coughing and struggling, produce a significant rise in IOP. Therefore, the ideal anaesthetic for an open eye injury should avoid any rise in IOP by smooth induction, excellent intubation conditions and blunting of the haemodynamic response to laryngoscopy and intubation.[31,32]

The risk of pulmonary aspiration is greatest when the airway is unprotected and consciousness is impaired. The optimal anaesthetic is a rapid sequence induction with preoxygenation and cricoid pressure, which will minimize the time between loss of protective airway reflexes and tracheal intubation. Alternative approaches to anaesthesia in this case would have to include awake intubation, regional anaesthesia or gaseous induction with cricoid pressure.[33] Finally, not attempting anaesthesia until the stomach is empty must be considered, and may be appropriate if the eye is not viable. However, after traumatic injuries, particularly if opioid analgesia has been used, the emptying of the stomach is delayed.[34,35] The obesity adds several problems, including potential airway difficulties, both ventilation and intubation, increased risk of regurgitation, problems estimating the appropriate drug dosages and difficult venous access.

In this case, a rapid sequence intravenous induction with propofol, alfentanil and rocuronium was used. The decision to use rocuronium raises two issues. Firstly, how much rocuronium to use and should the dose be modified in obesity? The adult rapid-onset dose of rocuronium is 0.6 $mg.kg^{-1}$, based upon two times the ED95 (effective dose in 95% of subjects), which is 0.3 $mg.kg^{-1}$.[36] The ED95 in children varies with age; in neonates and small infants, it is 0.25 $mg.kg^{-1}$, while in children it is 0.41 $mg.kg^{-1}$.[37] This may explain the variation in intubating conditions reported with 0.6 $mg.kg^{-1}$, when compared to suxamethonium.[38,39] Rocuronium 0.9 $mg.kg^{-1}$ produces more consistent intubating conditions.[40,41] Unlike vecuronium, which lasts up to 50% longer in obesity, the duration of action of rocuronium does not appear to be altered by obesity.[42,43] The dose should be calculated on the obese weight, just as with suxamethonium, rather than on an estimated lean weight.[36,44]

Secondly, the use of a long-acting, compared with suxamethonium, neuromuscular blocking agent in a rapid sequence induction is a balance of risks. Rocuronium does not cause a rise in IOP and, in this case, there was a high likelihood of successful intubation. The use of alfentanil obtunds the rise in IOP secondary to laryngoscopy and intubation. The operation would last at least an hour so the large dose of rocuronium would not have delayed recovery. Had there been doubt about the ability to intubate or that effective ventilation might have proved difficult in the event of a failed intubation, then suxamethonium would have been a safer choice.

Both suxamethonium and rocuronium, in an appropriate dose, produce a rapid onset of good/excellent intubating conditions.[38,40,41] The extent and significance of the rise in IOP caused by suxamethonium is still debated.[32,45,46] Many studies have relied upon intermittent measurements of IOP and may have missed short lived, but nonetheless significant rises, particularly at laryngoscopy and intubation, when access to the patient would have been restricted. Where IOP is measured continuously, and suxamethonium is given immediately after thiopentone (5 $mg.kg^{-1}$), there is a small (10%) rise above baseline.[47] Laryngoscopy produces a much greater (nearly 50%) rise above baseline, which is larger with propofol than thiopentone.[47] These rises in IOP may be controlled by either pretreatment with a non-depolarizing neuromuscular blocker, such as rocuronium 0.1 $mg.kg^{-1}$, or by modifying the response to laryngoscopy and intubation with lignocaine (1.5 $mg.kg^{-1}$) or alfentanil (15–40 $\mu g.kg^{-1}$).[48–55] Provided an adequate dose of induction agent is used and the response to laryngoscopy is obtunded, there is little to choose between the two muscle relaxants with regard to IOP. It would seem that the choice between a non-depolarizing neuromuscular blocker and suxamethonium should be decided by the airway and laryngoscopy requirements of the patient rather than concerns about increases in IOP.

Learning points

- Preoperative anxiety can often be predicted.
- Management of the environment, the parents and the child is necessary if controlling the child's anxiety is to be successful.
- The early intervention by experienced staff may stabilize a deteriorating situation.
- Midazolam, either orally or intranasally, is effective at alleviating anxiety.
- Simple anxiety-reducing techniques, such as distraction, focusing, imagery and positive reinforcement, are easily learnt and may be quickly applied.
- Attempts to minimize rises in intraocular pressure are essential in suspected open eye injury.
- The choice of neuromuscular blocking agent in the unfasted open eye injury should be guided by the needs of the airway.

References

1. Holm-Knudsen RJ, Carlin JB, McKenzie IM. Distress at induction of anaesthesia in children. A survey of incidence, associated factors and recovery characteristics. *Paediatr Anaesth* 1998; 8: 383–392.
2. McCann ME, Kain ZN. The management of preoperative anxiety in children: an update. *Anesth Analg* 2001; 93: 98–105.
3. Braet C, Mervielde I, Vandereycken W. Psychological aspects of childhood obesity: a controlled study in a clinical and nonclinical sample. *J Pediatr Psychol* 1997; 22: 59–71.
4. Strauss RS, Rodzilsky D, Burack G, Colin M. Pyschosocial correlates of physical activity in healthy children. *Arch Pediatr Adolesc Med* 2001; 155: 897–902.
5. Pastore DR, Fisher M, Friedman SB. Abnormalities in weight status, eating attitudes, and eating behaviors among urban high school students: correlations with self-esteem and anxiety. *J Adolesc Health* 1996; 18: 312–319.
6. Humphrey GB, Boon CMJ, van Linden van den Heuvell GF, van de Wiel HB. The occurrence of high levels of acute behavioral distress in children and adolescents undergoing routine venipunctures. *Pediatrics* 1992; 90: 87–91.
7. Kolk AM, van Hoof R, Fiedeldij Dop MJ. Preparing children for venepuncture. The effect of an integrated intervention on distress before and during venepuncture. *Child Care Health Dev* 2000; 26: 251–260.
8. Kain ZN, Mayes LC, O'Connor TZ, Cicchetti DV. Preoperative anxiety in children – predictors and outcomes. *Arch Pediatr Adolesc Med* 1996; 150: 1238–1245.
9. Lumley MA, Melamed BG, Abeles LA. Predicting children's presurgical anxiety and subsequent behavior changes. *J Pediatr Psychol* 1993; 18: 481–497.
10. Frank NC, Blount RL, Smith AJ et al. Parent and staff behavior, previous child medical experience, and maternal anxiety as they relate to child procedural distress and coping. *J Pediatr Psychol* 1995; 20: 277–289.
11. McGraw T. Preparing children for the operating room: psychological issues. *Can J Anaesth* 1994; 41: 1094–1103.
12. Kain ZN, Mayes LC, Weisman SJ, Hofstadter MB. Social adaptability, cognitive abilities, and other predictors for children's reactions to surgery. *J Clin Anesth* 2000; 12: 549–554.
13. Bevan JC, Johnston C, Haig MJ et al. Preoperative parental anxiety predicts behavioural and emotional responses to induction of anaesthesia in children. *Can J Anaesth* 1990; 37: 177–182.
14. Walker-Andrews AS. Emotions and social development: infants' recognition of emotions in others. *Pediatrics* 1998; 102: 1268–1271.
15. Bellew M, Atkinson KR, Dixon G, Yates A. The introduction of a paediatric anaesthesia information leaflet: an audit of its impact on parental anxiety and satisfaction. *Paediatr Anaesth* 2002; 12: 124–130.
16. Cameron JA, Bond MJ, Pointer SC. Reducing the anxiety of children undergoing surgery: parental presence during anaesthetic induction. *J Paediatr Child Health* 1996; 32: 51–56 .
17. Kam PCA, Voss TJV, Gold PD, Pitkin J. Behaviour of children associated with parental participation during induction of general anaesthesia. *J Paediatr Child Health* 1998; 34: 29–31.
18. Chen E, Joseph MH, Zeltzer LK. Behavioral and cognitive interventions in the treatment of pain in children. *Pediatr Clin North Am* 2000; 47: 513–525.
19. Powers SW. Empirically supported treatments in pediatric psychology: procedure-related pain. *J Pediatr Psychol* 1999; 24: 131–145.
20. McGraw T, Kendrick A. Oral midazolam premedication and postoperative behaviour in children. *Paediatr Anaesth* 1998; 8: 117–121.
21. Khahil S, Philbrook L, Rabb M et al. Sublingual midazolam premedication in children: a dose response study. *Paediatr Anaesth* 1998; 8: 461–465.
22. Lammers CR, Rosner JL, Crockett DE et al. Oral midazolam with an antacid may increase the speed of onset of sedation in children prior to general anaesthesia. *Paediatr Anaesth* 2002; 12: 26–28.
23. Weldon BC, Watcha NF, White PF. Oral midazolam in children: effect of time and adjunctive therapy. *Anesth Analg* 1992; 75: 51–55.
24. Fazi L, Jantzen EC, Rose JB et al. A comparison of oral clonidine and oral midazolam as preanesthetic medications in the pediatric tonsillectomy patient. *Anesth Analg* 2001; 92: 56–61.

25. Griffith N, Howell S, Mason DG. Intranasal midazolam for premedication of children undergoing day-case anaesthesia: comparison of two delivery systems with assessment of intra-observer variability. *Br J Anaesth* 1998; 81: 865–869.
26. Theroux MC, West DW, Corddry DH et al. Efficacy of intranasal midazolam in facilitating suturing of lacerations in preschool children in the emergency department. *Pediatrics* 1993; 91: 624–627.
27. Tobias JD, Phipps S, Smith B, Mulhern RK. Oral ketamine premedication to alleviate the distress of invasive procedures in pediatric oncology patients. *Pediatrics* 1992; 90: 537–541.
28. Funk W, Jakob W, Riedl T, Taeger K. Oral preanaesthetic medication for children: double-blind randomized study of a combination of midazolam and ketamine vs midazolam or ketamine alone. *Br J Anaesth* 2000; 84: 335–340.
29. Henderson JM, Spence DG, Komocar LM et al. Administration of nitrous oxide to pediatric patients provides analgesia for venous cannulation. *Anesthesiology* 1990; 72: 269–271.
30. Edgar J, Morton NS, Pace NA. Review of ethics in paediatric anaesthesia: consent issues. *Paediatr Anaesth* 2001; 11: 355–359.
31. Hamid RKA, Newfield P. Pediatric eye emergencies. *Anesthesiol Clin North Am* 2001; 19: 257–264.
32. Cunningham AJ, Barry P. Intraocular pressure – physiology and implications for anaesthetic management. *Can Anaesth Soc J* 1986; 33: 195–208.
33. Simonson D. Retrobulbar block for open-eye injuries: a report of 19 cases. *CRNA* 1992; 3: 35–37.
34. Bricker SR, McLuckie A, Nightingale DA. Gastric aspirates after trauma in children. *Anaesthesia* 1989; 44: 721–724.
35. Schurizek BA, Rybro L, Boggild-Madsen NB, Juhl B. Gastric volume and pH in children for emergency surgery. *Acta Anaesthesiol Scand* 1986; 30: 404–408.
36. Puhringer FK, Keller C, Kleinsasser A et al. Pharmacokinetics of rocuronium bromide in obese female patients. *Eur J Anaesthesiol* 1999; 16: 507–510.
37. Taivainen T, Meretoja OA, Erkola O et al. Rocuronium in infants, children and adults during balanced anaesthesia. *Paediatr Anaesth* 1996; 6: 271–275.
38. Stoddart PA, Mather SJ. Onset of neuromuscular blockade and intubating conditions one minute after the administration of rocuronium in children. *Paediatr Anaesth* 1998; 8: 37–40.
39. Lee SK, Kim JR, Bai SJ et al. Effects of priming with pancuronium or rocuronium on intubation with rocuronium in children. *Yonsei Med J* 1999; 40: 327–330.
40. Chiu CL, Jaais F, Wang CY. Effect of rocuronium compared with succinylcholine on intraocular pressure during rapid sequence induction of anaesthesia. *Br J Anaesth* 1999; 82: 757–760.
41. Cheng CA, Aun CS, Gin T. Comparison of rocuronium and suxamethonium for rapid tracheal intubation in children. *Paediatr Anaesth* 2002; 12: 140–145.
42. Sinha S, Jain AK, Bhattacharya A. Effect of nutritional status on vecuronium induced neuromuscular blockade. *Anaesth Intens Care* 1998; 26: 392–395.
43. Schwartz AE, Matteo RS, Ornstein E et al. Pharmacokinetics and pharmacodynamics of vecuronium in the obese surgical patient. *Anesth Analg* 1992; 74: 515–518.
44. Rose JB, Theroux MC, Katz MS. The potency of succinylcholine in obese adolescents. *Anesth Analg* 2000; 90: 576–578.
45. Edmondson L, Lindsay SL, Lanigan LP et al. Intraocular pressure changes during rapid sequence induction of anaesthesia. A comparison between thiopentone and suxamethonium and thiopentone and atracurium. *Anaesthesia* 1988; 43: 1005–1010.
46. Calobrisi BL, Lebowitz P. Muscle relaxants and the open globe. *Int Anesthesiol Clin* 1990; 28: 83–88.
47. Zimmerman AA, Funk KJ, Tidwell JL. Propofol and alfentanil prevent the increase in intraocular pressure caused by succinylcholine and endotracheal intubation during a rapid sequence induction of anesthesia. *Anesth Analg* 1996; 83: 814–817.
48. Tsui BC, Reid S, Gupta S et al. A rapid precurarization technique using rocuronium. *Can J Anaesth* 1998; 45: 397–401.
49. Chiu CL, Lang CC, Wong PK et al. The effect of mivacurium pretreatment on intra-ocular pressure changes induced by suxamethonium. *Anaesthesia* 1998; 53: 501–505.
50. Martin R, Carrier J, Pirlet M et al. Rocuronium is the best non-depolarizing relaxant to prevent succinylcholine fasciculations and myalgia. *Can J Anaesth* 1998; 45: 521–525.
51. Grover VK, Lata K, Sharma S et al. Efficacy of lignocaine in the suppression of the intra-ocular pressure response to suxamethonium and tracheal intubation. *Anaesthesia* 1989; 44: 22–25.
52. Polarz H, Böhrer H, Fleischer F et al. Effects of thiopentone/suxamethonium on intraocular pressure after pretreatment with alfentanil. *Eur J Clin Pharmacol* 1992; 43: 311–313.
53. Polarz H, Böhrer H, Martin E et al. Oral clonidine premedication prevents the rise in intraocular pressure following succinylcholine administration. *German J Ophthalmol* 1993; 2: 97–99.
54. Drenger B, Pe'er J. Attenuation of ocular and systemic responses to tracheal intubation by intravenous lignocaine. *Br J Ophthalmol* 1987; 71: 546–548.
55. Morton NS, Hamilton WF. Alfentanil in an anaesthetic technique for penetrating eye injuries. *Anaesthesia* 1986; 41: 1148–1151.

25

Anaesthesia for strabismus surgery

Stephen J Mather

Introduction

Strabismus surgery is a common procedure undertaken in young children often before they start school. It is usually performed outside paediatric centres with the anaesthesia provided by a non-specialist paediatric anaesthetist. The following history illustrates some of the potential pitfalls and difficulties that may occur especially in the hands of the inexperienced or unwary.

Case history

A 5-year-old boy was scheduled for strabismus surgery, requiring repositioning of two muscles on the left eye. A second year specialist registrar was rostered to provide anaesthesia without consultant supervision. She had recently obtained her final FRCA diploma and received an aggregate of 3 months' training in paediatric anaesthesia. She had not worked in an eye theatre since she had been a senior house officer.

The preoperative visit revealed nothing remarkable. The child was fit and weighed 19 kg. Clinical examination was normal. There were no allergies and he took no medication. The doctor prescribed local anaesthetic cream, which was applied to the dorsum of both hands. One and a half hours later the boy was escorted to the anaesthetic room by his mother and a nurse. The boy was well behaved and a cannula easily placed in a vein on the hand.

An induction sequence of fentanyl 15 μg and propofol 70 mg was given. A size 2 reinforced laryngeal mask airway was inserted with ease and the anaesthetic maintained with air, oxygen and isoflurane. On transfer to the theatre, ECG, blood pressure, saturation monitors were attached and a gas analyser connected. The child was allowed to breathe spontaneously and the end-tidal isoflurane concentration maintained in a circle system at 1.2–1.4%.

The surgeon was invited to proceed but while exerting traction on the medial rectus muscle the heart rate fell to 25 min^{-1} instantaneously. The registrar had followed good practice and previously had prepared syringes of atropine and suxamethonium in the anaesthetic room. However, because glycopyrrolate was immediately available at the anaesthetic workstation, she gave approximately 10 $\mu g.kg^{-1}$ (200 μg) glycopyrrolate. The isoflurane concentration was reduced to 0% in the fresh gas flow. After 1 minute the heart rate was still 30 min^{-1} and she realized the surgeon was still operating. She asked him to stop. By now she was very stressed and asked an assistant to call for senior help. There was a pulse wave form shown by the pulse oximeter but the rate was still very slow. She gave a further 100 μg glycopyrrolate. At 3 minutes the heart rate was still only 60 min^{-1} but the oscillometer gave the blood pressure as 70/30. The child was now ventilated and the oxygen concentration in the fresh gas flow increased. Within another minute the heart rate had increased to 140 min^{-1} with a blood pressure of 140/90. The end-tidal concentration of isoflurane was now 0.5% with FiO_2 of 0.8.

A further dose of 15 μg fentanyl was given and the child allowed to resume spontaneous breathing at an end-tidal isoflurane concentration of 1%. The surgeon asked if he could continue. The anaesthetist agreed. The surgeon complained that he could not perform a forced duction test because of Bell's reflex.[1,2] The anaesthetist had not heard of this reflex before so the surgeon explained that the eyes deviate either up or down in gaze under anaesthesia and so he asked if the muscles could be paralysed. Rocuronium 10 mg was given, the end-tidal isoflurane concentration increased to 1.2% and surgery to correct the squint proceeded uneventfully. Forty-five minutes after beginning surgery the relaxant was reversed and the child allowed to wake up on his side with the laryngeal mask airway in situ. Observations at this time, after a standard dose of reversal agents (glycopyrrolate 10 μg.kg^{-1} and neostigmine 50 μg.kg^{-1}) revealed a heart rate of 130 min^{-1} and blood pressure of 120/80.

As the child began to reject the laryngeal mask airway he vomited. The mask was removed and the mouth aspirated with a sucker. The child vomited twice more in the recovery area and subsequently on the ward. He complained that his eye was sore despite 20 mg.kg^{-1} paracetamol being given rectally. His intravenous cannula was still in situ and so he was given 1.5 mg morphine. He vomited again 30 minutes later and so he was kept in hospital overnight. No intravenous fluid had been given. On the ward he was disinclined to drink and when seen the next morning it transpired he had vomited again at midnight. He had not passed urine by 9.00 am.

Discussion

There are specific surgical requirements for strabismus surgery and this 5-year-old should not have been given a simple 'keep still' anaesthetic. It could be considered that the Anaesthetic Department rotamaker was at fault in asking an inexperienced registrar to do an ophthalmic case with no recent exposure to this kind of work even though she had fulfilled paediatric training requirements according to the Royal College of Anaesthetists syllabus.

Although not all squints require a forced duction test, an experienced ophthalmic anaesthetist would probably have discussed this with the surgeon or provided for it by giving neuromuscular blockade at the outset.

Both oculocardiac and oculoemetic reflexes exist. Vomiting is provoked by squint surgery even if no opioids are given. The use of opioids significantly increases the incidence of postoperative vomiting as does a car journey. Most ophthalmic anaesthetists would consider prophylaxis against the oculocardiac reflex rather than treat it when it occurs. Profound bradycardia with loss of cardiac output can occur within a few seconds. In small children a sinus arrest is not infrequent. If an anticholinergic is used to prophylactically block the oculocardiac reflex, glycopyrrolate is preferred as it is a quaternary compound and does not cross the blood–brain barrier. It is slow in onset however but the duration of action is longer than that of atropine and a single dose of 5–10 μg.kg^{-1} will cover most squint operations, certainly up to 1 hour of surgery.

Atropine however is preferred to treat established bradycardia as its onset is more rapid. Small doses may increase the tendency to dysrhythmia so it should not be given incrementally but rather as a single large dose of 20 μg.kg^{-1}. The cardiac output is rate-dependent in smaller children and so it is essential to relieve bradycardia urgently. Sinus arrest, unless transient, may require cardiac massage. A large dose of atropine always results eventually in tachycardia but children tolerate this well. The reflex fatigues and the stimulus to bradycardia upon surgical reintervention is less subsequently.

It is vital to ask the surgeon to stop operating while the bradycardia is treated

The reflex can also be blocked by a single medial canthal injection of local anaesthetic (1% lidocaine 2–2.5 ml depending on age).[3] (Figure 25.1) Bupivacaine is best avoided as it can produce long-lasting postoperative ptosis). This also provides good postoperative analgesia and is a very safe technique, performed with a 12.5 mm, 27 swg hypodermic needle. Such a block may also prevent the oculoemetic reflex but this is less certain.

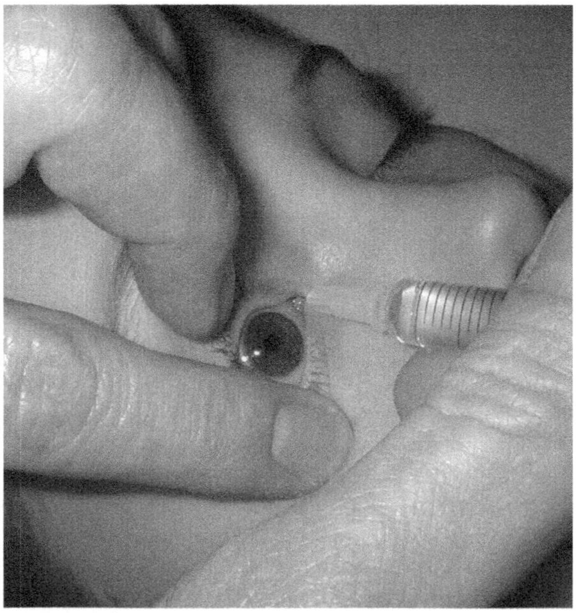

Figure 25.1
Medial canthal injection of local anaesthetic.

The great advantage of using a regional technique is that opioids can be given in minimal quantities or avoided altogether. Other drugs that predispose to vomiting, like thiopentone, should also not be used. Propofol is preferred for induction.[4–6] Nitrous oxide does not seem to cause much nausea in children compared with adults but is often used as a reversible analgesic to minimize the amount of opioid given. The best results are obtained with total intravenous anaesthesia with propofol and a regional block. However, propofol infusion is not licensed in children under 3 years of age. Any non-depolarizing neuromuscular blocking agent may be used and can be chosen to suit the expected duration of the operation.

Many attempts have been made to reduce postoperative nausea and vomiting (PONV) by the use of antiemetic drugs.[7] No one antiemetic is entirely efficacious. Ondansetron and granisetron appear to be useful in strabismus surgery although evidence is conflicting. Other older antiemetics such as antihistamines, metoclopramide and phenothiazines are still used. The efficacy of metoclopramide is reduced by opioids and the side effects of both metoclopramide and phenothiazines such as restlessness and possible dystonic reactions may outweigh their benefit.

It is probable that patients who are prone to motion sickness are more prone to PONV. It should be pointed out to parents and carers that violent cornering on the car journey home may provoke PONV which might not have occurred with a gentle driving technique.

With the use of paracetamol premedication, pre- or peroperative non-steroidal anti-inflammatory drugs (NSAIDs), e.g. diclofenac, and local anaesthesia, there is virtually no requirement for postoperative analgesic medication other than paracetamol. Very occasionally a small dose of opioid is required, sometimes after second or third strabismus operations, where there is much fibrosis and dissection to find the muscle is more extensive. In this instance repeated small incremental doses of opioid can be given intravenously in the recovery room, just sufficient to provide adequate analgesia. The aim should be to give as little opioid as possible. Tramadol and codeine or other weak opioids are frequently used in older children and adults often combined with paracetamol but these may also cause nausea, particularly at the higher strengths.

The use of diclofenac eye drops has now found an established place in strabismus surgery[8] and these can be applied to the muscle insertions before the conjunctiva is closed. The use of these drops dramatically reduces the requirement for postoperative analgesia. It must also be remembered that adequate loading doses of paracetamol should be given, such as 30 mg.kg^{-1} orally 1 hour preoperatively. If this has not been possible a dose of 40 mg.kg^{-1} can be given rectally with induction. Intravenous fluid should be given to ensure adequate hydration.

Learning points

- There are specific surgical requirements for strabismus surgery; a forced duction test requires neuromuscular blockade.
- Prophylaxis against the oculocardiac reflex is desirable:
  Glycopyrrolate 5–10 μg.kg^{-1}
  Peribulbar block (medial canthal single point injection).
- Treatment of profound bradycardia:
  Tell surgeon to desist
  Large dose (20 μg.kg^{-1} atropine) not glycopyrrolate
  Severe cases (sinus arrest) may require cardiac massage.
- Vomiting is very common if untreated:
  Always give an antiemetic
  Use minimal doses of opioid
  Use of peribulbar block minimizes opioid requirement and may block the oculoemetic reflex.
- Use of diclofenac eye drops and regional block results in very little postoperative pain.
- Preoperative paracetamol 30 μg.kg^{-1} oral + NSAID significantly reduce postoperative pain.

References

1. Casternera de Molina A, Giner-Munoz ML. Ocular alignment under general anaesthesia in congenital esotropia. *J Paediatr Ophthalmol Strabis* 1991; 28: 278–282.
2. McCall LC, Isenber SJ, Apt L. The effect of torsional muscle dysfunction and surgery on eye position under general anaesthesia. *J Paediatr Ophthalmol Strabis* 1993; 30: 154–156.
3. Guerzider V, Creuzot-Garcher C, Dupont G et al. Combined general and caruncular anaesthesia for strabismus surgery in children. *Opthalmologie* 1998; 12: 137–140.
4. Snellen FT, Vanacker B, Van Aken H. Propofol–nitrous oxide v thiopental sodium–nitrous oxide–isoflurane for strabismus surgery in children. *J Clin Anaesth* 1993; 5: 37–41.

5. Larrson S, Asgeirsson B, Magnusson J. Propofol–fentanyl anaesthesia compared to thiopental–halothane with special reference to recovery and vomiting after pediatric strabismus surgery. *Acta Anaesth Scand* 1992; 36: 182–186.
6. Tramer MR, Sansonetti A, Fuchs-Buder T et al. Oculocardiac reflex and post-operative vomiting in paediatric strabismus surgery. A randomised controlled trial comparing four anaesthetic techniques. *Acta Anaesth Scand* 1998; 42: 117–123.
7. Fuji Y, Toyooka H, Tanaka H. Anti-emetic efficacy of granisetron and metoclopramide in children undergoing ophthalmic or ENT surgery. *Can J Anaesth* 1996; 43: 1095–1099.
8. Morton NS, Benham SW, Lawson RA et al. Diclofenac v oxybuprocaine eye drops for analgesia in paediatric strabismus surgery. *Paediatr Anaesth* 1997; 7: 221–226.

26

Difficult intubation in an 18-month-old child

Ann E Black

Introduction

The vast majority of children undergoing anaesthesia will have an easy to manage airway and will not present difficulties with tracheal intubation. Unexpected difficult intubation in apparently normal children is very unusual. Most children with difficulties with their airway or intubation can be found in three main groups, those with facial abnormalities, those with temperomandibular joint (TMJ) fusion and those with soft tissue swelling. They therefore have an abnormality of the head or neck, or have syndromal features, which give the anaesthetist a warning of potential difficulties with airway management or intubation.[1]

However, assessment can be difficult and most tests used in adult practice including the Mallampati scoring[2] system and measurements of thyromental distance are not validated for the paediatric population, and are often not useful, particularly in the younger child. Attempts have been made to define what actually constitutes a difficult intubation. This has mainly been discussed with reference to the adult population and consists of either assessment of the number of attempts required to achieve tracheal intubation in a patient, (e.g. more than three attempts) the time required (e.g. more than 10 minutes) or the need to use specialized equipment such as specialized blades or the fibreoptic scope (FOS) to intubate the trachea.

Case history

An 18-month-old child weighing 11 kg presented to the maxillofacial surgeons for release of the left TMJ. He had been born at term but had suffered from repeated episodes of neonatal sepsis. One such event had resulted in a septic focus in the TMJ, which subsequently destroyed the joint resulting in permanent fusion with minimal movement by the age of 1 year. Despite this he had managed to feed adequately. He was known to have repeated respiratory infections but no specific cause had been found. He had a small ventricular septal defect (VSD), which was under review by the cardiology team. He required no medication and it was anticipated that the VSD would close spontaneously. Eating had become increasingly difficult in the past few months as his diet would be expected to include more solid foods which he had difficulty managing. There was no other past medical history; he had had no previous anaesthetics, no allergies, was on no medication and had no family history of problems with anaesthesia.

On examination he was a cheerful, active, well child. He had no symptoms of upper respiratory tract infection. He had minimal mouth opening, micrognathia, retrognathia and good neck movements. He snored mildly when asleep but had no apnoeas. Both nares appeared patent. He had no loose teeth. He was chubby and it was anticipated that provision of an intravenous cannula preoperatively might be difficult. His chest was clear on auscultation and the heart sounds revealed a systolic murmur.

Investigations

Preoperative investigations included a full blood count, and cross-match of two units of blood. A clotting screen was normal. There were no abnormalities on the ECG or chest X-ray. His oxygen saturation in air was 98%. A review by the cardiologist included an echocardiogram and this revealed only a small, non-significant VSD. Imaging for surgical planning had included a computed tomography scan, which confirmed destruction of the TMJ on the left.

He had had a sleep study, which indicated short periods of airway obstruction with a decrease in oxygen saturations to 90% on several occasions, these were self-limiting and there were no recorded apnoeas.

Management

The child was seen on the ward the day before surgery with his parents. At that time he was well, active and all investigation results were available. Premedication with atropine was prescribed orally and fasting guidelines implemented.

On the day of surgery he arrived in the anaesthetic room with his mother. Anaesthesia was induced with sevoflurane in oxygen while he sat on the trolley. Initial monitoring was with an ECG and pulse oximetry.

His mother left the anaesthetic room as he went to sleep. A peripheral intravenous cannula was inserted. Once he was laid down he developed marked obstruction to his airway, no adjustment to his jaw position was possible and it was not possible to put in an oral airway nor to grasp the tongue to manoeuvre it forward. There was insufficient mouth opening for use of a laryngeal mask. Continuous positive airway pressure (CPAP) by mask was ineffective in improving the situation and attempts at hand ventilation via the facemask were poorly effective. His airway obstruction caused compromise of ventilation and his SaO_2 decreased to 88%.

A nasal prong made from a cut Portex® tracheal tube was introduced into the left nares with immediate improvement in the airway. The anaesthetic circuit was connected to the prong and anaesthesia maintained with halothane in oxygen. It was possible to adequately inflate the child's chest with this circuit although there was considerable gas escape from the mouth. Spontaneous respiration was maintained. Monitoring included FiO_2, end-tidal CO_2, anaesthetic agent, non-invasive blood pressure and temperature. An additional peripheral intravenous cannula was placed and a radial arterial line inserted, the latter for blood pressure monitoring peroperatively and intermittent sampling for haemoglobin and blood gas analysis. Antibiotics for routine cardiac endocarditis prophylaxis were given.

The plan was to proceed to fibreoptic intubation. Ephedrine nasal drops were instilled into the right nares.

One anaesthetist was assigned primary care of the airway and deepened the anaesthetic using halothane in oxygen while maintaining spontaneous respiration. The fibreoptic equipment had been checked and a 4.5 flexometallic plain tracheal tube was mounted on the FOS. When the child was judged to be deeply asleep the FOS was introduced via the nose, the cords were identified and the FOS passed through and advanced until the carina was clearly identified. At this point suxamethonium $1\,mg.kg^{-1}$ was given. The tracheal tube was advanced over the scope and into the larynx. The tube position was confirmed as the scope was removed initially by direct visualization via the scope and then by identification of expired CO_2. Bilateral breath sounds were checked to confirm positioning of the tube above the carina. The tube size was suitable and a small gas leak was audible on ventilation. Ventilation was carefully checked and appeared adequate and a non-depolarizing muscle relaxant was given. It was not possible to use a pharyngeal pack. A nasogastric tube was passed.

Peroperatively anaesthesia was maintained with O_2, N_2O and isoflurane. A total of $7\,\mu g.kg^{-1}$ of fentanyl was given during the case. Local infiltration with 0.5% lignocaine, 1 : 200,000 epinephrine was used at the operation site and suppositories of paracetamol and diclofenac given. Dexamethasone and antibiotics were given as prescribed.

The operation proceeded uneventfully. Following surgical release of the TMJ mouth opening was immediately improved. The child did not require blood transfusion. Arterial gases were maintained within normal limits.

At the end of the procedure the child was extubated awake and with the use of a Guedel airway respiration and ventilation using a face mask was satisfactory. The child returned to the routine postoperative ward and no additional monitoring was used.

Discussion

TMJ ankylosis is one of the more common causes of difficulties with intubation.[3] It can be unilateral or bilateral, congenital or acquired. The reasons for acquired TMJ ankylosis include infection, trauma and juvenile rheumatoid arthritis. These children will require surgery as the condition progresses and feeding becomes more difficult. Other common causes of difficult intubation in children include hemifacial microsomia, Treacher–Collins syndrome, Pierre–Robin syndrome, mucopolysaccharidoses and facial burns.[4]

Although difficulties in intubation would be expected in this child it was unusual to have such early problems with actually maintaining an adequate airway. It is usual that airway maintenance is relatively easy in most children. The warning feature in this child's history was the presence of snoring implying a degree of airway obstruction during sleep. It is important that sedative premedication is avoided in this situation as obstruction may occur on the ward.

The assessment of the airway in children can be difficult. Blanco et al reported a series of 46 children who had fibreoptic intubation.[4] All were assessed with Mallampati scores, thyromental distance measurements and measurement of mouth opening with a limit of 4 cm being taken as a potential contributing factor to a difficult intubation. Twenty-six of the 46 patients had TMJ ankylosis and of these 17 had mouth opening ≤15 mm which practically was likely to increase the difficulty of intubation using conventional laryngoscopy. They assessed each child following induction using Cormack and Lehanes's classification of glottic exposure.[6] Vas and Sawant in their review, reported a series of 14 children with TMJ ankylosis and mouth opening < 10 mm; all were managed with a semi-blind nasal intubation technique.[7]

Management of any child with a history of cardiac abnormalities is important. The presence of a murmur on preoperative review indicates that efforts must be made to clarify the nature of the murmur and decide whether it is significant. Many paediatric syndromes are associated with cardiac abnormalities and the combination of airway abnormalities and cardiac disease is not unusual.[8] Any syndrome should be reviewed in the specialist books devoted to this area of paediatrics so that associated conditions can be identified. Most murmurs are innocent; however, in this case the presence of a small, physiologically non-significant VSD still requires correct antibiotic prophylaxis to avoid the risk of bacterial endocarditis. In the situation where non-urgent major surgery is being planned it is important to exclude significant cardiac disease.

Premedication with atropine is usually given orally in a dose of 20 µg.kg^{-1}. Atropine is useful as a drying agent, which helps when using fibreoptic equipment as secretions obscure the view, and also as a vagolytic agent to avoid bradycardia and ensure maintenance of cardiac output during deepening of the anaesthetic.

In constructing an anaesthetic plan for this child the first question is how to manage induction of anaesthesia. Gaseous induction is useful when difficulties with the airway are predicted. Sevoflurane is pleasant and rapidly effective; however, high concentrations are associated with apnoeas and hypotension. It has been used successfully for difficult intubations in paediatric practice as have halothane and propofol infusions as reported by Blanco et al.[5] The combination of induction of anaesthesia with sevoflurane and deepening and maintenance with halothane is a very safe technique. If spontaneous respirations are established, increasing the concentration of halothane to 5% slowly is cardiovascularly well tolerated and apnoea rarely occurs. Ventricular ectopics are not uncommon but usually well tolerated. If the child had compromised cardiac function this would not be the agent to use and isoflurane may be better, but care must be taken to increase the concentration slowly as airway irritation is common. Induction with sevoflurane and the deepening of the anaesthetic with sevflurane to allow fibreoptic intubation is another useful technique. Long experience with the use of halothane in paediatric practice has shown that it is a safe agent in the majority of children and the possibility of halothane hepatitis occurring is very remote. These issues have been discussed in Wark's editorial[9] and Hatch's article[10] on the use of inhalational agents in paediatric anaesthesia. Unfortunately in this case the child's airway became obstructed very early after induction. Provision of an adequate airway becomes imperative. The decision to wake the child up may be made at this point; however, this may not be uneventful as with poor ventilation, in the obstructed airway, elimination of the anaesthetic is delayed and oxygenation may be difficult and the situation becomes urgent. The development of an anaesthetic plan must take into account this possibility. The hope that the amount of mouth opening will be increased after the relaxation that accompanies the induction of anaesthesia is optimistic as in TMJ ankylosis the condition is often relatively fixed. In this particular child, the mouth opening remained minimal and insertion of a nasal prong was used successfully in restoring adequate ventilation and allowing anaesthesia to proceed. Other manoeuvres that can be tried are aimed at adjusting the airway, advancing the jaw, extending the neck, altering the child's position, for instance turning them on their side, advancing the tongue, or if there is sufficient mouth opening, inserting some form of oral airway such as a Guedel and trying different sizes. In larger children nasopharyngeal airways are suitable. In the six out of 15 patients in Vas and Sawant's series,[7] who similarly could not maintain their airway following induction, repositioning by turning the child on the side and use of a nasal airway was most effective. Frequently a laryngeal mask airway (LMA) provides a good airway and intubation is not attempted. Aids to intubation such as different laryngoscope blades and external manipulations of the larynx in order to allow passage of either the tracheal tube or the bougie followed by a tube are helpful. The McCoy blade is available in paediatric sizes and the Bullard is popular, particularly in the USA. Most of these techniques are of no value in the child who has very limited mouth opening. Successful use of a paediatric light wand has been reported even with limited mouth opening. Other reported manoeuvres include retrograde passage of transtracheal catheters to allow passage of the tracheal tube into the airway. Vas and Sawant reported a review of the management of 15 paediatric patients with TMJ ankylosis detailing an alternative semi-blind method of management involving administration of local anaesthetic to the airway, induction with halothane and manipulation of the nasal tube into the trachea, in the spontaneously breathing child, using Magill forceps and an external fibreoptic light source.[4] While somewhat complicated these methods do have their place, particularly in areas where fibreoptic intubation equipment is not available.

Tracheostomy may be a key part of the anaesthetic plan in a child in whom it is not possible to pass a tracheal tube, or who, because of their condition or the type of surgery, will have a compromised airway postoperatively. While tracheostomy does have morbidity and mortality associated with it, it provides a safe airway. If a tracheostomy is likely to be in the anaesthetic plan it is important that staff and equipment are available to undertake this surgical procedure in theatre, and that consent has been obtained. During a tracheostomy the airway can be managed using mask anaesthesia, a nasal prong, a LMA or intubation with the child positioned to provide the best airway possible.

Transtracheal jet ventilation is also used in some centres. This has more risk factors in children than in adult practice. It is technically more difficult and use of high-pressure gases, although pressure-limited, is potentially dangerous in the small airways of the child. There is often inadequate ventilation and if there is any obstruction to expiration tension pneumothoraces may develop; therefore it is essential that adequate expiration will be possible.

Fibreoptic intubation was electively used in this child. It is a well established technique in paediatric practice. Specialist scopes are made including a 2.2 mm, which takes a 2.5-mm tracheal tube and is useful for small babies. Larger sizes include a 3.8-mm scope, which takes a 4.5 tube and a 3.1-mm, which takes a 3.5 tube. Difficulties with the smallest scope include lack of a suction channel and increased flexibility of the scope making manoeuvring of the equipment difficult. Both the larger scopes have suction channels and they can be used in two main ways, firstly, as in adult practice, by placing the correct sized tracheal tube on the scope and via mouth or nose, advancing the scope into the trachea and then feeding the tube off the scope into the trachea. Alternatively a 'Seldinger' method can be used. The scope is used to visualize the cords but not to advance through them. Then a wire is introduced through the suction channel of the scope and advanced into the trachea under view of the scope. The scope is then removed, the wire stiffened with a fine-bore catheter and then the tracheal tube is passed over the catheter and into the trachea. Fibreoptic scopes can be used either orally or nasally depending on the child's condition. They can also be used to intubate through a laryngeal mask, for example using the 'Seldinger' technique.

One of the potential difficulties with fibreoptic intubation in children is choosing the correct sized tube. If the tube is too small, and the pharynx can be packed, this is sometimes suitable; however in a case with limited mouth opening such as described here, this is impossible. A correct sized tube must be placed. It can be useful to use a small cuffed tracheal tube in this circumstance so that you do not need to change the tube but will have a suitable airway and adequate ventilation. There is increasing interest in the use of cuffed tubes in young children and as long as they are placed with scrupulous care below the cricoid they may have a useful role.

Complications of paediatric fibreoptic intubation include failure of technique, misplacement of the tube in the oesophagus, trauma, bleeding, coughing, oxygen desaturation, infection and thermal trauma.

One significant difference in paediatric practice is that although in the adult fibreoptic intubation can readily be done in the awake cooperative patient, this is rarely an option in the child. The anaesthetic plan must ensure the child is adequately ventilating and asleep during fibreoptic intubation. Use of a nasal prong is very beneficial as in this case. Spontaneous respiration was maintained until the point of advancement of the tracheal tube and then a depolarizing relaxant was used. This allows passage of the tube under ideal conditions without needing to use local anaesthesia on the larynx. The tracheal tube should be gently rotated in. Softer bevelled tubes pass more easily. Only after the tube position is confirmed and the tube is secured is a long-acting relaxant given.

The management of extubation is important. In this case the child's airway was improved immediately and mouth opening was excellent, thus allowing laryngoscopic assessment of the glottis. This revealed a grade 2 (Cormack and Lehane[6]) view and therefore the child could return to the ward safely after the surgery and should not provide problems in recovery. Children with potentially compromised airways postoperatively should be observed on the intensive care unit. The use of steroids is common and mild stridor postoperatively can usually be managed with nebulized epinephrine, oxygen and humidification. Postoperative pain is not usually a significant problem and can be managed with simple analgesics and if necessary intramuscular or oral codeine phosphate.

Learning points

- Difficult paediatric intubations are usually predictable.
- Preoperative assessment must include a review of all systems and an adequate workup is important.
- Premedication with atropine is useful and sedative medication should be avoided.
- An anaesthetic plan should be carefully formulated and discussed with the parents and the theatre team. Consent should be taken for tracheostomy if this is a potential event.
- Adequate expert help must be available and equipment present and checked.
- Awake fibreoptic intubation is rarely an option in paediatric patients and asleep fibreoptic intubation may take some time to achieve. The anaesthetic plan must involve a suitable method to allow anaesthesia and oxygenation during the intubation procedure.
- Spontaneous respiration should be maintained until safe management of the airway is assured.

References

1. Anesthesia implications of syndromes and unusual disorders. In: Stewart DJ (ed.). *Manual of Pediatric Anesthesia,* 4th edn. New York: Churchill Livingstone 1995: 433–494.
2. Mallampati SR, Gatt SP, Guggino LD et al. A clinical sign to predict difficult tracheal intubation: A prospective study. *Can Anaesth Soc J* 1985; 32: 429–34.
3. Frei FJ, Ummenhofer W. Difficult intubation in paediatrics. *Paediatr Anaesth* 1996; 6: 251–263.
4. Katz J, Steward DJ. *Anesthesia and Uncommon Paediatric Diseases*. Place Saunders 1987.
5. Blanco G, Melman E, Cuairan V, et al. Fiberoptic nasal intubation in children with anticipated and unanticipated difficult intubation. *Paediatric Anaesth* 2001; 11: 49–53.
6. Cormack RS, Lehane J. Difficult tracheal intubation in obstetrics. *Anaesthesia* 1984; 39: 1105–11.
7. Vas L, Sawant P. A review of anaesthetic technique in 15 paediatric patients with temperomandibular ankylosis. *Paediatr Anaesth* 2001; 11: 237–244.
8. Lynn A, Sasaki S. Chapter title. In: Sumner E, Hatch DJ (eds). *Paediatric Anaesthesia*, 2nd edn. London: Arnold, 2000: 535–564.
9. Wark H. Is there still a place for halothane in paediatric anaesthesia? *Paediatric Anaesthesia* 1997; 7: 359–361.
10. Hatch DJ. New inhalational agents in paediatric anaesthesia. *Br J Anaesth* 1999; 83: 42–49.

27

Foreign body aspiration

Patricia M Weir

Introduction

Foreign body aspiration remains a common problem, especially in small children. Early diagnosis and treatment decrease morbidity. Early rigid bronchoscopy under general anaesthesia is the treatment of choice.

Case history

A 21-month-old boy was brought to the Accident and Emergency (A&E) department at 10 pm. Four hours previously, just after his evening meal, he had choked while playing with some peanuts his elder brothers were eating. Since then he had been coughing intermittently and would not settle to sleep. He was apparently completely well prior to this with no history of respiratory symptoms.

On examination, he was pink and playing happily. On chest auscultation, air entry was heard bilaterally with no added sounds. However, he coughed frequently during examination. A plain chest X-ray was normal. When reviewed by the radiologist, fluoroscopic screening was suggested. Screening showed air trapping with delayed exhalation from the right lung.

Inhalation of a peanut was strongly suspected, and it was decided to take him to theatre for a rigid bronchoscopy. He was reviewed in A&E by the anaesthetic specialist registrar (SpR). He asked the consultant on call for assistance. No premedication was prescribed. He weighed 12 kg. The SpR went to the operating room where he checked the anaesthetic equipment and familiarized himself with the Storz bronchoscope. About 30 minutes later, the child was taken to the anaesthetic room where an inhalation induction was performed using 100% O_2 and 8% sevoflurane via a facemask and Ayres T-piece circuit. ECG and pulse oximetry were applied and when he was sufficiently deeply anaesthetized to tolerate it, a 22G cannula was inserted in the dorsum of his right hand.

When he was breathing shallowly, pupils small and central, he was assessed as being sufficiently deeply anaesthetized and laryngoscopy was performed. His vocal cords and upper trachea were sprayed with 2 ml of 2% lignocaine. There was no coughing. Sevoflurane via facemask was then continued and he was transferred to the operating room. After establishing full monitoring (ECG, non-invasive blood pressure, SaO_2, end-tidal CO_2, FiO_2, Fiagent), the airway was handed over to the paediatric surgeon, who inserted a size 4.0 Storz rigid bronchoscope through the vocal cords uneventfully. The T-piece circuit was connected to the side arm of the bronchoscope and spontaneous ventilation maintained. The sevoflurane was decreased stepwise as the respiration was shallow.

On bronchoscopy the trachea was normal, but a piece of particulate matter was seen in the left main stem bronchus. The surgeon was able to grasp this with forceps passed through the bronchoscope and remove the object. Further inspection of both main stem and lobar bronchi revealed no further foreign bodies. The bronchoscope was removed, the patient turned on his side and switched to 100% O_2 via a tight-fitting facemask. A repeat chest X-ray, performed in recovery, was normal and showed no signs of collapse, consolidation, or pneumothorax.

He was discharged home on the following day.

Discussion

Foreign body aspiration remains common in small children because they:

- put things in their mouths
- run/shout/play with objects in their mouths

- have no molars and therefore cannot chew food adequately.

In patients arriving at hospital with incomplete airway obstruction, a history of choking is the most important pointer to diagnosis. There may also be coughing, wheezing, or stridor. Signs on chest auscultation, e.g. decrease air entry unilaterally, become more common with a delay in diagnosis.

In the most severe cases complete upper airway obstruction occurs, which requires the immediate instigation of resuscitation in the form of back slaps, followed by chest or abdomen thrusts (according to Advanced Paediatric Life Support guidelines[1]). In cases presenting alive to A&E, the obstruction will be partial and any manoeuvre that may move the object to position where it may cause complete obstruction should be discouraged.

Organic foodstuffs such as peanuts or seeds are the commonest objects to be aspirated. Foreign body aspiration is more common in boys than in girls. A high index of suspicion should be entertained if a history of a choking episode is elicited followed by any signs or symptoms of respiratory distress or respiratory irritation, e.g. cough, wheeze, stridor, or recession. Some experts advocate bronchoscopy in all children presenting to hospital with a history of choking.

If the diagnosis is delayed, then the presentation may be with signs or symptoms of pneumonia namely fever, decreased air entry and changes on chest X-ray. Plain anteroposterior chest films are commonly normal in acute presentation, as most foreign bodies are radiolucent. Inspiratory and expiratory films (Figures 27.1 and 27.2) can be helpful, as around 90% of foreign bodies will be lodged in a main bronchus (slightly more commonly on the right than the left). The expiratory film may show air trapping on expiration on the affected side. More recently, fluoroscopy has been advocated in cases with a significant index of suspicion and a normal chest X-ray.[2] If clinical suspicion persists, a bronchoscopy should be performed, as delay in diagnosis increases morbidity.

Preanaesthetic assessment

Preanaesthetic assessment should include history of aspiration, time since food ingestion, and consideration of premedication use, such as atropine for vagolysis or midazolam for anxiolysis. Signs of respiratory distress should be sought.

Anaesthetic management

The technique of choice remains rigid bronchoscopy using a Storz bronchoscope (Figure 27.3), under deep inhalational anaesthesia. In cases of a recent aspiration or potential tracheal foreign body, attempts should be

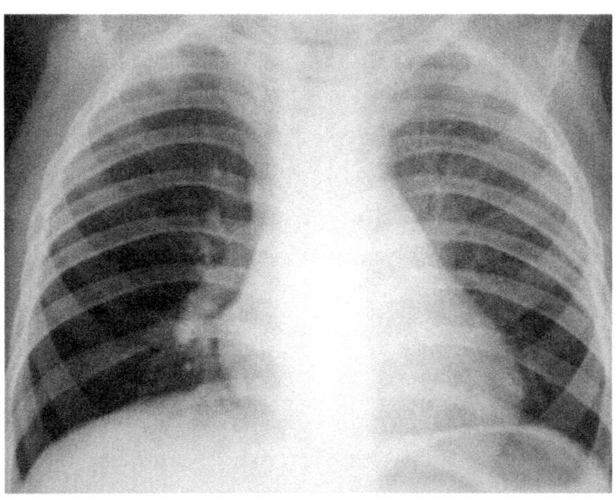

Figure 27.1
Inspiratory Chest X-ray.

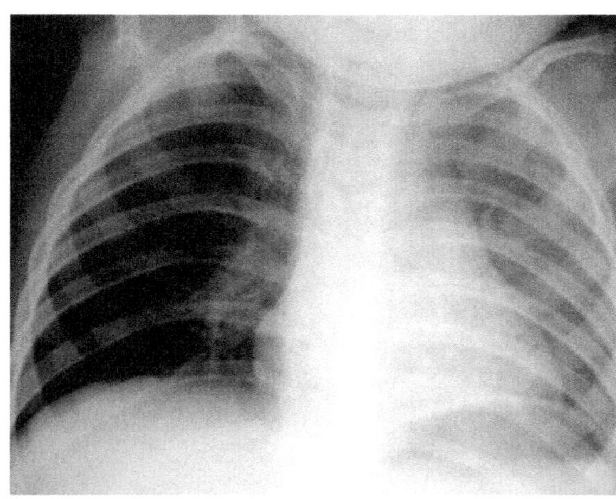

Figure 27.2
Expiratory Chest X-ray.

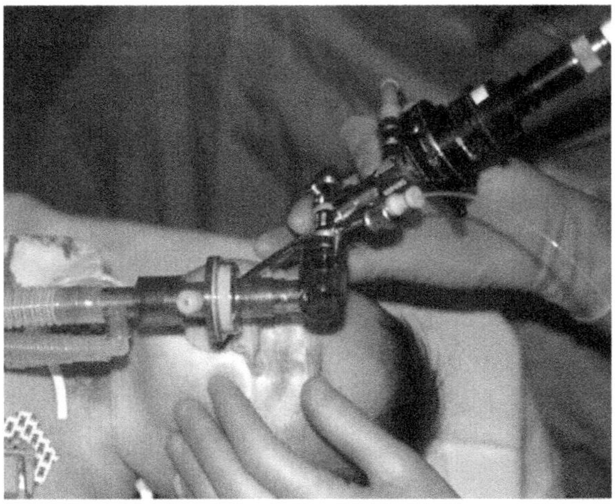

Figure 27.3
Storz bronchoscope with Ayres T-piece attached to side arm.

made to keep the child calm to prevent the foreign body from moving further and potentially causing complete obstruction. Senior paediatric anaesthetic help should be sought, and the bronchoscopist should be an experienced operator. This would usually be either a paediatric or ENT surgeon.

Inhalation induction and maintenance of spontaneous ventilation is the method of choice regardless of starvation time, as it prevents the possibility of pushing the foreign body further into the airway with positive pressure ventilation. The agent of choice will depend on the experience of the anaesthetist. The most commonly used agent at present, in the UK, for inhalation induction is sevoflurane. There are some advantages to using halothane, but they may well be outweighed now by lack of anaesthetist familiarity with the agent (see Table 27.1). The selected agent should be introduced in 100% oxygen. Nitrous oxide is contraindicated especially if there is extensive gas trapping. Where there is any degree of upper airway obstruction, then the induction time can be significantly prolonged. Signs of adequate depth of anaesthesia should be sought before instrumentation of the airway, namely pattern and depth of respiration, pupil size and position, abdominal wall tone, heart rate and blood pressure. Heart rate is decreased when using halothane. This can be a useful sign of depth of anaesthesia, however, bradycardia is poorly tolerated in infants due to their relatively fixed stroke volume, thus bradycardia leads to a decreased cardiac output. Atropine 10–20 $\mu g.kg^{-1}$ IV can be useful in preventing the bradycardia associated with deep halothane anaesthesia. When adequate depth of anaesthesia is achieved, laryngoscopy can be performed. The larynx can be sprayed with lignocaine (3–4 $mg.kg^{-1}$), either through a specific spray device or by using an IV cannula to drop local anaesthetic onto the larynx and upper trachea. The use of local anaesthetic will decrease the potential for coughing upon introduction of the bronchoscope. It also provides a good assessment of whether the depth of anaesthesia is adequate for bronchoscopy.

Anaesthetic	*Advantages*	*Disadvantages*
Halothane	• Smooth induction • Easy to gauge depth of anaesthesia • Relatively cheap • Easier to maintain depth of anaesthesia	• Moderate incidence of dysrhythmias • Lack of experience with its use • 'Halothane hepatitis' • Slower recovery
Sevoflurane	• Smooth induction • Familiarity • Relative CVS stability	• Rapid recovery • Less easy to maintain smooth intraoperative anaesthesia during bronchoscopy

Table 27.1
Comparison of halothane and sevoflurane

Preoxygenation with 100% O_2 agent should precede airway instrumentation. When ready, the airway is handed over to the surgeon. It is vitally important that the bronchoscopic equipment has been checked and that the T-piece fits onto the side arm. The aim is to maintain spontaneous ventilation for two reasons, firstly, to prevent the dissemination of foreign material (as mentioned before). Secondly, if the foreign body is more distal, then the bronchoscope could be in a single lobe of lung for some time and it is easier to keep spontaneously breathing patients well-saturated in this situation, as they will be entraining an O_2-enriched gas mixture around the bronchoscope. It can, however, be difficult to remain adequately anaesthetized in this situation and an agent that does not wear off rapidly (e.g. halothane) can be an advantage.

The list of potential complications is long (see Table 27.2). Fortunately, they are rare (5–8%).[3,4] Attention to detail and smooth anaesthesia decrease the chance of tracheal trauma from the bronchoscope. Death is usually related to acute complete airway obstruction, and is rare but well described following attempts at bronchoscope removal. Steroids (e.g. dexamethsone 0.25 $mg.kg^{-1}$ IV) are commonly given in an attempt to decrease oedema secondary to instrumentation, although there is little documented evidence for their efficacy. Failure to remove the foreign body occurs in up to 7% of cases. This may necessitate a thoracotomy, although mediastonoscopy has been described as an alternative.[5] A repeat chest X-ray should be performed after rigid bronchoscopy to look for pneumothorax/ pneumomediastinum, atelactasis or collapse.

- Hypoxia
- Failure to remove foreign body (2–7%)
- Coughing
- Laryngeal/tracheal/bronchial trauma, including tracheal perforation (may be related to coughing)
- Pneumothorax
- Loss of airway necessitating tracheostomy
- Need for continued ventilation
- Pneumonia
- Cardiac arrest
- Death

Table 27.2
Potential complications of bronchoscopy

Learning points

- A history of choking should give a high index of suspicion of presence of a foreign body and bronchoscopy should be considered.
- Delay in diagnosis increases morbidity.
- In the presence of a normal chest X-ray, fluoroscopy can assist in making the diagnosis.
- Inhalation induction and rigid bronchoscopy remain the techniques of choice.
- The anaesthesia and bronchoscopy should be undertaken by experienced physicians.
- Always check bronchoscopy equipment and connections before starting.
- Inhalation induction will be slow in the presence of upper airway obstruction.
- Ensure adequate depth of anaesthesia before instrumentation.
- Local anaesthetic to larynx and upper trachea will decrease stimulation from the bronchoscope.

References

1. *APLS: The Practical Approach*. 3rd edn. BMJ Publishing Group, 2000.
2. Tan HK, Brown K, McGill T et al. Airway foreign bodies (FB): a 10-year review. *Int J Pediatr Otorhinolaryngol* 2000; 56: 91–99.
3. Zaytoun GM, Rouadi PW, Baki DH. Endoscopic management of foreign bodies in the tracheobronchial tree: predictive factors for complications. *Otolaryngol Head Neck Surg* 2000; 123: 311–316.
4. Oguzkaya F, Akcali Y, Kahraman C et al. Tracheobronchial foreign body aspirations in childhood: a 10-year experience. *Eur J Cardiothorac Surg* 1998; 14: 388–392.
5. Lynch JB, Kerschner JE, Aiken JJ. Use of mediastinoscopy for foreign body removal. *Int J Pediatr Otorhinolaryngol* 1999; 50: 225–228.

Suggested reading

Rovin JD, Rodgers BM. Pediatric foreign body aspiration. *Paediatr Rev* 2000; 21: 86–90.

28

Major orthopaedic surgery in a child of Jehovah's Witness parents

Gillian R Lauder

Introduction

Major elective surgery for the child of Jehovah's Witness parents presents problems that need to be resolved well in advance of the planned surgery. The following case focuses on the preoperative planning and consent. The discussion outlines some of the dilemmas involved in planning major surgery in a child of Jehovah's Witness parents.

Case history

An 11-year-old girl with cerebral palsy and bilateral dislocated hips is referred for pre-operative anaesthetic assessment. The hips are increasingly painful and the surgical plan is for major pelvic reconstruction including open reduction of both hips, bilateral femoral osteotomies and bilateral acetabular osteotomies. This procedure will involve significant and possibly major haemorrhage. The child's parents are Jehovah's Witnesses and refuse to allow their daughter to have a blood transfusion. Preoperative assessment revealed findings documented in Table 28.1.

A case conference involving the referring paediatrician, the consultant paediatric orthopaedic surgeon and the consultant paediatric anaesthetist concluded that surgery would improve the child's quality of life despite the potential problems with the case.

A meeting with the parents was arranged well in advance of the planned surgery to discuss the benefits and risks of bilateral hip surgery in their child. At this meeting the parents reiterated their request that no blood products be transfused into their daughter; they also detailed what intravenous therapies they considered acceptable. The surgeon explained that the procedure would be done in stages; at each stage the decision to continue with the rest of the planned procedure would be dependent on the ongoing blood loss. The important aspects of the anaesthesia were explained to the parents. The potential for major haemorrhage was emphasized. The consequences of a non-life-threatening anaemia were described. The parents were reassured that all efforts would be made to adhere to their request to not transfuse blood products. However, they were made aware of Section 8 of the Children's Act 1989; and told that if it became necessary to save their child's life from life-threatening blood loss the child would be made a ward of the Court to authorize transfusion of blood or blood products. The strategies that would be adopted to optimize their daughter's condition preoperatively and conserve blood perioperatively were explained. The planned postoperative analgesia was described. The parents were warned of the potential need and reasons for ventilation in the postoperative period. The family signed a Jehovah's Witness consent form that was witnessed by the consultant surgeon and anaesthetist. These discussions were documented in the clinical notes. A letter summarizing this consultation was sent to the parents and the hospital solicitor. The child was referred to a haematologist to instigate preoperative iron, vitamin and erythropoietin therapy. The child awaits surgery but some important anaesthetic issues are discussed.

Discussion

Jehovah's Witness

The Jehovah's Witness movement, a Christian denomination, was founded in the late 1870s by Charles Russell in Pittsburg, Pennsylvania. Jehovah's Witnesses believe the bible to be the word of God,

Past medical history	Cerebral palsy; no seizures	
ASA grade	II	
Regular medications	None	
Allergies	None known	
Examination	Alert No comprehensive speech Spastic quadriplegia Normal airway Chest clear SaO_2 98% in air Normal heart sounds, pulse 90 bpm, BP 100/50 mmHg	
Investigations	*Weight*	39 kg
	FBC	Hb 12.0 $g.dl^{-1}$, Plat $264 \times 10^9 l^{-1}$, WBC $7.3 \times 10^9 l^{-1}$
	Clotting	PT 12.4, INR 1.0, APPT 22.9, fibrinogen 3.8 gl^{-1}
	U+Es	Na^+ 135 $mmol.l^{-1}$, K^+ 3.9 $mmol.l^{-1}$, Urea 4.4 $mmol.l^{-1}$, creatinine 40 $\mu mol.l^{-1}$
	ECG	NAD
	Chest X-ray	Lung fields clear

Table 28.1
Preoperative assessment findings

which should be obeyed. They named themselves Jehovah's Witnesses in 1931 on the basis of Isaiah (Isaiah: 43:10,11) where God (Jehovah) declares to his people 'ye are my witnesses'. Jehovah's Witnesses believe in the imminent end of this world and that a new world will be created by God; in this new world only those who have been faithful will have eternal life.[1] The Jehovah's Witness movement disseminates the concept that followers of the faith should not receive transfused blood or blood products, based on Genesis 9:3,4, Levicticus 17:11,12 and Acts 15:28,29, all of which describe the prohibition of the consumption of blood. This initially applied to the consumption of meat that had not been exsanguinated but from 1945 onwards was applied to blood transfusions. The prohibition of blood transfusion is a deeply held core value. Jehovah's Witnesses will not accept a transfusion of whole blood or any blood products including fresh frozen plasma, packed cells, white blood cells or platelets.

The decision to perform major elective surgery on a child of Jehovah's Witness parents should be made by an appropriate team including a consultant surgeon and a consultant anaesthetist because of the ethical and legal implications involved. The risk–benefit analysis, timing of surgery, staging of surgery, type of surgery and type of anaesthesia need to be carefully considered and planned. The most experienced surgeon and anaesthetist should then manage the case as this may influence the outcome. An individual doctor can elect not to become involved in elective surgery on a child of Jehovah's Witness parents but must ensure the continued care of the patient by another colleague willing to take on the case.

There is variability between individual Jehovah's Witnesses regarding the extent to which they adhere to the transfusion principles. Infusions of albumin, immunoglobulins and concentrates of clotting factors are not strictly forbidden. Haemodilution is acceptable to some Jehovah's Witness patients but only if the blood that is withdrawn remains in continuity with the circulation and keeps moving.[2] Cell salvage of blood intraoperatively is acceptable to most Jehovah's Witnesses even though the technique does not fulfill the criteria of blood remaining in continuity with the body. The views of each individual Jehovah's Witness should be determined preoperatively.

The family should be consulted to establish what blood products, if any, they would deem acceptable for their child. This consultation should occur without relatives or other members of the Jehovah's Witness community so that the family will not feel inhibited in expressing their acceptance of blood or blood products. Later involvement of an Elder of the Jehovah's Witness hospital liaison committee in these discussions will enable the development of trust between the child, parents and the doctor. The family must be made aware of Section 8 of the Children Act 1989; in order to save a child's life the child would be made a ward of the Court if it became necessary to transfuse blood against the parents' wishes. The outcome of these discussions needs to be documented in the clinical notes. The hospital solicitor and the Jehovah's Witness hospital liaison committee should be involved in difficult areas of consent.

A competent adult has the absolute right to decline medical treatment (except for compulsory treatment of mental disorder or illness under the Mental Health Act 1983). A competent Jehovah's Witness adult may freely refuse blood transfusion. The consequences of their refusal must be explained to the patient. This refusal must be documented on the Jehovah's Witness consent form and witnessed by a second doctor.[3] It is unlawful and unethical to transfuse an adult patient against their express wishes. The situation in a child is more complex.

In English law if a child is of sound mind and aged above 12 years then they are mature enough to give informed consent to treatment. A child who demonstrates 'Gillick-competence'[4] may consent to blood transfusion despite parental opposition. Competent patients of 16–18 years can consent to procedures in their own right; this consent takes precedence over any parental objections. The courts have ruled that children cannot refuse blood in life-threatening situations.[4] The Children and Young Persons Act 1933 states that parents have a duty of care to their children. Refusal of an essential blood transfusion constitutes wilful neglect. A doctor must act in the best interests of a child therefore the well-being of any child below the age of 16 years overrides the religious beliefs of the parents. If it becomes necessary to transfuse a child when the parents refuse to give permission then a 'Specific Issue Order', under Section 8 of the Children Act 1989 via the courts, needs to be sought prior to transfusion. The Association of Anaesthetists booklet[5] details the procedure to follow in this situation. Before this order is sought two consultant doctors need to sign in the patient's notes to declare that the blood transfusion is essential to save the child's life. The parents need to be kept fully informed at all times during this procedure.

Transfusion of blood to the child of Jehovah's Witness parents against the express wishes of the parents should not result in rejection of that child from their family although it has been reported.[6] Nor should it result in the rejection of the family from the local Jehovah's Witness community as long as the family displays a repentant attitude.[7] Transfusion of blood to a child may however result in psychological and spiritual upset for that Jehovah's Witness family. It is important to honour the parental wishes where it does not constitute a life-threatening risk for the child. The Association of Anaesthetists of Great Britain and Ireland has prepared a booklet to advise on the anaesthetic management of Jehovah's Witness patients.[5] Information and advice can also be sought from the Elder of the local 'Hospital Liaison Committee for Jehovah's Witnesses'.

Conservation of haemoglobin

Blood loss during elective surgery is the best predictor of mortality in Jehovah's Witness patients.[8] It is therefore vital to conserve blood throughout the whole perioperative period. This requires good preoperative assessment and planning. Preoperative conservation involves optimization of haemoglobin levels and limiting preoperative blood sampling. Optimization of haemoglobin levels can be achieved with oral iron, folate and vitamin B12 a number of weeks prior to elective surgery supplemented with parenteral erythropoietin. Case reports highlight the use of erythropoietin to increase both the pre- and postoperative haemoglobin concentrations in Jehovah's Witness patients.[9,10] Goodnough states that in patients for whom blood is contraindicated the use of erythropoietin has become a standard of care.[11] Selby and Lerman aim for a maximum preoperative haematocrit of 50%.[12] This preoperative optimization should be achieved under the direction of a haematologist to minimize the associated side effects reported in renal patients.[13]

Autologous blood transfusion is not usually acceptable to the Jehovah's Witness patient; however, it has been reported that 18% of Spanish pregnant women predonating blood in the third trimester are Jehovah's Witness patients.[14] There is a significant risk that should a Jehovah's Witness patient allow predonation of blood to be performed they will subsequently refuse for that blood to be reinfused, resulting in an iatrogenically anaemic patient presenting for surgery.

There are several strategies for blood conservation during surgery and anaesthesia for elective surgery. These have been extensively reviewed.[15–19] They include acute normovolaemic haemodilution, good surgical technique with careful haemostasis, correct positioning of the patient to minimize venous congestion in the surgical field, tourniquets where appropriate, hypotensive anaesthesia, cell salvage of blood, antifibrinolytic therapy with transenamic acid[20] or aprotonin,[15,21,22] prevention of hypothermia and regional techniques. Cell salvage with the 'bowl' technique has been limited in paediatric patients by the need for a specific volume requirement before any blood can then be washed and returned to the patient. Continuous autotransfusion systems that are fast, require small volumes for processing, eliminate fat and yield not only high haematocrit blood but platelets as well will revolutionize paediatric practice. The reviews suggest there is insufficient evidence to prove that these techniques are safe and/or effective in the paediatric population. Hence, the cost-effectiveness, the logistics and the risks involved for each one of these blood salvage techniques needs to be carefully considered for each individual case.

If predicted blood loss exceeds expectations the surgical procedure can be staged to allow the patient's haemoglobin level to recover between stages. If the haemoglobin level at the end of the procedure is less than 6.5 $g.dl^{-1}$ the patient will need to be electively sedated and ventilated to maximize oxygen delivery and minimize oxygen consumption. Careful observation of the wound postoperatively is essential; a pressure dressing may be required to minimize continued oozing of blood.

Religious beliefs prohibit the transfusion of blood in a Jehovah's Witness patient but there are other reasons to avoid homologous blood transfusion. Possible risks include viral contamination, bacterial contamination, parasitic contamination, Creutzfeldt–Jacob disease, alloimmunization, immunomodulation, graft versus host disease, metabolic imbalance and ABO incompatability from human error.[9,20] The current risk of transfusion-transmitted infections in the United Kingdom is very small[23] but there are significant risks from human error. The Serious Hazards of Transfusion (SHOT) scheme revealed a 52% incidence of human error in the 366 incidents reported over 2 years.[24] Even autologous blood transfusion is not without risk; reactions to autologous donations occur in 4% of patients.[18] Blood salvage in children has extra benefits beyond those seen in the adult population. Acquired blood-borne diseases such as cytomegalovirus cause acute illness and harmful effects on growth and development in infants and children. In addition prevention of sensitization becomes more important the younger the patient.

Growing medical and parental concern about the potential hazards of blood transfusion necessitates the need to avoid or at least minimize homologous blood transfusion in all children undergoing elective surgery, not just the children of Jehovah's Witness parents. The Jehovah's Witness movement has forced the issue of blood conservation into the medical domain. The techniques and principles utilized to avoid blood transfusion in Jehovah's Witness patients are now increasingly adopted for all paediatric patients to minimize the risks associated with homologous blood transfusion.

Learning points

- Surgery with the potential for major blood loss in a child of Jehovah's Witness parents raises a spectrum of age-related ethical and legal issues.
- Careful preoperative evaluation of the patient is required to weigh up the risk–benefit ratio of performing major surgery in a child of Jehovah's Witness parents.
- The parents, child and the medical team need to meet preoperatively to discuss and agree the management plan. The parents must be made aware of Section 8 of the Children Act 1989.
- Difficult areas of consent should involve the trust solicitor and an Elder of the local 'Jehovah's Witness Hospital Liaison Committee'.
- The results of the preoperative consultation need to be documented in the patient's notes.
- The parents should sign a Jehovah's Witness consent form.
- The medical team should respect the wishes of Jehovah's Witness parents when there is no risk to the life of their child.
- The child's haemoglobin should be optimized preoperatively to a safe level under the direction of a haematologist.

- All appropriate strategies should be adopted to minimize blood loss before, during and after surgery.
- In the situation of life-threatening anaemia the doctor must act in the best interests of the child.
- Blood transfusion against parental wishes during elective surgery should only be administered in a life-threatening situation. It requires prior application to the courts for a 'Specific Issue Order', under Section 8 of the Children Act 1989.
- Safe and effective blood conservation strategies should be adopted in all paediatric patients presenting for elective surgery.

References

1. Watch Tower Bible and Tract Society of Pennsylvania. Jehovah's Witnesses in the Twentieth Century, 2nd edn. Watchtower Bible and Tract Society of New York, Inc., 1989.
2. Schaller RT, Scaller J, Morgan A, Furman EB. Haemodilution anaesthesia: a valuable aid to major cancer surgery in children. *Am J Surg* 1983; 146: 79–84.
3. British Medical Association. Rights and Responsibilities of Doctors. British Medical Association, 1992.
4. Gilmartin G. Jehovah's Witnesses. In: Scott WE, Vickers MD, Draper H (eds.). Ethical Issues in Anaesthesia. Butterworth Heinemann, 1994; 105–113.
5. Management of Anaesthesia for Jehovah's Witnesses. The Association of Anaesthetists of Great Britain and Ireland. March 1999.
6. Wilson JR, Gaedeke MK. Blood conservation in neonatal and pediatric populations. *AACN Clin Iss* 1996; 7: 229–237.
7. Malyon D. Transfusion-free treatment of Jehovah's Witnesses: respecting the autonomous patient motives. *J Med Ethics* 1998; 24: 376–381.
8. Spence RK, Carson JA, Poses R et al. Elective surgery without transfusion: influence of pre-operative hemoglobin level and blood loss on mortality. *Am J Surg* 1990; 159: 320–324.
9. Snook NJ, O'Beirne HA, Enright S et al. Use of recombinant human erythropoietin to facilitate liver transplantation in a Jehovah's Witness. *Br J Anaesth* 1996; 76: 740–743.
10. Rothstein P, Roye D, Verdisco L, Stern L. Preoperative use of Erythropoietin in an adolescent Jehovah's Witness. *Anesthesiology* 1990; 73: 568–570.
11. Goodnough LT. Recombinant human erythropoietin therapy in patients for whom blood is contra-indicated. P99-103. Bloodless Surgery. Surgical and anaesthetic perspectives. Legal and ethical issues. Arnette Blackwell.
12. Selby IR, Lerman J. Anaesthesia for Jehovah's Witnesses. *Anaesthesia* 1996; 51: 95–96.
13. Ersley AJ. Erythropoietin. *N Engl J Med* 1991; 324: 1339–1344.
14. Majiluf-Cruz AS, Marin-Lopez A, Luis A. Autotransfusion and pregnancy. *Sangre (Barc)* 1993; 38: 207–210.
15. De Ville A. Blood saving in paediatric anaesthesia. *Paediatr Anaesth* 1997; 7: 181–182.
16. De Ville A, Govaerts MJM. Blood saving in paediatric surgery, 4th European Congress of Paediatric Anaesthesia. Paris, 1997.
17. Mazzerello G, Lampugnani E, Carbone M et al. Blood saving in children. *Anaesthesia* 1998; 53: 30–32.
18. Canadian Medical Association. Guidelines for red blood cell and plasma transfusion for adults and children. *Can Med Assoc J* 1997; 156(11S): 1S–23S.
19. Mertes N, Booke M, Van Aken H. Strategies to reduce the need for peri-operative blood transfusion. *Eur J Anesthesiol* 1997; 14: 24–34.
20. Yassen KA, Bellamy MC, Sadek SA, Webster NR. Transenamic acid reduces blood loss during orthoptic liver transplantation. *Clin Transplant* 1993; 7: 453–458.
21. Herynhopf F, Lucchese F, Pereira E. Aprotonin in children undergoing correction of congenital heart defects. A double blind pilot study. *J Thor Cardiovasc Surg* 1994; 108: 517–521.
22. Capdevila X, Calvet Y, Biboulet P et al. Aprotonin decreases blood loss and homologous transfusions in patients undergoing major orthopedic surgery. *Anesthesiology* 1998; 88: 50–57.
23. Regan FAM, Hewitt P, Barbara JAJ, Conteras M. Prospective investigation of transfusion transmitted infection in recipients of over 20 000 units of blood. *BMJ* 2000; 320: 403–406.

24 Williamson LM, Lowe S, Love EM et al. Serious Hazards of Transfusion (SHOT) initiative: analysis of the first two annual reports. *BMJ* 1999; 319: 16–19.

29

Revision ventriculoperitoneal shunt in a child with spina bifida (complicated by latex allergy)

Deborah J Harris

Introduction

Shunt procedures are the commonest paediatric neurosurgical operations, and frequently occur in the neonatal period. It is essential for the anaesthetist to be aware of all the possible complications associated with both the surgery and the underlying condition. Some of these complications are illustrated by the following case presentation.

Case history

A 2-year-old girl weighing 10 kg was admitted to the paediatric ward complaining of increasing headache over the previous 3 days. This had been associated with nausea and one episode of vomiting on the day of admission. Medical history, examination and investigations are presented in Table 29.1.

Past medical history	Born at 39/40 by elective Caesarean section Meningomyelocoele repaired day 2 Ventriculoperitoneal (VP) shunt inserted day 5 for hydrocephalus Infected shunt revised aged 9 months Blocked shunt revised aged 12 months
ASA grade	III
Regular medications	None
Allergies	None known
Examination	Quiet, pale child lying head up in bed BP 80/55 p 90 regular Chest clear Development: not dry day or night; can stand and take a few steps with support. Speech: good range of words, no sentences; no change in neurology since beginning of this illness
Investigations	Computed tomography – hydrocephalus Shunt series (anteroposterior and lateral skull and abdominal or chest X-ray) – no disconnection or kinks visible
Diagnosis	Blocked VP shunt requiring revision

Table 29.1
History and presentation

Management

The child was premedicated with 20 mg.kg^{-1} paracetamol orally an hour prior to surgery. She came to theatre on her bed in her own pyjamas and accompanied by her mother. Previous experiences in the anaesthetic room had led the parents to request an inhalational induction. A pulse oximeter probe and ECG electrodes were applied. Anaesthesia was induced with sevoflurane, oxygen and nitrous oxide. As soon as the patient was asleep and the mother had left the anaesthetic room a 20G intravenous cannula was inserted and connected to an infusion of Hartmann's solution at 40 ml.hr^{-1}, the blood pressure was recorded and ECG and end-tidal carbon dioxide monitoring were attached. Alfentanil 30 µg.kg^{-1} and atracurium 0.5 mg.kg^{-1} were administered intravenously and the trachea intubated with a 4.5 non-cuffed RAE™ endotracheal tube. The position of the tube was confirmed by auscultation and end-tidal carbon dioxide monitoring. There was a small leak around the endotracheal tube. The patient was ventilated with oxygen, nitrous oxide and isoflurane (to an end-tidal isoflurane concentration of 1% and an end-tidal carbon dioxide concentration of 30 mmHg), using a Penlon Nuffield 300 ventilator with a Newton valve and an Ayre's T-piece. Cefuroxime 30 mg.kg^{-1} was given intravenously as antibiotic prophylaxis.

The shunt was to be sited in the left lateral ventricle and tunnelled down the left side of the neck hence the endotracheal tube was fixed on the right side of the mouth with zinc oxide plaster. The child was then positioned on the operating table, under the supervision of the surgeon with a roll under the shoulders and the head turned to the right, on a paediatric head ring. A warm air-blowing sheet was applied to the torso of the child leaving the left thorax and abdomen exposed. An oesophageal temperature probe was inserted and taped to the right side of the neck.

The surgical area was prepared and draped and the scalp incision infiltrated with 5 ml 0.25% bupivacaine with adrenaline. Surgery commenced and anaesthesia was uneventful throughout the procedure, though a further bolus of alfentanil 10 µg.kg^{-1} was required at the time of the subcutaneous tunnelling. No further doses of muscle relaxant were needed.

The pulse and blood pressure remained stable until closure of the abdominal wound, 70 minutes after induction. The systolic blood pressure was suddenly noted to have dropped from 80 to 45 mmHg, the pulse rate had risen to 140 min^{-1} and the oxygen saturation had fallen to 88% with a normal capillary refill time.

In response to these findings the isoflurane anaesthesia was discontinued and the patient ventilated by hand with 100% oxygen. The chest compliance was noted to be poor. As the surgery had finished the drapes were removed completely to enable inspection and examination of the child. The differential diagnoses considered at this time included hypovolaemia, bowel perforation, pneumothorax and anaphylaxis. The surgery had been straightforward up until this moment and there was no evidence either of bleeding nor of perforation. Air entry was detected equally in both hemithoraces but associated with bilateral expiratory wheeze. Anaphylaxis was then considered to be the most likely diagnosis and 20 ml.kg^{-1} of colloid solution was infused with little response. Adrenaline 10 µg.kg^{-1} was administered intravenously and an immediate improvement was seen in all the vital signs. The child then developed a widespread rash. The improvement was short-lived, however, and further doses of adrenaline and boluses of colloid were required. The child was resedated and an adrenaline infusion was started at 0.1 µg.kg^{-1}.min^{-1}. Hydrocortisone 3 mg.kg^{-1} iv and a salbutamol (1.25 mg) nebulizer were administered and she was transferred to the Paediatric Intensive Care Unit (PICU). She improved rapidly over the afternoon, the adrenaline was weaned and she was extubated 6 hours after the episode.

Blood serum was sent for mast cell tryptase and complement levels on admission to PICU and again 3 and 8 hours later. A rise in mast cell tryptase above baseline was demonstrated which was highest in the 3-hour sample. This was suggestive of anaphylaxis and the follow up samples taken 6 weeks later were strongly positive for specific IgE antibodies to latex.

Discussion

Ventriculoperitoneal shunts

Shunt procedures for hydrocephalus are the most frequent operations performed in paediatric neurosurgical units. The incidence of congenital hydrocephalus is quoted as being between 0.2–3.5/1000 births.[1] Congenital hydrocephalus accounts for approximately 67% of cases of hydrocephalus in the paediatric population. Other causes include infection, haemorrhage, neoplastic and non-neoplastic (mainly vascular) obstruction and posterior fossa surgery. Hydrocephalus can be classified functionally as either communicating or non-communicating depending on whether the cerebrospinal fluid (CSF) circulation is blocked at the level of the arachnoid granulations or proximal to them. In the infant, although the skull sutures may still be open, a rapid rise in volume of CSF can cause a high intracranial pressure due to the relative rigidity of the dura mater.[2] Symptoms include irritability, nausea and vomiting, engorgement of scalp veins and irregular respiration. In older children, slowly enlarging ventricles may be asymptomatic or can be the cause of poor school performance. More specific signs and symptoms include headache, nausea and vomiting, gait change and altered vision or papilloedema. The classical presentation of sixth nerve palsy and 'setting sun sign' are signs of advanced hydrocephalus.

The goals of therapy are to achieve normal intracranial pressure and thus optimal neurological function and cosmesis. Post-haemorrhagic hydrocephalus may only be transient and serial CSF taps may be sufficient. Other treatment options include shunting, choroid plexus coagulation and third ventriculostomy. The most commonly used shunt is VP, usually from the lateral ventricle tunnelled subcutaneously down the neck and anterior chest wall to the abdomen.[1] If a long peritoneal catheter is used, the shunt may not need to be revised as the child grows. An alternative in those patients who have had, for example, multiple abdominal procedures would be a ventriculoatrial shunt.

The anaesthetic considerations of shunt surgery over and above those for surgery of other types include:

Difficult intubation
The large head may lead to difficulties in positioning the child for intubation. Usually this can be overcome by having an assistant supporting the head hanging over the end of the bed or trolley.

Positioning
The child should be positioned so as to allow the straight insertion of the surgical tunnelling device thus reducing the chance of tunnelling complications such as disruption of the major vessels and pneumothorax (Table 29.2).

Temperature control
Even with the ambient temperature in theatre raised, the surgical technique requires a large proportion of the child, including the head, to be exposed and prepared with antiseptic. The smaller the child the more significant this heat loss will be, and the more care should be taken to preserve temperature using hot air mattresses and wrapping the limbs in bubble wrap or wadding.

Hypotension at the time of CSF tap
Dysrhythmias at the time of ventricular catheter insertion
Pneumothorax at the time of tunnelling
Bowel perforation
Disruption of major vessels

Table 29.2
Intraoperative complications of shunt surgery

Bleeding
Bleeding should not be a problem in shunt surgery, although extreme rotation of the head may raise the venous pressure. Nevertheless, with the close proximity of major vessels in the neck and the risk of tunnelling through the ribs, it is wise to have blood available for smaller children and babies.

Pain control
It is worth noting that the scalp incision is essentially made under local anaesthesia and that undoubtedly the most surgically stimulating manoeuvre is the subcutaneous tunnelling. This is of particular interest in the preterm neonate in whom the aim may be to limit the use of opiates. Postoperatively most patients are comfortable with paracetamol with or without non-steroidal anti-inflammatory medication. Codeine phosphate 1 $mg.kg^{-1}$ or morphine 0.3 $mg.kg^{-1}$ orally can be used as rescue analgesia.

Postoperative care
Rapid draining of CSF can predispose to the formation of a subdural haematoma. Sometimes, therefore, it is preferable to drain the CSF slowly and allow the patient to sit up gradually over a period of a few days. Neonates and other small babies who cannot turn themselves should not lie on the side of the shunt for extended periods as pressure necrosis can occur over the cranial end of the shunt.

Meningomyelocoele

Approximately 10–20% of the general population will have spina bifida occulta, which is a congenital absence of a spinous process and variable amounts of lamina.[2] This is usually of no clinical significance. Spina bifida cystica has an incidence of 1/1000 live births in the

United Kingdom but this is falling, possibly due to earlier antenatal diagnosis and the administration of folic acid. The risk is greater if the parents have one or two previous children affected. The majority of defects occur in the lumbosacral area, 20% are meningocoeles 80% are myelomeningocoeles and the neurological signs are usually consistent with the level of the lesion. Hydrocephalus develops in approximately 80% of patients with myelomeningocoele and this will be clinically evident at birth in 5–10%. Most myelomeningocoele patients have an associated Type 2 Chiari malformation. Closure of the myelomeningocoele defect should take place within 24 hours of birth to reduce the risk of infection. In patients with clinically overt hydrocephalus at birth, closure and shunting may be performed simultaneously without increasing the risk of infection, with a shorter period of hospitalization and possibly reducing the risk of breakdown of the wound. Closure may convert latent hydrocephalus into active hydrocephalus, in which case shunting is usually performed at least 3 days later as in this patient.[3] With modern treatment 85% of infants with myelomeningocoele survive. Early deaths are related to complications of the Chiari malformation and late deaths to shunt malfunction. Eighty per cent of affected children will have a normal IQ, in the other 20% mental retardation is most closely related to repeated shunt infections. Over 50% will be ambulatory although many will use a wheelchair for ease and most will need intermittent catheterization or urinary diversion.

Latex allergy

This patient was diagnosed as having an anaphylactic reaction and responded clinically to the appropriate treatment. The delay in cardiorespiratory collapse from the time of induction is typical of latex allergy and indeed makes a reaction to one of the anaesthetic drugs unlikely. Delayed, type IV, cell-mediated contact dermatitis to latex has been described for several decades whereas immediate, type I or IgE-mediated reactions which present clinically with anything from hives to full blown anaphylaxis have only been described since the 1970s and are on the increase.[4] Why this should be so is unclear. Various theories have been put forward including the introduction of universal precautions related to HIV, changes in the production methods of latex gloves and the use of cornstarch which is a latex carrier and remains airborne when used as a glove powder, acting as a latex-aeroallergen in operating theatres.[5]

Spina bifida patients have a prevalence of latex sensitization of up to 80% and are at high risk of clinical latex allergy.[6] The incidence of latex sensitization increases with the number of surgical episodes but it has been suggested that the incidence is still out of proportion to other conditions which require repeated surgery. Szepfalusi et al compared 21 children with spina bifida with 32 children who had VP shunts for posthaemorrhagic or congenital hydrocephalus.[6] There was a significantly higher incidence of latex sensitization in the spina bifida group, even when the self-catheterizing patients were excluded. Whether this represents a genetic predisposition or is related to age at first contact with latex, has not been established.

This patient responded well to the standard treatment of anaphylaxis. The clinical picture can be much more severe, however, and curiously the severe reactions reported have tended to occur in clusters in the same institutions. This may be related to the surgical technique or materials used.

In cases of suspected anaphylaxis the anaesthetist is responsible for ensuring adequate investigation after the treatment of the emergency has been completed. Serum (at least 1 ml) should be sent for mast cell tryptase and complement levels. In practice the first sample is usually taken once the patient is clinically stable. Further samples should be taken at 3–6 hours and 24 hours (the latter acts as a baseline level if no preoperative sample is available). Normal mast cell tryptase level is less than approximately $10\,\mu g.l^{-1}$ (depending on the laboratory). A raised level that peaks between 1 and 6 hours is suggestive of anaphylaxis. If the level is equivocal, total IgG levels may be measured in the samples to enable the laboratory to correct for the haemodilution that may have occurred during resuscitation. Post event skin testing and specific IgE antibody to latex levels are recommended to provide the diagnosis. It is usually performed 4–6 weeks after the suspected reaction. Specific IgE antibodies to latex are measured on a grade of 0–6, with 4 or above being 'strongly positive'. They may not be raised during the acute reaction and a low titre at that time may be misleading. There is, however, some cross-reactivity, particularly with foods, plants and other related allergens. Skin prick testing is reasonably sensitive and specific and has the advantage that the weal and flare response acts as a predictor of clinical response.[7] It has a high negative predictive value and thus a negative reaction will virtually exclude latex allergy. In contrast, it should be noted that false positive reactions may occur. Skin prick testing should only be performed by trained personnel with the appropriate resuscitative equipment. After the acute event patients confirmed to have had an anaphylactic reaction should be counselled, given a medi-alert bracelet and referred to an immunologist.

Those patients in whom one has a strong suspicion of latex allergy should be managed in a latex-free environment while in hospital and it has been suggested that this should also apply to any group of patients who are known to be at a high risk of becoming sensitized. Premedication with corticosteroids or antihistamines has not been shown to be of benefit but those who favour it argue that it may modify any reaction that does occur.

Cremer et al compared the sensitization to latex in spina bifida patients before and after the introduction of latex-free surgery and anaesthesia.[8] Three of eight children became sensitized before and zero of 12 became sensitized after the introduction of the measures. No special instructions were given to the parents to avoid latex products in every day life, so it appears that the main cause of sensitization was repeated surgery. Nearly all anaphylactic events related to latex allergy have been secondary to mucosal exposure during surgery or dental or vaginal examinations. The single most important precaution is the use of latex-free gloves, followed closely by the reduction of the level of aerosolized latex antigens by leaving the theatre unoccupied for at least 2 hours.[7]

All hospitals should have a latex-free policy with, at the very least, lists of latex-free equipment, equipment containing latex but which can be used with modification and equipment which cannot be used. Ideally a separate trolley should be available so that latex-free equipment is available in an emergency.

It has been pointed out in the literature that there is much less awareness and understanding of latex allergy in hospital areas outside the theatre suite and that exposure to latex is common during the postoperative care of these patients.[9] Although every attempt should be made to increase awareness of latex allergy on the ward, it is much more difficult to avoid latex altogether and this may well be less important.[8]

Learning points

- Hydrocephalus may present with vague symptomatology.
- Children undergoing shunt surgery are usually covered completely by surgical drapes and are therefore difficult to assess clinically.
- The onset of anaphylaxis to latex may be delayed.
- When latex allergy occurs it should be treated following well rehearsed algorithms.
- All theatre suites should have the capability of providing latex-free conditions.
- All spina bifida patients should be treated in a latex-free theatre environment from birth.

Acknowledgements

I would like to thank Mr Bob Lock, Principal Clinical Scientist, Department of Immunology, North Bristol NHS Trust, for his help in preparing this chapter.

References

1. Greenberg MS. *Handbook of Neurosurgery* 5th Edn. 2001; Ch 8 Hydrocephalus, Greenberg Graphics Inc.
2. Matta B, Menon D, Turner J. (Eds) *Textbook of Neuroanaesthesia and Critical Care* 2000; Ch 16 Principles of Paediatric Neuroanaesthesia. Greenwich Medical Media Ltd.
3. Greenberg MS. *Handbook of Neurosurgery* 5th Edn. 2001; Ch 6.7.2 Spinal Dsyraphism. Greenberg Graphics Inc.
4. Kelso JM. Latex allergy. *Ped Ann* 1998; 27: 736–739.
5. Frankland AW. Latex-allergic children. *Pediatr Allergy Immunol* 1999; 10: 152–159.
6. Szepfalusi Z, Seidl R, Bernert G et al. Latex sensitisation in spina bifida appears disease-associated. *J Pediatr* 1999; 134: 344–348.
7. Dakin MJ, Yentis SM. Latex allergy: a strategy for management. *Anaesthesia* 1998; 53: 774–781.
8. Cremer R, Kleine-Diepenbruck U, Hoppe A, Bläker F. Latex allergy in spina bifida patients – prevention by primary prophylaxis. *Allergy* 1998; 53: 709–711.
9. Craig A, Rawlings E, Morphett S. Latex allergy – further comment. *Anaesthesia* 2000; 55: 98–99.

30

Adenotonsillectomy in a 5-year-old child with obstructive sleep apnoea

Anthony Pickering and Alexander Mayor

Introduction

Obstructive sleep apnoea (OSA) syndrome was first described in children in 1976 and has become an increasingly recognized problem. In children it is commonly associated with adenotonsillar hypertrophy and can be treated successfully by adenotonsillectomy. The dangers of perioperative upper airway obstruction and potential cardiovascular collapse demand expertise and vigilance from all members of the team involved in the management of these children.

Case history

A 5-year-old boy weighing 16 kg presented for adenotonsillectomy under general anaesthesia for the treatment of OSA. The child's parents reported that his development had been normal up to 3 years of age. However, over the last 2 years they noticed he had a disturbed sleep pattern with increased wakening and occasional bed-wetting. They also complained that he had become hyperactive during the day with decreased ability to concentrate on tasks. Despite a reasonable appetite he had fallen from the 25th centile for weight age 3 years to below the 10th centile at age 5 years. He had been admitted to the paediatric ward 4 weeks previously for investigations (see Table 30.1).

The results of the investigations are indicative of OSA syndrome with early signs of right ventricular strain. The parents were informed of the risks and benefits of adenotonsillectomy for their child. The consultant anaesthetist was informed of the child's history and investigations by the ENT team prior to admission and a high dependency unit (HDU) bed for postoperative observation was requested. The child was

Presenting complaints	Failure to thrive, noisy breathing, apnoeas during sleep and daytime hyperactivity
Past medical history	Born at full term with normal delivery; recurrent upper respiratory tract infections
Medications	None
Examination	Small child (< 10th centile), adenotonsillar hypertrophy and pharyngeal mucosal thickening (see Figure 30.1)
Investigations	Hb 16 g.dl^{-1}; ECG – right axis deviation, P wave in II (3 mm), S wave in V6 (6 mm); chest X-ray – heart size upper limit of normal; frequent desaturations on nocturnal SpO_2 monitor

Table 30.1
Investigations

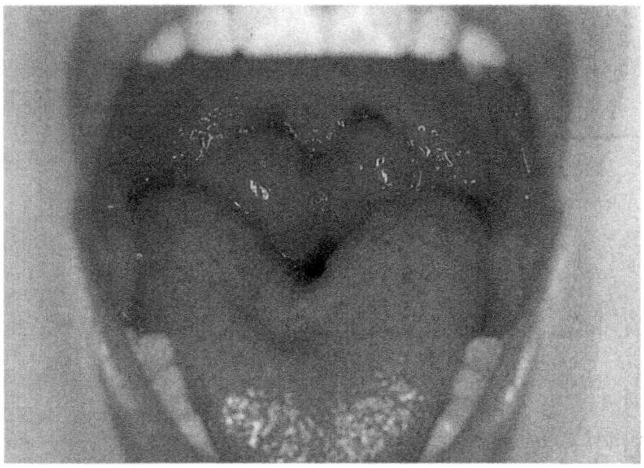

Figure 30.1
Tonsillar hypertrophy and pharyngeal mucosal thickening.

admitted on the morning of surgery; he was first on the operating list with extra time allotted for the case.

At the preoperative visit the anaesthetist assessed the child and explained to the parents that although adenotonsillectomy would improve his obstructive symptoms in time, there was a risk of early postoperative obstruction and therefore a HDU bed would be required. The process of induction of anaesthesia was explained to the child and one of the parents invited to be present for the induction. Consent was obtained for the administration of rectal diclofenac. Premedication, 1 hour before surgery, was local anaesthetic cream (Ametop®) to the dorsum of both hands and oral paracetamol ($35\,mg.kg^{-1}$). Sedative premedication was considered inappropriate.

On arrival in the anaesthetic room the child had a SpO_2 of 97% breathing air. A 22G intravenous cannula was inserted into a vein and anaesthesia induced with propofol $4\,mg.kg^{-1}$. Following insertion of a Guedel airway, bag and mask ventilation of the lungs was straightforward. It was therefore considered safe to give fentanyl $2\,\mu g.kg^{-1}$ and mivacurium $0.2\,mg.kg^{-1}$ to facilitate endotracheal intubation. On laryngoscopy, marked bilateral tonsillar hypertrophy was noted, but the vocal cords were easily seen and a size 5 uncuffed 'south facing' preformed RAE™ tube was passed into the trachea. A small leak around the tube was noted, but ventilation of the lungs easily achieved. Correct placement of the tube was confirmed by auscultation of the lung fields and end-tidal CO_2 monitoring. Rectal diclofenac $1–2\,mg.kg^{-1}$ was given before transfer into the operating theatre.

The lungs were ventilated with 35% oxygen to a tidal volume of $10\,ml.kg^{-1}$ at rate of $15\,min^{-1}$ to maintain normocapnoea. Anaesthesia was maintained with 2% end-tidal sevoflurane plus nitrous oxide. Intraoperative monitoring consisted of ECG, non-invasive blood pressure, pulse oximetry, inspired O_2, end-tidal CO_2 and end-tidal sevoflurane concentration. Intravenous fluids of 0.9% NaCl $10\,ml.kg^{-1}$ were administered.

At the end of surgery the pharynx was inspected using a laryngoscope to ensure haemostasis had been obtained. Recovery from mivacurium was confirmed using a peripheral nerve stimulator. The sevoflurane and nitrous oxide were discontinued. The child was positioned on his side with a slight head down tilt by positioning over a pillow. An awake extubation was performed when protective airway reflexes had returned. Supplemental oxygen was administered via a facemask during the initial recovery period.

The child was transferred to the HDU once alert and comfortable for a 24-hour period of one-to-one nursing care with monitoring of respiratory pattern and rate, oxygen saturation and ECG. Analgesia was provided with regular paracetamol elixir $15\,mg.kg^{-1}$ (max. $90\,mg.kg^{-1}.24\,h^{-1}$) and ibuprofen $5\,mg.kg^{-1}$ 6-hourly.

Discussion

The anaesthetic management of children with OSA for adenotonsillectomy is focused on the maintenance of a patent upper airway and the avoidance of cardiovascular collapse. Departments of Anaesthesia should develop guidelines for the perioperative management of children with OSA. The anaesthetic implications of paediatric OSA have recently been reviewed.[1]

Preoperative assessment

The epidemiology of children presenting for adenotonsillectomy is changing with fewer operations for recurrent tonsillitis and an increasing proportion of children with OSA. Therefore it is important to enquire specifically about sleeping habit and snoring in all children presenting for adenotonsillectomy. Examination of the child may reveal hypertrophic tonsils and evidence of chronic mouth breathing such as thickened pharyngeal mucosa, although these are by no means universal features.[2]

If the clinical features of OSA are present then baseline investigations of haematocrit (for polycythaemia), ECG and pulse oximetry are indicated. The ECG signs of cor pulmonale include a large P wave in leads II and V1, a large R wave in V1 and a deep S wave in V6. It has been shown that 3% of all children presenting for adenotonsillectomy have features of right ventricular strain on ECG.[3] Any ECG change suggestive of right ventricular hypertrophy merits further investigation. A chest X-ray is useful in assessing heart size and the presence of pulmonary oedema. Echocardiography can assess right ventricular function and cardiac catheterization may demonstrate pulmonary hypertension.

Polysomnography is considered to be the gold standard for diagnosing OSA. This technique utilizes multimodal monitoring (ECG, EEG, EOG, EMG, SpO_2, airflow and respiratory effort) to assess sleep patterns. On the basis of the polysomnographic findings children can be classified into mild, moderate or severe OSA depending on the number of apnoeas or hypopnoeas per hour. However, it is laborious to perform and requires co-operation from the subject and is consequently difficult to obtain data from children. If the clinical diagnosis of OSA is clear cut and the child is symptomatic then the child should proceed to adenotonsillectomy. An improvement in sleep pattern and polysomnography can be demonstrated following surgery.[4,5]

A retrospective analysis of 37 OSA cases (10 of which had complications) has identified the factors associated with postoperative morbidity:[6]

- age under 2 years
- cor pulmonale
- craniofacial abnormality
- morbid obesity
- failure to thrive
- previous airway trauma
- hypotonia
- high risk on polysomnography.

Anaesthetic management

The key to successful management of children with OSA is maintenance of airway patency. Even brief periods of airway obstruction can result in cardiovascular collapse and/or pulmonary oedema. Sedative drugs, anaesthetic agents and opioid analgesics can all worsen OSA by reducing pharyngeal muscle tone and inhibiting the central responses to hypoxia and hypercapnoea. Therefore these cases require careful planning, good technique and co-ordinated team working.

There is consensus that sedative premedications are contraindicated in children with OSA because of the risk of unobserved airway obstruction.[1] There is a rationale for the use of antisialagogues, such as glycopyrrolate, to reduce secretions and to protect against bradycardia, which can be particularly detrimental in children with OSA. The preoperative administration of an oral loading dose of paracetamol will assist with postoperative analgesia.

The induction of anaesthesia is a high-risk time for upper airway obstruction, particularly in children with craniofacial anomalies. The consequence of even brief periods of obstruction can be cardiac decompensation and pulmonary oedema. There are few controlled studies upon which to base practice in this area. Inhalational induction has been used effectively in severe cases of OSA syndrome with cor pulmonale.[7] It can provide a smooth induction while maintaining a patent airway and may allow a safe recovery should the child prove to be difficult to intubate. However, there have been reports of airway obstruction and consequent negative pressure pulmonary oedema during inhalational induction of children with OSA in the absence of significant cardiac pathology.[8,9] Furthermore high concentrations of volatile agent are required to allow intubation without muscle relaxants, which may cause significant cardiac and respiratory depression. The successful use of intravenous induction has also been reported in children with mild OSA.[5] This technique will usually result in the loss of spontaneous respiration. In the large majority of OSA cases (without craniofacial abnormalities) there should be little difficulty in either ventilation by hand or tracheal intubation.

It is traditional to use endotracheal intubation with an uncuffed RAE™ tube to secure a definitive airway for tonsillectomy and this is particularly recommended for OSA children. However, the reinforced laryngeal mask airway (LMA) is increasingly employed for 'straightforward' tonsillectomy.[10] Indeed, it has been reported that the use of the LMA is associated with fewer airway complications on recovery from anaesthesia than the endotracheal tube.[11] There is no data on the use of LMA in children with OSA and any such use requires extra vigilance to ensure that the airway does not become dislodged.

Intermittent positive pressure ventilation is used to reduce the concentration of volatile anaesthetic agent needed for surgery. The use of short-acting anaesthetic agents such as sevoflurane and nitrous oxide will facilitate rapid recovery of consciousness following surgery. Intraoperative analgesia for tonsillectomy is commonly provided with an opioid but for OSA the use of long-acting drugs such as morphine may increase the risk of postoperative respiratory depression and airway obstruction. The intraoperative use of $2\,\mu g.kg^{-1}$ fentanyl has been shown to be safe in children with mild OSA syndrome.[5] The use of non-steroidal anti-inflammatory drugs (NSAIDs) remains controversial because of worries over increased surgical bleeding associated with large intravenous doses of ketorolac; however, there is no evidence for increased bleeding with other NSAIDs.[12] As NSAIDs are effective analgesics for tonsillectomy and are opiate-sparing in the postoperative period we would advocate their use for children with OSA syndrome.

After surgery the children can be extubated in a deep or a light plane of anaesthesia. It has been suggested that deep extubation after tonsillectomy provides a smoother recovery with less coughing, bucking and hence less bleeding from the tonsillar beds. However, deep extubation would seem likely to increase the risk of airway obstruction in children with OSA. Therefore it is preferable to extubate in a light plane of anaesthesia, after confirmation of reversal of muscle relaxant.

Postoperative care

The recovery from surgery is an important period as the child remains at risk of obstruction, apnoea and hypoxia for several days, although an immediate improvement in polysomnography on the first postoperative night has been demonstrated.[5] Following surgery the child should be transferred to a high dependency care area with one-to-one nursing for the first postoperative night. Essential monitoring includes respiratory pattern and rate, pulse oximetry and ECG. Supplementary metered oxygen should be given if the arterial oxygen saturation falls below 90%.

Our suggested anaesthetic technique is just one of many possible safe techniques for this procedure. There is little evidence from controlled studies to suggest which is the optimal method of anaesthetic management.

Learning points

- OSA is increasingly commonly recognized in children.
- It may be associated with significant right heart strain and pulmonary hypertension.
- There is an increased risk of upper airway obstruction in the perioperative period.
- Maintenance of a patent upper airway is the key to successful management.
- Avoid sedative premedication.
- Use opioids with caution for analgesia.
- Postoperative HDU care is needed for children with significant sleep apnoea syndrome.

References

1. Warwick JP, Mason DG. Obstructive sleep apnoea syndrome in children. *Anaesthesia* 1998; 53: 571–519.
2. von-Someren VH, Hibbert J, Stothers JK et al. Identifying hypoxaemia in children admitted for adeno-tonsillectomy. *Br Med J* 1989; 298: 1076.
3. Wilkinson AR, McCormick MS, Freeland AP, Pickering D. Electrocardiographic signs of pulmonary hypertension in children who snore. *Br Med J* 1981; 282: 1579–1581.
4. Stradling JR, Thomas G, Warley AR et al. Effect of adenotonsillectomy on nocturnal hypoxaemia, sleep disturbance, and symptoms in snoring children. *Lancet* 1990; 335: 249–253.
5. Helfaer MA, McColley MD, Pyzik PL et al. Polysomnography after adenotonsillectomy in mild pediatric obstructive sleep apnea. *Crit Care Med* 1996; 24: 1323–1327.
6. Rosen GM, Muckle RP, Mahowald MW et al. Postoperative respiratory compromise in children with obstructive sleep apnoea syndrome: can it be anticipated? *Pediatrics* 1994; 93: 784–788.
7. Yates DW. Adenotonsillar hypertrophy and cor pulmonale. *Br J Anaesth* 1988; 61: 355–359.
8. Feinberg AN, Shabino CL. Acute pulmonary edema complicating tonsillectomy and adenoidectomy. *Pediatrics* 1985; 75: 112–114.
9. Motamed M, Djazaeri B, Marks R. Acute pulmonary oedema complicating adenotonsillectomy for obstructive sleep apnoea. *Int J Clin Pract* 1999; 53: 230–231.
10. Nair I, Bailey PM. Review of uses of the laryngeal mask in ENT anaesthesia. *Anaesthesia* 1995; 50: 898–900.
11. Williams PJ, Bailey PM. Comparison of the reinforced laryngeal mask airway and tracheal intubation for adeno-tonsillectomy. *Br J Anaesth* 1993; 70: 30–33.
12. Romsing J, Walther-Larsen S. Peri-operative use of nonsteroidal anti-inflammatory drugs in children: analgesic efficacy and bleeding. *Anaesthesia* 1997; 52: 673–683.

31

Bronchospasm complicating internal fixation of humerus in a 3-year-old asthmatic

Kathy Wilkinson

Introduction

Trauma is a frequent cause of emergency admission in early childhood. If surgery is urgent (within 24 hours of injury), anaesthesia is undertaken in the knowledge that the patient may have a full stomach. Asthma is also frequently encountered in the paediatric population and may be aggravated by viral airway infection. The management of bronchospasm following intubation in such a patient is discussed.

Case history

A 3-year-old boy presented with a displaced supracondylar fracture of the left humerus, following a fall from an upper bunk bed, requiring urgent reduction and internal fixation. The injury occurred 4 hours prior to the planned anaesthetic induction. Relevant findings on history and examination are detailed in Table 31.1 below.

The child had eaten approximately 1 hour before the injury. He was given morphine orally (Oramorph® 3 mg) on arrival in the Emergency department. At anaesthetic pre-assessment rapid sequence induction was discussed with the parents while the child was shown an anaesthetic mask and encouraged to play with it. Amethocaine (4%) gel was applied to the right hand and antecubital fossa. A consultant anaesthetist directly supervised induction by a trainee anaesthetist 45 minutes later. Anaesthesia was induced approximately 4 hours post injury and 5 hours after food. A 22g cannula was inserted painlessly into the dorsum of the right hand and flushed to check patency. An attempt was made to preoxygenate the child with 100% oxygen via a clear mask and the Jackson Rees modification of the Ayres T-piece. This was difficult as he cried and struggled. Thiopentone 80 mg followed immediately by suxamethonium 30 mg was given and the cannula flushed with saline. Cricoid pressure was applied at the time of loss of eyelash reflex. He was intubated easily with a 5-mm orotracheal tube which was secured at 13 cm at the lips. A moderate leak around the tube was noted and there was a brief period of desaturation after intubation to a minimum of 88%. This improved to 95% when ventilation was re-established (FiO2 1.0). Auscultation revealed bilateral wheeze and occasional coarse crackles in both lung fields. However, saturation and cardiovascular parameters remained stable and the child was given rocuronium 5 mg, fentanyl 30 µg and paracetamol 500 mg parenterally. Manual ventilation with an Ayres T-piece was continued (inspired isoflurane in nitrous oxide and oxygen). The child was transferred into theatre and connected to the ventilator (Penlon Nuffield series 200 with Newton valve attachment). The oxygen saturation deteriorated to 90% (FiO_2 0.5) and chest movement was noted to be poor. When airway pressures were increased saturations improved to 93%. A capnograph trace revealed an end-tidal CO_2 of 7.8 kPa. On examination there was now a large leak around the tracheal tube and bilateral wheeze was audible over both lung fields during both inspiration and exhalation. The child was given isoflurane in oxygen for 3 minutes, cricoid pressure was re-applied and he was re-intubated with a 5.5-mm tracheal tube. He was re-connected to the ventilator and airway pressures were increased to 25 cm H_2O. SaO_2 was maintained at 95% (FiO_2 0.5) but on auscultation wheeze and coarse crackles remained. Salbutamol (2.5 mg) was administered via the anaesthetic T-piece and an 'in line' nebulizer. Following this secretions were detected in the tracheal tube and a size 10 FG suction catheter was passed. A moderate amount of thick white mucus was aspirated with some improvement in chest compliance (as assessed

Asthma history	Asthma since the age of 10 months Precipitated by viral infections and exposure to cats One previous hospital admission aged 18 months managed with nebulized bronchodilators and oral steroids Required an increase in regular medication to control symptoms two weeks prior to this admission following an upper respiratory tract infection
ASA grade	II
Anaesthetic history	No previous surgery or general anaesthesia No family history of problems with anaesthesia
Regular medications	Beclomethasone 100 µg BD via spacer device Salbutamol 100 µg PRN via spacer device
Drug allergies	None known
Examination	Tearful child Apyrexial Normal airway Purulent nasal discharge Chest clear, transmitted sound from the upper airway SaO_2 97% in air Normal heart sounds Pulse 100 min^{-1} Displaced supracondylar fracture of left humerus No other injuries
Investigations	*Weight* 16 kg

Table 31.1
Relevant findings from history and examination

by manual ventilation) and oxygenation as judged by oximetry (SaO_2 98%, FiO_2 0.5). The child also developed a moderate tachycardia of 150 bpm. He was given 80 mg (approximately 4 $mg.kg^{-1}$) of hydrocortisone intravenously. Anaesthesia was maintained with nitrous oxide, oxygen and isoflurane (end-tidal concentration 0.8–1.0) with increments of rocuronium. SaO_2 remained between 96% and 98% (FiO_2 0.4) and end-tidal CO_2 6–6.5 kPa with ventilatory pressures of 20 cmH_2O at a rate of 12 breaths per minute. The child was then positioned for surgery which proceeded uneventfully over the next one and a quarter hours. Internal fixation of the humerus was confirmed with X-ray screening. At skin closure the wound was infiltrated with bupivacaine 0.25% 10 ml, the volatile anaesthetic was discontinued, and a back slab plaster applied.

The child was placed in a lateral position before reversal of muscle relaxants. He coughed forcefully on the tracheal tube before full awakening and vomited prior to extubation. His airway was protected by immediate suction and head down tilt.

Post extubation the child was tachypnoeic with a respiratory rate of 30 breaths per minute, moderate intercostal and subcostal recession and paroxysms of coughing. He was treated with a second dose of nebulized salbutamol (dose 2.5 mg in oxygen) with some improvement in cough and recession. Oxygen saturation remained stable at 96–97% in 4 $l.min^{-1}$ of face mask oxygen. His chest was clear on auscultation and a chest X-ray in the recovery room revealed no focal changes. He returned to the paediatric ward with oxygen administered through a simple (low flow) oxygen mask. Oxygen saturations were monitored and he required no further nebulizers overnight. He was discharged home well the following day on a tapering dose of oral steroids.

Discussion

This case poses a number of problems which are relatively common in emergency anaesthesia for small children. These include the management of a potentially full stomach, and an acute exacerbation of pre-existing significant asthma coincident with a recent viral infection.

Full stomach risk and rapid sequence induction

Skeletal trauma makes up 10–15% of childhood injuries[1] and is a common reason for hospital admission. Stomach emptying is delayed as a result of the autonomic response to pain and fear, with blood flow being diverted away from the visceral circulation. In many cases this leads to gastric stasis. Although current advice is that we allow clear fluids up to 2 hours before elective surgery,[2] it is well documented that large gastric volumes remain even many hours after significant trauma in childhood.[3,4] Opiate-based analgesia further delays stomach emptying and gut peristalsis.[5] At all times while the child is anaesthetized airway protection must be ensured, minimizing the chance of aspiration. The highest risk period in a recent retrospective review seemed to be at induction.[6] The method most widely practised in the UK to reduce the risks of pulmonary aspiration of gastric contents at induction is the rapid sequence induction.[7] Many would regard this type of induction as the 'gold standard' in emergency anaesthesia in children.[8] However, there may be problems including the difficulties of establishing venous access and performing effective preoxygenation. There is some diversity of opinion about the use of rapid sequence induction in all trauma situations in children.[9] This is in part due to a lack of certainty as to when the stomach can be relied upon to be empty. Even at 12 hours a substantial number will still have a high risk of aspiration[3] and each case therefore needs to be individually assessed. Despite its widespread use rapid sequence induction has been largely adopted without firm evidence of its efficacy. There are documented differences in the way UK anaesthetists currently conduct a rapid sequence induction.[10] However, the history in the scenario discussed would recommend the use of manoeuvres to protect against aspiration such as cricoid pressure. As mentioned, preoxygenation in small children is potentially difficult. Oxygen consumption is greater in the infant and small child compared with the adult and is further increased in a frightened struggling individual. However, in one study younger children (under 5 years) achieved an end-expired oxygen concentration of 0.9 more rapidly, and all children (aged 0–5 years plus) achieved this within 100 seconds.[11] The use of a clear mask impregnated with a pleasant smell may be useful, and masks can be obtained purpose built or can be sprayed individually.[12]

Asthma and anaesthesia

Despite work which demonstrates no significant effect of anaesthesia on respiratory function in stable childhood asthma[13] and low long-term morbidity and mortality,[14] others have shown an increased risk of respiratory complications in association with anaesthesia.[15,16] Risks in children are increased further by the presence of respiratory infection[17] and the need for intubation.[18] This child had a clear chest preoperatively. Nevertheless, the child has had a recent exacerbation of asthma in association with a respiratory infection and it may have been helpful to administer nebulized salbutamol preoperatively.[19] Thiopentone is a standard anaesthetic agent for rapid sequence induction but may be avoided by some in patients with asthma.[20] In adult asthmatics it has been associated with wheeze after intubation more frequently than propofol.[21] However, it remains the most commonly selected agent for rapid sequence induction,[10] perhaps because it provides a more definite end point and intravenous administration is painless. Nevertheless, propofol has also been shown to provide satisfactory conditions in this situation[22] and does not appear to alter respiratory mechanics in asthmatics.[23] If used in unpremedicated children a sufficiently high dose must be used.[24] Ketamine may have been another alternative because of its intrinsic bronchodilator properties.[25,26] However, its use as a sole induction agent, particularly during a rapid induction sequence, may be problematic as an end point may be difficult to judge. If venous access had proved impossible a modified rapid sequence induction using sevoflurane would have been possible with cricoid pressure applied and access gained by a second (experienced) anaesthetist as soon as the child was unconscious. Though a left lateral position has been recommended,[27] it may be impractical to implement and in fact a right lateral and or upright position has been shown to improve gastric emptying.[28] As an alternative to suxamethonium, rocuronium has been shown to provide equivalent conditions in a dose of 0.9 $mg.kg^{-1}$.[29] In some emergency situations the prolonged duration of this dose is inconvenient. It is the agent of choice in any child with suspected or actual suxamethonium sensitivity.

In the case presentation, lung compliance deteriorated following intubation and the child required increased ventilatory pressures and inspired oxygen concentration to maintain oxygenation. Bronchospasm may be precipitated by intubation (particularly if anaesthesia is insufficiently deep). However, the dose of thiopentone used was appropriate.[30] The subsequent need for increased ventilatory pressures resulted in a loss of minute ventilation around the uncuffed tube and this was improved with re-intubation with a larger tracheal tube. Airway instrumentation is always a risk in such patients but should be tolerated well if deep anaesthesia is maintained, the child is preoxygenated and the procedure is completed smoothly. The Penlon Nuffield ventilator with Newton valve in situ will not compensate for changes in resistance or compliance of the respiratory system,[31] and therefore should always be used with reliable end-tidal CO_2 monitoring. It is also important to ensure that ventilator circuit dead space is sufficiently large to prevent dilution of inspired gases with driving gas and should be at least equal to inspired tidal volume.[32] A slow respiratory rate (in this case 12 breaths per minute) with a long expiratory time is ideal in the asthmatic to provide good gas distribution and adequate emptying of overexpanded alveoli. Oxygenation is the priority and a relatively high end-tidal CO_2 ($ETCO_2$) should be tolerated (e.g. up to 8 kPa). Specific asthma treatment in the form of nebulized beta 2 adrenoreceptor stimulants led to further improvements in oxygenation, ventilatory indicators and chest signs. Other strategies to consider should include increasing the end-tidal concentration of volatile anaesthetic and more aggressive specific pharmacological treatment which might have included intravenous salbutamol, nebulized ipratropium bromide and intravenous theophylline (See Figure 31.1). Steroids were commenced but no improvement can be expected within 4 hours. However, they are recommended as a means of preventing relapse of symptoms in asthma after initial presentation. In the treatment of acute severe asthma in childhood their early use is supported by a grade A recommendation in a recent British Thoracic Society guideline.[33] In refractory cases nebulized or intravenous adrenaline has also been used (nebulized 1/1000 0.5 $ml.kg^{-1}$, maximum 6 ml, intravenous up to 0.05 $\mu g.kg^{-1}.min^{-1}$). In such cases it may be necessary to stop or delay surgery while treatment is instituted and some will need postoperative high dependency unit care.

In children with moderately severe asthma (i.e. those requiring continued prophylactic treatment) the use of non-steroidal anti-inflammatory drugs is controversial.[34] In practice, however, the number of asthmatic children who have had problems with this group of drugs is very small. Recent research has further demonstrated their relative safety.[35] However remote the chance of a severe reaction, it must be balanced against the benefits in terms of analgesia. In this situation the child will probably gain satisfactory pain relief with a combination of opiates, infiltration with local anaesthetic and paracetamol plus limb immobilization. A rectal dose of paracetamol of 30–40 $mg.kg^{-1}$ should provide a satisfactory blood level but a total daily dose of 90 $mg.kg^{-1}$ should not be exceeded.[36]

Anaesthesia was supervised by a consultant anaesthetist, recognizing that a trainee anaesthetist may have insufficient experience to deal with emergency anaesthesia in a small child. In 1989, the National Confidential Enquiry into Perioperative Deaths (NCEPOD) recommended that occasional practice in paediatric anaesthesia and surgery should be discouraged in an effort to further improve standards of care.[37] As a result of this report and many others in the interim some hospitals have decided not to admit children below a certain age for emergency surgery. The 1999 NCEPOD report[38] demonstrates that far less occasional practice in both anaesthesia and surgery now occurs particularly in very young children. A balance must be struck between leaving the district general hospital with an adequate service to treat the local population and the need to provide all children with a high standard of care.[39] Age criteria are in themselves insufficient and clearly the starvation status of the child, coincident disease, extent and risks of surgery and the distance from a specialist centre need to be taken in to account in a decision to transfer or involve senior staff.

In this case the child was properly prepared for extubation but vomited at this point – a relatively common event. Aspiration in this situation is unusual but is perhaps more of a risk with an uncuffed tube in situ. Fortunately, aspiration in children in the perioperative period would appear to be relatively benign,[40] which might be predicted from large adult surveys suggesting that death from aspiration occurs predominantly in those with associated medical problems.[6] Despite a stormy intraoperative course the child made

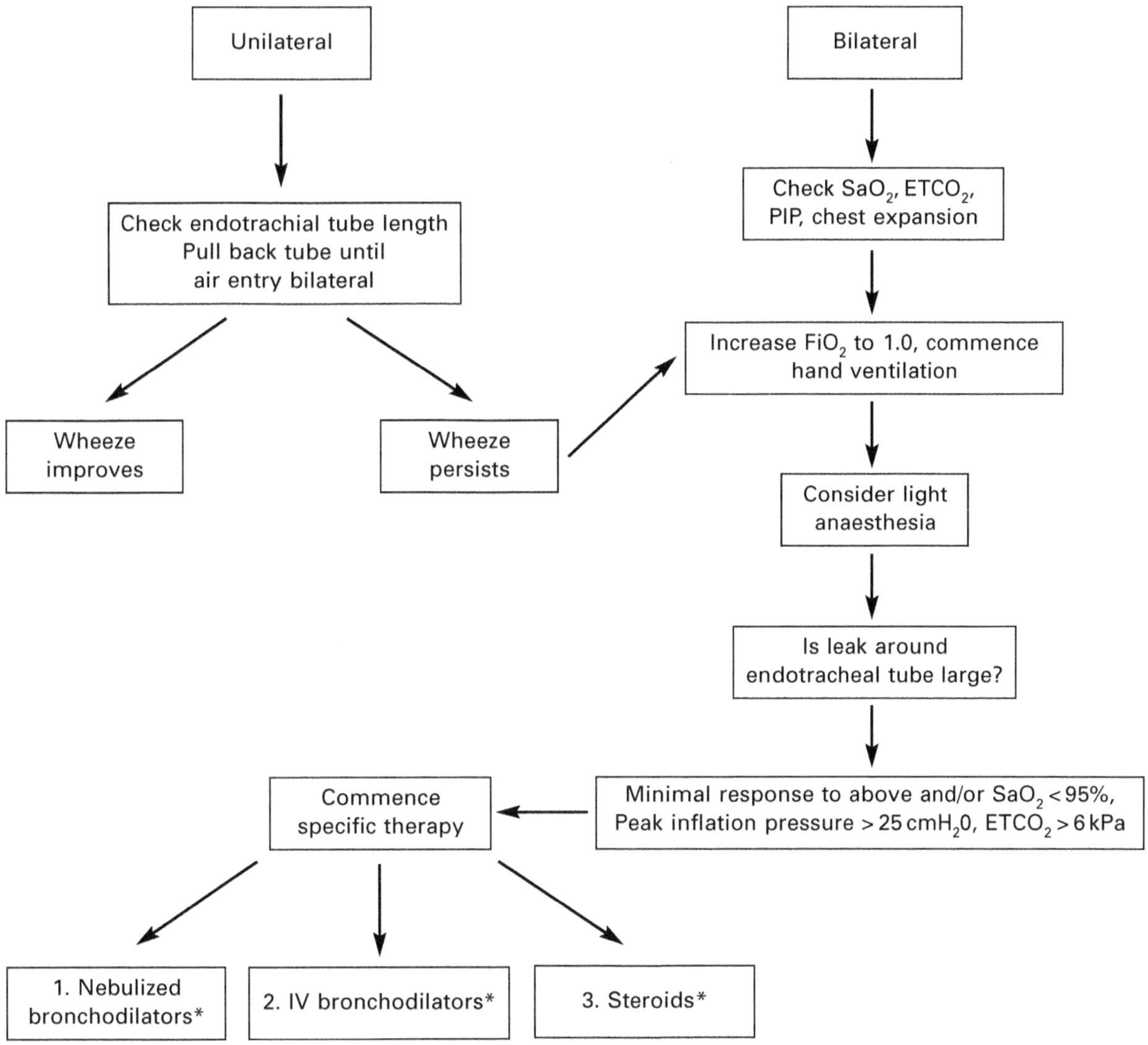

*** Doses:**
Nebulized salbutamol: 2.5 mg < 5 years, 5 mg > 5 years or 0.03 $ml.kg^{-1}$
Ipratropium bromide: 250 μg, may mix with salbutamol
!IV salbutamol: 15 $\mu g.kg^{-1}$, 1–5 μg $kg^{-1}.min^{-1}$
!IV aminophylline: 5 $mg.kg^{-1}$, 1 $mg.kg^{-1}.hour^{-1}$
IV steroid: hydrocortisone 4 $mg.kg^{-1}$

! Give boluses slowly over 15–20 mins with ECG control. Salbutamol may cause acute hypokalaemia. Bolus dose of aminophylline should be omitted if on maintenance therapy.
Step 1 should be considered prior to 2 and 3

Figure 31.1
Management of peri-operative wheeze in infants and children.

a satisfactory recovery. This is in keeping with published evidence which suggests that asthma, despite its frequency, does not usually result in serious long-term morbidity or mortality perioperatively.[14]

Learning points

- Trauma is a common reason for admission to hospital in early childhood.
- If urgent anaesthesia and surgery are required full precautions should be taken to avoid pulmonary aspiration of stomach contents as gastric emptying is prolonged and unreliable.
- Rapid sequence induction of anaesthesia poses special difficulties in the small child.
- Asthma in childhood is common and is often aggravated by viral upper respiratory infection, particularly in the preschool child.
- Intubation in a child with asthma and viral infection may result in bronchospasm that requires urgent diagnosis and appropriate management.
- Management of acute bronchospasm during anaesthesia needs to follow well rehearsed treatment algorithms.
- Anaesthesia in a child with asthma does not usually result in serious long-term sequelae.
- Use of non-steroidal anti-inflammatory drugs in asthmatic children remains controversial; each case deserves individual assessment but the incidence of problems would appear to be very low.

References

1. Advanced Paediatric Life Support Manual. Advanced Life Support Group, 3rd edn. BMJ Publishing, London, UK 2001.
2. Splinter WM, Schreiner MS. Preoperative fasting in children. *Anesth Analg* 1999; 89: 80–89.
3. Bricker SRW, McLuckie A, Nightingale DA. Gastric aspirates after trauma in children. *Anaesthesia* 1989; 44: 721–724.
4. Schurizek BA, Rybro L, Boggild NB et al. Gastric contents in children for emergency surgery. *Acta Anaesthesiol Scand* 1986; 30: 404–408.
5. Bailey PL, Egan TD, Stanley TH. Intravenous opioid anaesthetics. In: Miller RD (ed). *Anesthesia*, 5th edn. Churchill Livingstone, Philadelphia, 2000.
6. Kluger MT, Short TG. Aspiration during anaesthesia: a review of 133 cases from the Australian incident monitoring study (AIMS). *Anaesthesia* 1999; 52: 19–26.
7. Rasmussen G, Tobias JD. Paediatric anaesthesia. In: Adams AP, Hewitt PB, Grande CM, (eds) Textbook of *Emergency Anaesthesia* 2nd edn. Arnold, 1998.
8. Phillips S, Daborn K, Hatch DJ. Preoperative fasting for paediatric anaesthesia. *Br J Anaesth* 1994; 73: 529–536.
9. Marcus RJ, Thompson JP. Anaesthesia for manipulation of forearm fractures in children: a survey of current practice. *Paediatr Anaesth* 2000; 10: 273–277.
10. Morris J, Cook TM. Rapid sequence induction: a national survey of practice. *Anaesthesia* 2001; 56: 1090–1096.
11. Morrison JE, Friesen RH, Logan L. Pre-oxygenation before laryngoscopy in children: how long is long enough? *Paediatr Anaesth* 1998; 8: 293–298.
12. Maskumm bubble gum scented anaesthesia mask spray. Distrib. Trademark Medical, 1053 Headquarters Park, Fenton MO, 63026.
13. May HA, Smyth TL, Romer HC et al. Effect of anaesthesia on lung function in children with asthma. *Br J Anaesth* 1996; 77: 200–202.
14. Warner D, Warner MA, Barnes R et al. Perioperative respiratory complications in patients with asthma. *Anesthesiology* 1996; 85: 460–467.
15. Chung F, Mezei G, Tong D. Pre-existing medical conditions as predictors of adverse events in day surgery. *Br J Anaesth* 1999; 83: 262–270.
16. Bishop MJ. Cheney FW. Anesthesia for patients with asthma. Low risk but not no risk. *Anesthesiology* 1996; 85: 455–456.
17. Vener DF, Long T, Lerman J. Periop respiratory complications after general anaesthesia in children with asthma. *Can J Anaesth* 1994; 41: A55.
18. Cohen MM, Cameron CB. Should you cancel the operation when a child has an upper respiratory tract infection? *Anesth Analg* 1991; 72: 282–288.
19. Van der Walt J. Anaesthesia in children with viral respiratory tract infections. *Paediatr Anaesth* 1995; 5: 257–262.
20. Olsson GL. Bronchospasm during anaesthesia. A computer incidence study. *Acta Anaesth Scand* 1987; 31: 244–252.
21. Pizov R, Brown RH. Weiss MD et al. Wheezing during induction of anaesthesia – a randomized blinded trial. *Anesthesiology* 1995; 82: 1111–1116.
22. Dobson AP, McCluskey A, Meakin G, Baker RD. Effective time to satisfactory intubation conditions after administration of rocuronium in adults (comparison of thiopentone and propofol for rapid sequence induction of anaesthesia). *Anaesthesia* 1999; 54: 172–197.
23. Habre W, Matsumoto I, Sly PD. Propofol or halothane anaesthesia for children with asthma: effects on respiratory mechanics. *Br J Anaesth* 1996; 77: 739–743.
24. Aun CST, Short SM, Leung DHY, Oh TE. Induction dose–response of propofol in unpremedicated children. *Br J Anaesth* 1992; 68; 64–67.
25. Wilson LE, Hatch DJ, Rehder K. Mechanisms of the relaxant action of ketamine on isolated porcine trachealis muscle. *Br J Anaesth* 1993; 71: 544–550.

26. Sato T, Matsuki A, Zsigmond EK, Rabito SF. Ketamine relaxes airway smooth muscle contracted by endothelin. *Anesth Analg* 1997; 84: 900–906.
27. Surgical Emergencies and Trauma. In: Brown TCK, Fisk GC (eds). Anaesthesia for Children, 2nd edn. Blackwell Scientific Publications, Oxford, UK. 1992.
28. Villaneuva-Meyer J, Swischuk LE, Cesani F et al. Pediatric gastric emptying: value of right lateral and upright positioning. *J Nucl Med* 1996; 37: 1356–1358.
29. Mazurek A, Rae B, Hann S et al. Rocuronium versus succinylcholine: are they equally effective during rapid sequence induction of anaesthesia? *Anesth Analg* 1998; 87: 1259–1262.
30. Booker P, Intravenous agents. In: *Paediatric Anaesthesia* Sumner E, Hatch DJ (eds). 2nd edn. Arnold 2000, ISBN 0340 719427.
31. Hatch DJ, Chakrabarti MK, Whitwam JG et al. Comparison of two ventilators used with the T-piece in paediatric anaesthesia. *Br J Anaesth* 1990; 65: 262–267.
32. Wongprasartsuk P, Mason DG. The Newton valve revisited: an in-vitro study of ventilator circuit dead space. *Paediatr Anaesth* 2000; 10: 389–393.
33. British Guidelines on the Management of Asthma. BMJ Publications, Feb 2003. *Thorax* 2003; 58: supp.
34. Clinical guidelines for the use of non steroidal anti-inflammatory drugs in the peri-operative period. Royal College of Anaesthetists, London UK: April 1998.
35. Short JA, Barr CA, Palmer CD et al. Use in diclofenac in children with asthma. *Anaesthesia* 2000; 55: 334–337.
36. Shann F. Paracetamol: when and why and how much? *J Paediatr Child Health* 1993; 29: 84–85.
37. NCEPOD 1989. Campling EA, Devlin HB, Lunn JN. The Report of the National Confidential Enquiry into Perioperative deaths. 1989
38. Calum IG, Cray AJG, Hoile RW et al. NCEPOD 1999. The extremes of age. The 1999 Report of the National Confidential Enquiry into Perioperative Deaths.
39. McNichol R, Rollin AM. Paediatric anaesthesia – who should do it? *Anaesthesia* 1997; 52: 513–516.
40. Warner MA, Warner ME, Warner DO et al. Perioperative pulmonary aspiration in infants and children. *Anesthesiology* 1999; 90: 66–71.

32

Appendectomy in a child with insulin-dependent diabetes mellitus

Anna Johnson and Gillian R Lauder

Introduction

Diabetes mellitus is the commonest endocrine disorder in childhood and acute appendicitis is a common surgical emergency. The combination of the two may present a complex medical problem with potential for profound acidosis and severe dehydration. Management requires close liaison with paediatricians, anaesthetists and surgeons and may also necessitate paediatric intensive care support.

Case history

A 9-year-old child presented with a 3-day history of lower abdominal pain of increasing severity. Two days previously she had several bouts of diarrhoea. She had vomited several times in the last 12 hours. She had not passed urine for several hours. The surgical team had found acute tenderness in the left iliac fossa with guarding and made a presumptive diagnosis of acute appendicitis. They decided it was necessary to perform an emergency appendectomy. She was a known insulin-dependent diabetic on 15 IU of insulin day^{-1} and was previously fit and well with no other past medical history of note and no known allergies. A summary of her admission examination and investigations is shown in Table 32.1.

Management

Preoperative resuscitation

A diagnosis of diabetic ketoacidosis (DKA) was made and the child was admitted to the paediatric high dependency unit (HDU). Oxygen was administered via a face mask and initial fluid resuscitation was with $10\,ml.kg^{-1}$ of normal saline. The child was monitored with ECG and pulse oximetry. An insulin infusion was commenced at $3\,U.hr^{-1}$. The fluid requirements were calculated and a normal saline infusion was commenced at $265\,ml.hr^{-1}$. Paracetamol $30\,mg.kg^{-1}$ was administered as a suppository. A patient-controlled analgesia (PCA) pump with a morphine solution of $1\,mg.ml^{-1}$ was prescribed with a bolus dose of $20\,\mu g.kg^{-1}$, a lockout of 5 minutes and a background infusion of $2\,\mu g.kg^{-1}.hr^{-1}$. A nasogastric (NG) tube was passed.

An arterial line was successfully inserted after topical local anaesthetic had time to be effective at the left radial site. A femoral venous line was planned to be inserted but the child was not co-operative. Hourly urine output was monitored. Blood samples were repeated every hour. Hourly neurological observations were instituted.

Within 8 hours the child appeared much improved with normal respiration, normal capillary perfusion and the blood results depicted in Table 32.2. The rate of the insulin infusion was reduced after 8 hours to $0.05\,units.kg^{-1}.hr^{-1}$ as the blood glucose had reached $12\,mmol.l^{-1}$. The patient was again reviewed by the surgical team, who decided to proceed to appendicectomy.

Preoperative management

The child and her parents were given a full explanation as to what to expect in the anaesthetic room and recovery area. The child was comfortable using her PCA satisfactorily. No other premedication was prescribed.

Induction

All equipment and anaesthetic apparatus were checked. On arrival in the anaesthetic room full monitoring was

Examination	Flushed and unhappy, sleepy but easily rousable Extremely dehydrated; dry mucous membranes, loss of skin turgor Normal airway Noticeable ketotic smell Deep and sighing (Kussmaul's) respirations Chest clear, SaO_2 97% in air Heart rate, 132 beats per minute Capillary refill time prolonged at 4 seconds Normal heart sounds BP 95/60 mmHg	
Investigations	*Weight*	30 kg
	FBC	Hb 13.9 $g.dl^{-1}$
	WBC	WBC $23.5 \times 10^9 l^{-1}$
	U+Es	Urea 9.6 $mmol.l^{-1}$ Creatinine 57 $mmol.l^{-1}$ Sodium 131 $mmol.l^{-1}$ Potassium 3.9 $mmol.l^{-1}$
	Core temp	38.4°C
	ABGs	pH 7.16 $PaCO_2$ 3.4 kPa PaO_2 10.6 kPa HCO_3^- 15.4 $mmol.l^{-1}$ BE –8.5
	Blood glucose	35 $mmol.l^{-1}$
	Urinary glucose and ketones	Glucose +++ Ketones +++
	MSU	Sent to microbiology for culture
	Blood culture	Sent to microbiology for culture

Table 32.1
A summary of admission examination and investigations

instituted including the invasive arterial blood pressure from the radial arterial line. The NG tube was aspirated and left on free drainage. After preoxygenation using a transparent mask and a Bain's circuit with a flow of 10 $l.min^{-1}$ oxygen a rapid sequence induction was performed using propofol 5 $mg.kg^{-1}$ and suxamethonium 1 $mg.kg^{-1}$. The child was intubated with an uncuffed 6.5 endotracheal tube cut at 17 cm. After securing the tube and auscultating the chest to ascertain the correct tube position cricoid pressure was removed.

Fentanyl 1 $\mu g.kg^{-1}$ was given and as soon as it appeared that the suxamethonium was no longer causing full paralysis atracurium 0.5 $mg.kg^{-1}$ was administered. The patient's eyes were taped. A triple lumen central venous catheter was inserted into her left femoral vein.

Maintenance

Anaesthesia was maintained with isoflurane in 33% O_2 and 66% N_2O and ventilated at a rate of 12 breaths per

U+Es	Urea	5.8 $mmol.l^{-1}$
	Creatinine	51 $mmol.l^{-1}$
	Sodium	136 $mmol.l^{-1}$
	Potassium	4.3 $mmol.l^{-1}$
Blood glucose	12 $mmol.l^{-1}$	
Blood gases	pH 7.36	
	$paCO_2$ 5.4 kPa	
	paO_2 11.6 kPa	
	HCO_3^- 25.4 $mmol.l^{-1}$	

Table 32.2
Subsequent preoperative tests

min with tidal volumes of 7–10 $ml.kg^{-1}$ to maintain normocapnia. Boluses of fentanyl 0.5 $\mu g.kg^{-1}$ were administered as required. The crystalloid fluid of 0.45% saline/2.5% glucose was continued at 172 $ml.hr^{-1}$ and a further bolus of colloid of 20 $ml.kg^{-1}$ was given to maintain heart rate and capillary perfusion.

Reversal

At the end of the surgical procedure 10 ml of 0.25% bupivacaine was infiltrated subcutaneously around the incision. Neostigmine 50 $\mu g.kg^{-1}$ and glycopyrrolate 10 $\mu g.kg^{-1}$ were given to reverse the atracurium and 100% O_2 administered. The child was extubated on her side once awake and taken to the recovery area with 4 $l.min^{-1}$ of O_2 via a face mask.

Postoperative management

The patient was returned to the HDU for postoperative care so that careful monitoring of fluid status, blood glucose and U&Es could be continued.

O_2 (4 $l.min^{-1}$) was administered via a face mask to keep O_2 saturation levels greater than 96%. The PCA was continued as was the regular administration of paracetamol which kept the child pain free.

The crystalloid fluid of 0.45% saline/2.5% glucose with 40 $mmol.l^{-1}$ of KCl was continued at 172 $ml.hr^{-1}$ and the insulin infusion was adjusted to maintain a blood glucose level of between 6 and 10 $mmol.l^{-1}$. During the next 6 hours two further doses of 20 $ml.kg^{-1}$ of colloid were given in response to increasing heart rate and decreasing urinary output.

Oral fluids were introduced gradually the following day and fluid requirements were adjusted accordingly to provide a normal maintenance regime of 70 $ml.hr^{-1}$. Once free fluids were tolerated a light diet was started and the insulin was converted to short-acting insulin given three times daily.

By the fourth postoperative day the child was on her normal diet and normal insulin and fully mobile and she was discharged home on the following day.

Discussion

The management of these complex cases entails careful assessment, treatment and monitoring. Patients with diabetic ketoacidosis may present with abdominal pain which resolves with treatment. Gastric dilatation can also mimic an acute abdomen and makes the placement of an NG tube essential. Pneumonia should be excluded as this may also present with abdominal signs.

Assessment, investigations and treatment must be continuous and repetitive. Management aims to improve the patient's condition prior to surgery. This includes careful fluid therapy, insulin infusion and antibiotics while preventing cerebral oedema.

Fluid management

Fluid management requires calculation of the estimated fluid deficits and replacing these over a 24-hour period. Fluid replacement is aimed at providing normal maintenance fluid, replacing the estimated deficits, replacing ongoing losses (allowing an extra 10% for fever) and replacing urinary losses above 2 $ml.kg^{-1}.hr^{-1}$.

The child in the case described was clinically about 10% dehydrated; this equates with a 3.0 l fluid deficit. Fifty per cent of this needed to be replaced in the first 8 hours, i.e. 187.5 $ml.hr^{-1}$. Her maintenance fluids were calculated using the formula below:

Weight	*$ml.kg^{-1}.day^{-1}$ of fluid*
1st 10 kg	100
2nd 10 kg	50
Each subsequent kg	20

Maintenance = 1700 ml

10% added for fever = 1870 ml

Hourly maintenance $= \frac{1870}{24} = 78\ ml.hr^{-1}$

Therefore to correct her fluid deficit and to provide adequate maintenance the fluid requirement for the first 8 hours was 78 + 187 = 265 $ml.hr^{-1}$ and for the next 16 hours was 78 + 94 = 172 $ml.hr^{-1}$. The deficit was replaced with 0.9% saline but once the blood glucose reached 12 $mmol.l^{-1}$ then this was replaced with 0.45% saline/2.5% glucose. After the first hour and after ensuring adequate urine output potassium was added at 40 $mmol.l^{-1}$.

In DKA the total body potassium will be depleted despite adequate plasma levels and as the acidosis is corrected more potassium will move intracellularly. Patients with DKA die from hypokalaemia so potassium should only be omitted if the plasma level is above 6.0 $mmol.l^{-1}$ or the patient is anuric.

Detailed monitoring of the serum electrolytes and glucose is necessary to decide on the correct intravenous fluid replacement. Sudden changes in osmolality may result in cerebral oedema so great care must be taken to avoid altering sodium levels and the serum glucose too quickly. Serum glucose should be reduced by a maximum of 5 $mmol.hr^{-1}$.

Insulin

Intravenous insulin was given by an intravenous infusion of 0.1 $U.kg^{-1}.hr^{-1}$. The aim was to decrease the blood glucose at a rate of less than 5 $mmol.hr^{-1}$ and the blood osmolality at a rate of 0.5–1.0 $mOsmol.hr^{-1}$. A bolus of insulin should not be given as this may cause a sudden decrease in the serum glucose. The rate of the insulin infusion was reduced after 8 hours to 0.05 $U.kg^{-1}.hr^{-1}$ as the blood glucose had reached 12 $mmol.l^{-1}$. The insulin infusion was then adjusted according to need which was reduced further over the next 3 hours stabilizing at 0.8 $U.h^{-1}$ per hour. The insulin requirements may be very variable so again close monitoring is essential to prevent too rapid a decrease in glucose levels. Rapid changes in blood osmolality can cause cerebral oedema.

Prevention of cerebral oedema

Cerebral oedema in DKA is exclusively a complication of childhood. It is unpredictable but occurs more frequently in younger children. Cerebral oedema in DKA has 25% mortality.

As ketoacidosis develops the serum osmolality increases partly due to the increasing glucose but also due to the dehydration occurring from the glycosuria. The intracellular osmolality rises simultaneously. However, when treatment is instituted the serum osmolality may fall rapidly, thus water will move intracellularly causing oedema. The intracranial pressure will rise leading to decreased cerebral perfusion with resulting decrease in consciousness, this usually occurs 4–12 hours from the start of treatment. If the pressure continues to rise untreated then it will result in herniation of the brain and death.

Signs and symptoms of cerebral oedema include headache, confusion, irritability, decreased conscious level, fits, small pupils, increasing blood pressure with slowing pulse, respiratory change and/or papilloedema (late sign).

If any of these signs occur it is also important to exclude hypoglycaemia.

The aim of treating DKA is to prevent cerebral oedema occurring with careful attention to gradual glucose and electrolyte correction. Neurological observations need to be documented carefully and any changes (for example decreasing conscious level, behaviour change or headache) must be acted on immediately.

If cerebral oedema occurs it should be treated with intravenous mannitol 0.5–1.0 $g.kg^{-1}$ followed by intubation and ventilation. Fluids should be restricted to two-thirds maintenance. The head of the patient's bed should be elevated to 20–30 degrees. The patient will require a computed tomography head scan to rule out any other pathology.

Analgesia

The above patient received regular paracetamol, patient-controlled morphine analgesia and local infiltration of the wound with local anaesthetic. Non-steroidal anti-inflammatory agents were avoided because of the preoperative dehydrated state of the patient and the potential risk of acute renal failure.

Learning points

- Diabetic ketoacidosis can present with acute abdominal pain which resolves with treatment of the acidosis.
- In acute appendicitis it is important wherever possible to correct the metabolic derangements prior to surgery.
- Good communication between the surgeon, the paediatrician and the anaesthetist will help ascertain the optimum time for surgery.
- Dehydration can be severe and requires careful calculation of the fluid deficits.

- If there is cardiovascular compromise then a 20 ml.kg^{-1} bolus of colloid solution should be administered.
- Initially the crystalloid replacement is 0.9% NaCl; this may need to be changed to 0.45% NaCl with 2.5% dextrose when the serum glucose decreases beyond 12 mmol.l^{-1}.
- The insulin requirements may be very high initially and subsequently vary so regular monitoring of the blood glucose is essential; the dose administered must be adjusted according to need.
- The maximum rate of fall of blood glucose is 5 mmol.hr^{-1}; higher than this will cause too rapid a change in blood osmolality and may result in cerebral oedema.
- The patient must have regular neurological observations; any changes must be treated immediately.
- Cerebral oedema should be treated with mannitol, intubation and ventilation and a head up tilt.
- Non-steroidal anti-inflammatory agents should not be used in the sick dehydrated patient as there is a risk of inducing acute renal failure.

Further reading

Advanced Paediatric Life Support. The Practical Approach, 3rd edn. BMJ Books. 2001; 274–276.

Charalambous C, Schofield I, Malik R. Acute diabetic emergencies and their management. *Care Crit Ill* 1999; 15: 132–135.

Diabetes UK. Guidelines for the management of diabetic ketoacidosis in children and adolescents. www.diabetes.org.uk

Hammond P, Wallis S. Cerebral oedema in diabetic ketoacidosis. *Br Med J* 1992; 305: 203–204.

Hillman K. Fluid resuscitation in diabetic emergencies. *Intens Care Med* 1987; 13: 4–8.

Hillman K. The management of acute diabetic emergencies. *Clin Intens Care* 1991; 2: 154–162.

Royal College of Anaesthetists Guidelines for the use of non steroidal anti inflammatory drugs in the perioperative period. Quick reference guide. Jan 1998.

33

Cholycystectomy in a child with sickle cell disease

Isabeau Walker

Introduction

Sickle cell disease (SCD) describes a group of disorders associated with chronic haemolytic anaemia, acute vaso-occlusive crisis (leading to progressive end-organ damage) and infection. It is due to the inheritance of the sickle β haemoglobin gene which results in a single point mutation on the β globin chain. When deoxygenated, sickle haemoglobin (HbS) becomes insoluble and if present in sufficient quantity, will polymerise to form rigid fibres. The red cells become distorted and less deformable (typically sickle-shaped cells). Sickle cells have reduced survival and are responsible for the vaso-occlusion which is the hallmark of the disease.

The sickle mutation arose in multiple sites across Equatorial Africa and India, probably some 2000–4000 years ago, coincident with the advent of agriculture and the emergence of malaria as an endemic disease in these regions. Infection of sickle trait red cells with the malarial parasite causes the cells to sickle and results in splenic clearance of the parasite from the circulation. The persistence of the gene appears to be an example of balanced polymorphism in which the healthy heterozygous state has conferred an advantage to balance the significantly increased mortality associated with the homozygous state. Under normal circumstances in sickle cell trait, sickle globin is present in insufficient quantity to cause symptomatic disease. Population movement has resulted in the spread of the sickle gene mutation widely throughout Africa, the Middle East, Mediterranean countries and more recently, the Caribbean, North America and Northern Europe. The number of patients with SCD in the United Kingdom was estimated to be 10,000 in the year 2000, with most patients living in urban areas.[1]

The severity of SCD varies enormously between individuals. The most common and severe sickling disorder is homozygous sickle cell disease (HbSS), also known as sickle cell anaemia. It is a debilitating disorder with a significantly reduced life expectancy (median 42 years for men and 48 years for women in developed countries).[26] However, some individuals with HbSS can have a less severe illness and a near normal life expectancy. SCD can occur as a result of co-inheritance of the β^S gene with another abnormal β gene such as haemoglobin C (HbSC), β thalassaemia (HbS/β^+ thal or HbSS/β^0 thal) or haemoglobin D Punjab (HbSD). In general, individuals with HbSS and HbS/β^0 thalassaemia and HbSD Punjab tend to follow a severe clinical course, HbSC disease, HbS/β^+ thalassaemia follow a milder course.[2] α thalassaemia is also common in populations in which SCD occurs. Patients with α thalassaemia and SCD may have a mild clinical course in childhood, but α thalassaemia is thought to be an increased risk factor for mortality in adults with SCD.[3] Sickle cell trait (HbAS) is a clinically insignificant condition.

The clinical features of SS include those due to haemolysis (chronic haemolytic anaemia, pigment gallstones), those due to vaso-occlusion (acute painful crisis, stroke, acute sickle chest syndrome, splenic sequestration, splenic atrophy, priapism, leg ulcers, chronic renal insufficiency, retinopathy, chronic sickle lung disease, delayed growth and development) and those due to infection (pneumococcal sepsis, haemophilus infection, aplastic crisis associated with parvovirus B19). Pigment gallstones are very common in patients with SCD and cholycystectomy is the most frequently performed surgical procedure in this group.[1]

The perioperative period is a time of increased risk for patients with SCD. Unfortunately, many of the factors known to promote the polymerization of deoxygenated HbS are commonly encountered (dehydration, hypoxia, acidosis) and meticulous care is required to avoid sickle-related complications. The complex case history of a child with homozygous sickle cell disease (HbSS) presenting for cholycystectomy will be discussed in this chapter.

Case history

A 13-year-old Jamaican boy with sickle cell anaemia presented with a history of recurrent right upper quadrant pain associated with nausea. He experienced pain every 2–3 weeks and was having difficulty keeping up at school. He was admitted to hospital on several occasions for pain control. Abdominal ultrasound demonstrated the presence of multiple gallstones. He also had signs and symptoms of severe obstructive sleep apnoea (OSA), with snoring, intermittent apnoea, morning headaches and daytime somnolence, confirmed on sleep study. He was referred for adenotonsillectomy and cholycystectomy. A transcranial Doppler ultrasound was performed to screen for cerebrovascular disease and was normal. Past medical history included frequent painful episodes in infancy and operation for orchidopexy at 6 months of age – this was performed in Jamaica without preoperative blood transfusion. He had received immunization against pneumococcal infection and was taking long-term penicillin V prophylaxis. In view of the severity of his upper airway obstruction, it was decided to proceed with adenotonsillectomy as a matter of some urgency, prior to cholycystectomy.

After discussion between the referring paediatrician, haematologist, anaesthetist and the child's family, the child was prepared for adenotonsillectomy with a simple top-up transfusion to raise his haemoglobin level to greater than 10 $g.dl^{-1}$ (avoiding overtransfusion). The operation was uneventful and he suffered no complications.

Three months after adenotonsillectomy he was prepared for laparoscopic cholycystectomy. Again, the issue of preoperative transfusion was discussed widely. A decision was made to prepare for surgery with a more aggressive transfusion regimen, planned to increase his haemoglobin to 9–11 $g.dl^{-1}$ (but < 12 $g.dl^{-1}$) and reduce his HbS fraction to < 30%. This was achieved by several top-up transfusions in the 3 weeks prior to admission to hospital for surgery. All transfusions were with phenotypically matched leucodepleted blood.

Preoperative investigations revealed Hb 9.6 $g.dl^{-1}$, HbS fraction of 11%, HbA_2 3.4%, HbF 1.1% (pre-exchange, Hb 8.5 $g.dl^{-1}$, HbS 55%, reflecting previous transfusion for adenotonsillectomy) (see Table 33.1).

The child was admitted to hospital the day before surgery. Two units of blood were cross-matched for surgery and were also available to be used in the event of a sickle-related crisis. The child was extremely needle phobic so preoperative hydration was with oral fluids – free clear fluids were given up until 2 hours preoperatively. Temazepam 15 mg was given 1 hour preoperatively as premedication. The child requested an inhalational induction. Induction was uneventful, with nitrous oxide and oxygen followed by incremental sevoflurane to 8%. Two intravenous cannulae were inserted, the child paralysed with atracurium, intubated with a cuffed oral tube and anaesthesia continued with isoflurane in air and oxygen. Standard non-invasive monitoring was used throughout. A hot air warming mattress was used to maintain body temperature which was monitored using a nasopharyngeal temperature probe. Analgesia consisted of fentanyl 3 $\mu g.kg^{-1}$ iv, paracetamol 40 $mg.kg^{-1}$ pr and diclofenac 1 $mg.kg^{-1}$ pr given at the start of surgery. Bupivacaine 0.25% 1 $ml.kg^{-1}$ was used (rectus sheath block and local infiltration to port sites). A standard laparoscopic cholycystectomy was performed with carbon dioxide insufflation to 12 mmHg. Ventilation was adjusted to maintain normocarbia throughout. The surgery took approximately 120 minutes. Blood loss during surgery was minimal and hydration was maintained with Hartmann's solution. A total of 30 $ml.kg^{-1}$ fluid was given during the procedure and full maintenance fluids continued postoperatively. A loading dose of morphine (0.1 $mg.kg^{-1}$) was given towards the end of surgery and postoperative analgesia continued with morphine via a patient-controlled analgesia pump (PCA) – bolus dose morphine 20 $\mu g.kg^{-1}$, lockout 5 minutes, and no background infusion.

The child was extubated at the end of the procedure and saturation monitoring continued in recovery and on the ward. Facemask oxygen was prescribed to maintain oxygen saturation > 95%, but was not required after the first hour postoperatively. Postoperative analgesia requirements were minimal and the PCA was discontinued the following morning. Analgesia was continued with paracetamol and diclofenac. The child started taking clear fluids 10 hours postoperatively and the intravenous fluids were discontinued the following morning. The child was well and discharged home from hospital 2 days after surgery. He was seen in the surgical outpatients clinic 4 weeks later when the surgical scars were well healed and he had had no further pain.

The child became acutely unwell 4 months after surgery. He was admitted from home with a history of

Past medical history	HbSS diagnosed on routine screening aged 6 months Routine orchidopexy aged 6 months (no transfusion) Dactylitis in infancy OSA on sleep study (baseline saturation 90%, dips to 80%) Frequent episodes of right upper abdominal pain
Regular medications	Penicillin V
Examination	Mild jaundice Tender right upper quadrant
Investigations	Hb 9.6 $g.dl^{-1}$, WBC $14.9 \times 10^9 l^{-1}$, platelets $411 \times 10^9 l^{-1}$ HbS 11%, HbA_2 3.4%, HbF 1.1% Na 141 $mmol.l^{-1}$, K 3.8 $mmol.l^{-1}$, urea 3.8 $mmol.l^{-1}$, creatinine 62 $\mu mol.l^{-1}$ Bilirubin 84 $\mu mol.l^{-1}$ *Chest X-ray* – no focal lesion *Abdominal ultrasound* – three gallstones within dilated gallbladder; kidneys of normal size with loss of corticomedullary differentiation; small shrunken spleen *Transcranial Doppler ultrasound* – normal result

Table 33.1
Preoperative investigations

chest pain and breathlessness. He was noted to be anaemic with a Hb of 8.0 $g.dl^{-1}$, and elevated white cell count of $27.3 \times 10^9 l^{-1}$. Oxygen saturation was 83% in air and chest X-ray showed bilateral pulmonary consolidation. A diagnosis of acute sickle chest syndrome was made, probably associated with mycoplasma infection. Treatment consisted of oxygen, intravenous hydration and antibiotics (although he remained culture negative). He underwent an emergency exchange transfusion to reduce his HbS to < 30%. His condition deteriorated and he required mechanical ventilation for a period of 5 days. After extubation he was noted to have developed a left hemiplegia – a computed tomography scan revealed an infarct in the posterior parietal region. He remains well and is now on a programme of regular transfusions to maintain his HbS level < 20%.

Discussion

The case report describes the complex history of a child with severe SS who nevertheless underwent successful cholycystectomy under general anaesthesia. Children with SCD undergoing surgery are at high risk of perioperative complications and meticulous anaesthetic care is required.[15,24]

Clinical features have been identified which predict the severity of SCD and may be useful to identify those at increased risk in the perioperative period. SCD in childhood is associated with periods of well-being interspersed with episodes of acute illness.[4] Dactylitis (pain in hands or feet), severe anaemia and leukocytosis during infancy have been shown to be predictive of severe SCD in later life.[5] Twenty per cent of children have a painful crisis requiring hospitalization during childhood and the frequency of painful crises increases after puberty.[14] Frequent painful episodes (more than three per year) are a marker of clinical severity and correlate with early death in patients over the age of 20 years.[13]

Cerebral vasculopathy with cerebral infarction is first seen during childhood. Stroke occurs by the age of 20 years in 11% of patients with SCD and is recurrent in 60% if untreated. A further 17% may have changes on magnetic resonance imaging (MRI) suggestive of infarction or ischaemia in the absence of stroke. Risk factors for 'silent' cerebral infarction in children are a history of seizure, raised white cell count, low pain event rate and low HbF. Silent infarction can be associated with a low haemoglobin and has a distribution suggestive of a watershed perfusion injury.[6] Profound anaemia may trigger stroke and haemoglobin levels below 5 $g.dl^{-1}$ should be avoided, especially in children.[7] Transcranial Doppler has been used to screen children at risk for stroke. Long-term blood transfusion programmes have been shown to reduce the incidence of recurrent stroke and first stroke in children with abnormal transcranial Doppler results. Children receive 4-weekly transfusions aimed to maintain the HbS level $< 30\%$.[8]

Acute sickle chest syndrome is associated with sickling and ischaemia in lung tissue. It is seen at all ages but in young children is frequently associated with infection and tends to follow a milder course than in older children and adults. Five per cent of patients require hospitalization for acute sickle chest syndrome during mid-childhood and adolescence. Acute sickle chest syndrome is both predictive of shortened survival and is one of the most frequent causes of death in SCD regardless of age.[26] Recurrent episodes lead to chronic lung disease.[9] Acute sickle chest syndrome in the postoperative period has a peak occurrence at 48 hours after operation.[14]

The pathophysiology of the disease at a cellular level is interesting with respect to perioperative management. The polymerization (gellation) of deoxy HbS within red cells is the primary event in the molecular pathogenesis of SCD.[10] The deoxy HbS polymers aggregate to form fibres that distort the red cells; on reoxygenation the polymers 'melt' and the red cells regain their shape. Sickling of red cells is not an acute event as the result of an episode of sudden deoxygenation; it is a chronic ongoing process for each red blood cell as it is exposed to hypoxic conditions every time it passes through the microcirculation. Each cell is estimated to sickle to some extent an average of 6000 times per day.[11] There is an important delay between the formation of deoxy HbS and the generation of polymer – most red cells do not become distorted until they have passed through the capillaries into the venous system where they are no longer in danger of causing vascular occlusion. Factors that delay red cell transit time, such as vasoconstriction, increases in blood viscosity or increased stickiness of the HbSS red cells to vascular endothelium, will increase the probability of vascular occlusion. Repeated episodes of red cell sickling and unsickling result in damage to the red cell membrane causing dehydration and the formation of irreversibly sickled cells. These cells demonstrate increased adhesion to vascular endothelium and are responsible for vaso-occlusion. A sickle crisis can both activate and result from the action of the inflammatory cascade (possibly triggered by infection) involving the production of inflammatory mediators interleukins 1 and 6 (IL-1, IL-6) and tumour necrosis factor (TNFα), activation of the haemostatic system and neutrophils and the binding of sickle reticulocytes to vascular endothelium in the postcapillary venule. Activated neutrophils cause endothelial damage and the formation of fibrin clot. Sickle reticulocytes and irreversibly sickled cells build up proximal to the fibrin clot so microvascular occlusion occurs.[12] A high neutrophil cell count is predictive of higher mortality in SCD.

Foetal haemoglobin is an important modulator of the severity of SCD. The beneficial effects are due to dilution of HbS within the red cell so that the HbF interferes with HbS polymerization. In normal individuals HbF ($\alpha2\gamma2$) predominates through gestation. Adult haemoglobin production begins midway during gestation and from birth increases rapidly to become the predominant haemoglobin. By 6 months of age, erythrocytes of normal individuals contain their final complement of haemoglobins, HbA ($\alpha2\beta2$) 96%, HbA_2 ($\alpha2\beta2$) 2–3% and HbF $< 1\%$. Normal levels of HbF of 60–80% at birth decline slowly in children with SCD, reaching a nadir by 5–7 years. Individuals with HbSS in central India and the Eastern Province of Saudi Arabia have high levels of HbF, mild anaemia and less severe clinical disease. It is thought that HbF levels of 7% or higher may have an ameliorating effect on the severity of sickle disease.[13] The chemotherapeutic agent, hydroxyurea, has been noted to increase HbF levels in patients with SCD and reduce the incidence of complications. It is used in adults with severe disease but unknown long-term adverse effects (carcinogenicity, mutagenicity) mean it is used only exceptionally at present in children. Hydroxyurea may exert its beneficial effect in part by a reduction in neutrophils.[14]

Various factors under the anaesthetist's control may reduce sickling. Hyperosmolar dehydration is poorly tolerated as red cells are perfect osmometers – intracellular haemoglobin concentration rises if the patient becomes dehydrated and the tendency of red cells to sickle is increased. Patients with SCD are particularly prone to clinical dehydration as the environment of the renal medulla makes it extremely vulnerable to sickle vaso-occlusion and even patients with sickle trait have impaired urine-concentrating ability. Children with SCD demonstrate renal tubular concentration defects from the age of 2 years. It is important to ensure that patients are well hydrated at all times, including in the preoperative period. Some have suggested at least

8 hours of intravenous hydration preoperatively,[15] others suggest intravenous hydration from the night before surgery with 1.5 times maintenance fluids.[16] Our patient demonstrated a problem common to many children with SCD in that they have poor veins, are subjected to multiple blood tests/transfusions and become extremely needle phobic. Intravenous therapy is preferable but if opting for oral hydration preoperatively, care should be taken that the fluid intake is adequate. Intravenous fluids should continue into the postoperative period until the child is able to tolerate full oral fluids again.

Obviously, hypoxia should be avoided as a risk factor for sickling although the role of isolated alveolar hypoxia in the absence of dehydration or acidosis as a trigger for a sickle crisis is not clear. Of note, 20–30% of individuals with SCD develop painful crises when flying at altitude in unpressurized aircraft.[17] Oxygen therapy should be given in the postoperative period as indicated by continuous oxygen saturation monitoring. Our patient had a diagnosis of OSA made at the same time as he was referred for cholycystectomy. OSA secondary to adenotonsillar hypertrophy is common in children with SCD. The peak incidence of childhood OSA coincides with the peak incidence of painful crisis and stroke in children[2] and OSA may be a potential risk factor for the development of stroke in children with sickle disease.[3] Cerebrovascular disease is often subclinical in this age group.[8] Although OSA improves in the months following surgery,[18] clinical experience indicates that severe OSA is not improved immediately following surgery.[19] It has been shown that adenotonsillectomy carries a high risk of postoperative complications relative to other operations in children with SCD.[20] Given all these factors, it was decided to proceed to adenotonsillectomy in the months before cholycystectomy in this child, both to reduce the risks associated with a combined procedure, and to reduce the risks associated with OSA post cholycystectomy. If prior adenotonsillectomy had not been possible, then facemask continuous positive airway pressure (CPAP) may have been required in the immediate postoperative period. Early ambulation, incentive spirometry and chest physiotherapy in the postoperative period are indicated to reduce postoperative hypoventilation and atelectasis and hence the likelihood of postoperative hypoxia and acute sickle chest syndrome.[16]

Systemic acidosis causes a left shift of the oxygen dissociation curve, reduces the affinity of haemoglobin for oxygen and increases the amount of deoxy HbS formed, thus increasing the likelihood of sickling. Obviously, avoidance of acidosis is part of routine anaesthetic management; it is poorly tolerated by these patients. Routine alkalinization has not been shown to be of benefit.[21] With respect to intraoperative management, meticulous fluid balance is required, with monitoring of blood loss and replacement when necessary. Ventilation should be controlled to avoid hypercarbia. End-tidal carbon dioxide ($ETCO_2$) concentrations rise during laparoscopic surgery with carbon dioxide insufflation – ventilation should be adjusted to maintain a normal $ETCO_2$ at all times. Hypocarbia should be avoided so as not to compromise cerebral blood flow.

Cold may be one of the triggers for a painful crisis in some individuals and should be avoided at all times. Intraoperative hypothermia will induce vasoconstriction and postoperative shivering with greatly increased oxygen consumption. Body temperature should be recorded during surgery with measures taken to maintain a normal temperature (warming mattress, humidified gases and warmed fluids).

In terms of the anaesthetic technique employed, an observational study has suggested that regional anaesthesia is associated with a higher incidence of sickle-related problems, mainly pain, in the postoperative period.[22] This may have been due to factors associated with the type of surgery (mainly Caesarean sections), but may be related to hypotension or alterations in regional blood flow associated with epidural anaesthesia (compensatory vasoconstriction in unblocked areas). It is our practice to employ a standard general anaesthetic technique combined with regional anaesthesia as indicated by the nature of the surgery undertaken. Good postoperative analgesia is of paramount importance.

The question of perioperative transfusion in patients with SCD remains controversial. The rationale behind preoperative transfusion is to reduce the likelihood of sickle-related complications occurring in the perioperative period, the most feared of which are acute sickle chest syndrome and stroke. The aim is to improve oxygen delivery to the tissues by correcting anaemia, to improve blood viscosity and flow by reducing the proportion of sickle erythrocytes present and to reduce the erythropoietic drive by increasing the haematocrit.[23] Sickle red cells are poorly deformable and even oxygenated sickle blood is more viscous than normal HbA blood. Tissue blood flow is critically affected by blood viscosity. In vitro studies indicate that blood viscosity depends both on the percentage of sickle cells present and the haematocrit. At a fixed haematocrit, viscosity increases with the fraction of sickle cells; above a sickle percentage of 30–40% viscosity increases abruptly. Conversely, at a fixed fraction of sickle cells, viscosity increases abruptly with haematocrit values above 35%.[7] This is the basis for traditional exchange transfusion practices, aiming to reduce the sickle percentage below a given value (usually 30%), but avoiding an increase in haematocrit above 35%. Great care must be taken when transfusing sickle patients not to raise haematocrit levels excessively; painful crisis and stroke may be precipitated.[23]

There are concerns about blood transfusions. Complications include alloimmunization with the development of new clinically important red cell antibodies, transfusion reactions, transmission of infection, iron overload, problems with venous access, and precipitation of crisis by rapid transfusion of cold, acidotic bank blood. Alloimmunization is a serious and common problem in patients with SCD in North America and Europe due to the differences in red cell phenotype between the recipient population (predominantly Caribbean or African) and the donor population (predominantly Caucasian). Alloimmunization causes difficulties with cross-matching and delayed transfusion reactions which may be life threatening. Unnecessary blood transfusions in the perioperative period are therefore to be avoided.

The issue of preoperative transfusion for SCD patients, including those undergoing cholycystectomy, has been addressed in a prospective multicentre study from the Preoperative Transfusion in Sickle Cell Disease Study Group. Patients of all ages were randomly assigned to receive either an aggressive transfusion regimen (exchange), designed to obtain a preoperative haemoglobin of $10\,g.dl^{-1}$ ($9–11\,g.dl^{-1}$) and reduce the HbS level to < 30%, or a conservative regimen (top-up), designed to increase the haemoglobin level to $10\,g.dl^{-1}$ ($9–11\,g.dl^{-1}$), irrespective of the HbS level.[15,24] There was no non-transfusion arm in the randomization. The median preoperative HbS level was 31% in the aggressively transfused group and 59% in the conservative group. The frequency of serious complications was high but similar in the two groups, but there were only half as many transfusion-associated complications in the conservatively transfused group, thought to be due to the lower exposure to transfused units. The authors concluded that conservative transfusion regimens were as effective as aggressive transfusion regimens and should be advocated to reduce the incidence of transfusion-related complications. The acute chest syndrome developed in 10% of patients in both groups and was predicted by higher risk surgery (such as abdominal surgery) and a history of pulmonary disease.

The cholycystectomy study also included a small group of non-randomized, non-transfused patients who had the highest incidence of sickle-related events of all groups and concluded that transfusion did reduce the incidence of perioperative sickle-related events in patients undergoing cholycystectomy. Other studies have also indicated the benefit of preoperative transfusion in patients with SCD undergoing surgery,[20,22] although transfusion versus no transfusion has not been investigated by a randomized controlled study.

A retrospective study from Duke University considered their experience in the paediatric age range using an aggressive preoperative transfusion regimen. Their overall incidence of complications, including transfusion-related complications, was very low. Most patients received two to three simple phenotypically matched transfusions over a 3–4-week period preoperatively; a few were treated by exchange transfusion. The mean Hb was $11\,g.dl^{-1}$ and mean HbS 21%. They concluded that the benefits of an aggressive transfusion regimen in the perioperative period in children outweighed the risks.[16]

In considering preoperative transfusion practice, the anaesthetist managing a child with severe SCD is faced with a difficult problem, whether to reduce short-term risk (minimize the HbS level by transfusion), or long-term risk (reduce exposure to possible complications of transfusion). Moreover, exchange transfusion in a young child is time-consuming and traumatic for the child. However, if the child does develop a significant complication in the postoperative period (stroke or chest crisis), definitive treatment includes emergency exchange transfusion. Our personal practice in deciding preoperative transfusion strategy is to consider each child on an individual basis, in the light of their past medical history, risk factors for complications and the planned surgical procedure. Decisions about preoperative transfusion are made after discussion between the paediatrician, haematologist, anaesthetist and the child's family. Preparation takes place in the weeks prior to surgery. Transfused blood is always leucodepleted and fully phenotypically matched (Rh compatible, Kell negative). Blood is always cross-matched for surgery and standing by in case of perioperative complications. We adopt a four-tiered approach to preoperative transfusion, tailored to suit the individual case.

1. Children with no special risk factors, who are currently well, having short procedures with minimal risk of perioperative complications, e.g. insertion of grommets, are given a top-up transfusion to correct anaemia only ($Hb > 7\,g.dl^{-1}$).

2. Children with no special risk factors, having intermediate risk surgery, e.g. body surface surgery such as herniorrhaphy, or tonsillectomy in older children with mild to moderate OSA, receive a top-up transfusion to raise the haemoglobin to 9–11 $g.dl^{-1}$ (but not > 12 $g.dl^{-1}$).
3. Children who have had a chest crisis or suffer frequent painful crises, or children undergoing major surgery, such as intra-abdominal surgery (including laparoscopic surgery) or tonsillectomy in children < 5 years of age, receive preoperative transfusions to reduce the HbS level to < 30% (but maintaining Hb < 12 $g.dl^{-1}$).
4. Children who have had a stroke (usually on a regular transfusion programme), or who are undergoing high-risk major surgery, e.g. thoracic or neurosurgery, receive preoperative transfusions to reduce the HbS level to < 20% (but maintaining the Hb < 12 $g.dl^{-1}$).

In the case described here, the child underwent two surgical procedures at our hospital. His general health was good, although he had suffered from frequent painful crises in infancy and currently suffered from frequent episodes of abdominal pain, due to his gall bladder disease. He was noted to have a low HbF level (1.1%). A top-up transfusion was given prior to tonsillectomy. A more aggressive approach was taken prior to cholycystectomy, in light of the higher-risk operative procedure to be undertaken. Laparoscopic surgery (as compared with open surgery) has not been shown to be protective with respect to the development of acute sickle chest syndrome in children, despite the predicted advantages of reduced postoperative pain.[25] Several small top-up transfusions were required to raise the haemoglobin to 9.6 $g.dl^{-1}$ and reduce the HbS fraction to < 30%. Fortunately, he made an uneventful recovery after both surgical procedures. The severe nature of this child's SCD was revealed in his subsequent clinical course when he unfortunately developed severe acute sickle chest crisis requiring ventilation and complicated by a stroke. He remains well on a long-term transfusion programme.

Learning points

- SCD describes a group of disorders associated with the inheritance of the sickle β globin gene. It is characterized by a chronic haemolytic anaemia, episodic acute vaso-occlusive crises and chronic end-organ damage.
- There are marked phenotypic variations between individuals sharing the same HbS genotype, due to environmental, socioeconomic and genetic factors. Some individuals have mild disease, others severe disease with greatly reduced life expectancy.
- The fundamental molecular abnormality in SCD is the ability of HbS to form polymers when deoxygenated. Polymerization depends on the intracellular concentration of deoxy HbS and the concentration of other haemoglobins, particularly HbF. It results in the distortion of red cells to form sickle cells.
- Sickle cells are formed continuously in the circulation. Factors that increase the intracellular concentration of deoxy HbS (acidosis, hypoxia, dehydration), or increase the transit time of red cells through the microcirculation (vasoconstriction, increased blood viscosity, activation of inflammatory mediators) will promote vaso-occlusion by sickle cells.
- Factors which predict severe disease include dactylitis in infancy, severe anaemia, leucoytosis, frequent painful episodes, previous acute chest crisis, previous stroke, seizures and low HbF. Transcranial Doppler and MRI may identify asymptomatic children at risk for stroke.
- Children with SCD undergoing major surgery have a high incidence of sickle-related complications. Perioperative care must be meticulous. Dehydration, hypoxia, acidosis, pain and hypothermia must be avoided.
- Preoperative transfusion to raise the haemoglobin to 10 $g.dl^{-1}$ may be indicated prior to all except the most minor surgery.
- Debate surrounds the use of aggressive perioperative transfusion regimes. Our practice is to reduce the HbS level to < 30% for high-risk cases.
- All children must receive leucodepleted, phenotypically matched blood to reduce transfusion reactions. Over-transfusion must be avoided.
- Blood must be available in the event of an acute complication such as stroke, when exchange transfusion is indicated.

Acknowledgements

I am very grateful to Professor Sally Davies for her helpful comments in reviewing this manuscript.

References

1. Davies S, Oni L. Fortnightly review: management of patients with sickle cell disease. *BMJ* 1997; 315: 656–660.
2. Sergeant G. Sickle cell disease. *Lancet* 1997; 350: 725–730.
3. Chui D, Dover G. Sickle cell disease: no longer a single gene disorder. *Curr Opin Pediatr* 2001; 13: 22–27.
4. Powars D. Natural history of disease: the first two decades. In: Embury S, Hebbel R, Mohandas N, Steinberg M (eds). *Sickle Cell Disease. Basic Principles and Clinical Practice.* New York: Raven Press Ltd., 1994.
5. Millar S, Sleeper L, Pegelow C et al. Prediction of adverse outcomes in children with sickle cell disease. *N Engl J Med* 2000; 342: 83–89.
6. Kinney T, Sleeper L, Wang W et al. Silent infarcts in sickle cell anaemia: a risk factor analysis. *Pediatrics* 1999; 103: 640–645.
7. Vichinsky E. Transfusion therapy. In: Embury S, Hebbel R, Mohandas N, Steinberg M (eds). *Sickle Cell Disease. Basic Principles and Clinical Practice.* New York: Raven Press Ltd., 1994.
8. Adams R, McKie V, Hsu L et al. Prevention of a first stroke by transfusions in children with sickle cell anaemia and abnormal results on transcranial Doppler ultrasonography. *N Engl J Med* 1998; 339: 5–11.
9. Vichinsky E, Styles L, Colangelo L et al. Acute chest syndrome in sickle cell disease: clinical presentation and course. *Blood* 1997; 89: 1787–1792.
10. Bunn F. Pathogenesis and treatment of sickle cell disease. *N Engl J Med* 1997; 337: 762–769.
11. Embury S, Hebbel R, Steinberg M, Mohandas N. Pathogenesis of vasoocclusion. In: Embury S, Hebbel R, Mohandas N, Steinberg M (eds). *Sickle Cell Disease. Basic Principles and Clinical Practice.* New York: Raven Press Ltd., 1994.
12. Vivay V, Cavenagh J, Yate P. The anaesthetist's role in acute sickle cell crisis. *Br J Anaesth* 1998; 80: 820–828.
13. Platt O, Thorington B, Brambilla D et al. Pain in sickle cell disease. Rates and risk factors. *N Engl J Med* 1991; 325: 11–16.
14. Steinberg M. Management of sickle cell disease. *N Engl J Med* 1999; 340: 1021–1030.
15. Vichinsky E, Haberkern C, Neumeyer L et al. A comparison of conservative and aggressive transfusion regimens in the perioperative management of sickle cell disease. *N Eng J Med* 1995; 333: 206–213.
16. Adams D, Ware R, Schultz WH et al. Successful surgical outcome in children with sickle hemaglobinopathies: the Duke University experience. *J Pediatr Surg* 1998; 33: 428–432.
17. Mahony B, Githens J. Sickling crisis and altitude: occurrence in the Colorado population. *Clin Pediatr* 1979; 18: 431–438.
18. Samuels M, Stebbens V, Davies S et al. Sleep related upper airway obstruction and hypoxaemia in sickle cell disease. *Arch Dis Child* 1992; 67: 925–929.
19. Gerber M, O'Connor D, Adler E et al. Selected risk factors in pediatric adenotonsillectomy. *Arch Otolaryngol Head Neck Surg* 1996; 122: 811–814.
20. Griffen T, Buchanan G. Elective surgery in children with sickle cell disease without preoperative blood transfusion. *J Ped Surgery* 1993; 28: 681–685.
21. Scott-Connor C, Brunson C. The pathophysiology of the sickle hemaglobinopathies and implications for perioperative management. *Am J Surg* 1994; 168: 268–274.
22. Koshy M, Weiner S, Miller S et al. Surgery and anesthesia in sickle cell disease. *Blood* 1995; 10: 3676–3684.
23. Davies S. Blood transfusion in sickle cell disease. *Curr Opin Hematol* 1996; 3: 485–491.
24. Haberkern C, Neumeyer L, Orringer E et al. Cholycystectomy in sickle cell anemia patients: perioperative outcome of 364 cases from the National Perioperative Transfusion Study. *Blood* 1997; 89: 1522–1542.
25. Delatte S, Hebra A, Tagge E et al. Acute chest syndrome in the postoperative sickle cell patient. *J Pediatr Surg* 1999; 34: 188–192.
26. Platt OS, Brambilla DJ, Rosse WF et al. Mortality in sickle cell disease. Life expectancy and risk factors for early death. *N Engl J Med* 1994; 330: 1639–1644.

34

Management of head injury in a child

Lauren Barker and Peter J Murphy

Introduction

The severity of a head injury depends on the extent of neuronal damage at the time of injury, but also on secondary insults such as hypoxia, hypercapnia, hypotension and sustained raised intracranial pressure. The aim of clinical management is to prevent these secondary insults. Many patients with head injuries (10–40%) will have associated injuries such as intra-abdominal trauma and fractured long bones requiring surgery. In addition in adults with moderate to severe head injury the incidence of cervical spine injury is 5.4%.[1]

Case history

A 9-year-old boy fell off the roof of a house and sustained a moderately severe head injury as well as a compound fracture of his right femur. History, initial examination findings and investigations are shown in Table 34.1 below.

Examination

The child was brought, by the paramedics, into A&E on a spine board with his neck stabilized in a hard cervical collar and his head fixed with sandbags and tape. 15 $l.min^{-1}$ of oxygen was administered by facemask. He was breathing spontaneously with an unobstructed airway. Auscultation of the chest revealed bilateral air entry. Intravenous access was secured with an 18G cannula in his right antecubital fossa. Blood was sent for FBC, U&E, glucose and a group and save. A fluid bolus of 500 ml of 0.9% saline was given, following which his blood pressure increased to 100/60 and heart rate decreased to 125 min^{-1}. Glasgow coma score (GCS) was assessed as 10/15 (E2 M5 V3) as he was talking but extremely confused, groaning and crying out in pain whenever his leg was moved; he localized to pain and he opened his eyes in response to painful stimuli. Prior to log-rolling him 1 mg morphine was administered intravenously and a femoral nerve block was performed with 20 ml 0.25% bupivacaine by the on-call anaesthetic consultant. The patient was log-rolled uneventfully and a splint was applied to his right leg. No other injuries were clinically apparent. Further investigations included X-rays of his chest, pelvis, cervical spine and right femur. No abnormalities were detected on the chest, pelvic and lateral C-spine X-rays, but a femoral shaft fracture was confirmed. Cervical spine immobilization was maintained throughout.

The wound on the boy's right leg was dirty and the orthopaedic surgeons wanted to take the boy to the operating room as soon as possible to debride it and fix the fracture. Prior to going to the operating room, the boy was reassessed by the anaesthetic consultant and antibiotics (cefuroxime 25 $mg.kg^{-1}$) were given. Haemodynamic observations were stable, but he had become more difficult to rouse and it was uncertain if this was due to the morphine given or to the effect of the head injury. A decision was made to perform a computed tomography scan of his brain before going to surgery. The boy had eaten 1 hour prior to the accident and was therefore assumed to have a full stomach. The cervical collar was loosened and in-line cervical stabilization was applied by an A&E sister who was trained in Advanced Paediatric Life Support (APLS). Thiopentone 100 mg and suxamethonium 30 mg were given into a cannula with a rapidly running drip attached and cricoid pressure applied. The patient was successfully intubated by the anaesthetic registrar with an oral endotracheal tube size 6,

Past medical history	Fit and well Previous admission to A&E with a Colles fracture, age 7 years	
ASA grade	III	
Regular medications	None	
Allergies	None known	
Examination	Opens eyes only in response to pain Airway clear, cervical spine immobilized, face mask oxygen Chest clear, bilateral air entry, SaO_2 99% Respiratory rate 16 min^{-1} Normal heart sounds, pulse 140 min^{-1}, BP 85/50 mmHg Capillary refill time = 5 secs Compound fracture of right femur	
Investigations	*Weight*	25 kg
	FBC	Hb 11.0 $g.dl^{-1}$, Plat $298 \times 10^9 l^{-1}$, WBC $10.2 \times 10^9 l^{-1}$
	U+Es	Na^+ 134 $mmol.l^{-1}$, K^+ 4.9 $mmol.l^{-1}$, Urea 4.0 $mmol.l^{-1}$, creatinine 45 $\mu mol.l^{-1}$
	BM Stix	6.0
	Chest X-ray	Lung fields clear No pneumothorax
	C-spine X-ray	No abnormality detected
	Pelvic X-ray	No fracture
	Rt femur X-ray	Shaft of femur fracture
	Glasgow coma scale	10/15 (E2 M5 V3)

Table 34.1
Findings on admission

which was secured at 16.5 cm at his lips. He was ventilated using a Penlon Nuffield ventilator on an air–oxygen mix, pressures of 20/3 and a respiratory rate of 20 breaths per minute. An orogastric tube was inserted and a 22G arterial line was sited in his right radial artery for accurate blood pressure monitoring and for CO_2 measurement. Sedation (morphine and midazolam) was given by continuous intravenous infusion and he was paralysed with pancuronium 2.5 mg for transfer to the CT scanner. During this time he was fully monitored with oxygen saturation, ECG and end-tidal CO_2. The CT scan of his head revealed a small subdural haematoma in the right temporo-occipital region with no evidence of raised intracranial pressure (Figure 34.1). The case was discussed with the neurosurgeons who reviewed the films and their opinion was that no surgical intervention was required for the subdural haematoma at this time. They advised insertion of an intracranial pressure (ICP) monitor prior to commencement of the surgical procedure. A Codman intraparenchymal ICP monitor was inserted uneventfully and the initial ICP reading was 12 mmHg.

The boy was transferred to the operating room where he was moved to the operating table while cervi-

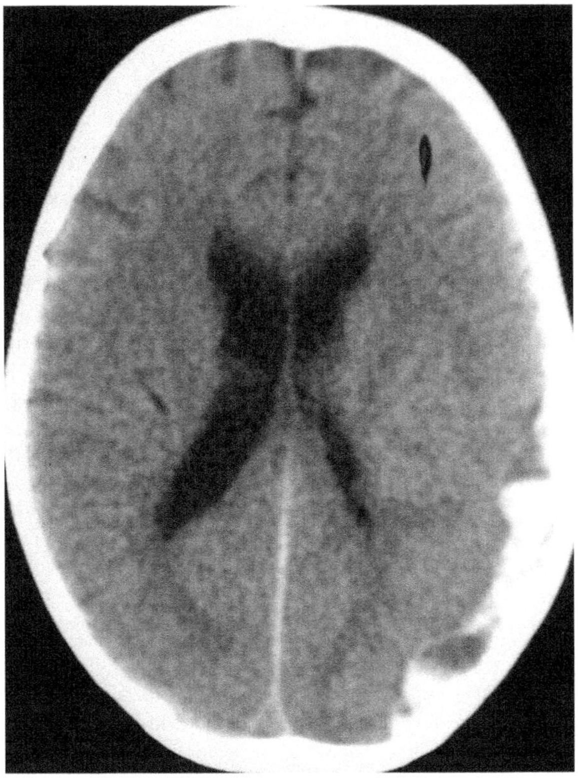

Figure 34.1
One cut from CT scan of brain showing a right subdural haematoma.

cal spine immobilization was maintained. The table was positioned with a 15 degree head up tilt to aid venous drainage from his head. Sedation was continued and isoflurane was commenced (end-tidal isoflurane 1.2%) with air–oxygen mix. A subclavian central line was inserted by the anaesthetic consultant and the patient was catheterized. It was then noticed that the boy's blood pressure had fallen to 80/60, the central venous pressure was 0–1 mmHg and the haemoglobin concentration was 10 g.dl^{-1}. Human albumin solution 4.5% (500 ml) was transfused over 30 minutes in addition to a normal saline infusion, which was infusing at 52 ml.h^{-1} (80% fluid restriction). Ventilation was adjusted to maintain end-tidal CO_2 at 30–35 mmHg. Thirty minutes into the operation, the boy's blood pressure dropped again to 80/55 with a central venous pressure reading of 2 mmHg. Haemoglobin concentration on an arterial blood gas sample had now fallen to 7.5 g.dl^{-1}. A colloid fluid bolus, 250 ml blood, was given over 10–15 minutes and a noradrenaline (norepinephrine) infusion was commenced to maintain a mean arterial blood pressure of 70–80 mmHg.

Just as the surgeons were closing the wound after 2 hours, the patient became hypertensive (BP 180/100) and bradycardic (HR 55/minute) in spite of end-tidal isoflurane of 1.2% and a loading dose of morphine, 3 mg, which was given in increments 15 minutes previously. The ICP had risen to 22 mmHg. His pupils remained small, equal and reactive. The patient was hyperventilated to an end-tidal CO_2 of 26 mmHg using a Bains Circuit and mannitol, 12.5 g, was given. Blood pressure and heart rate returned to normal and ICP decreased to 15 mmHg.

The patient's CT brain scan was repeated following the surgical procedure. This revealed no enlargement of the haematoma and no further clinical deterioration was noted. He was then transferred to the Paediatric Intensive Care Unit (PICU) where his subsequent brain injury management followed the hospital protocol (Appendices 1 and 2).

Progress in Paediatric Intensive Care Unit

His subsequent management on PICU for the following 24 hours was relatively uncomplicated. He was sedated with morphine (40 µg.kg^{-1}.hr^{-1}) and midazolam (100 µg.kg^{-1}.hr^{-1}) and paralysed using a vecuronium infusion (60 µg.kg^{-1}.hr^{-1}). His $PaCO_2$ was kept between 30 and 35 mmHg. Ventilation was not problematic and he remained well oxygenated with an FiO_2 of 0.35.

Cardiovascularly he was very stable and it was possible to maintain a cerebral perfusion pressure in excess of 60 mmHg despite weaning off the noradrenaline (norepinephrine) infusion.

Normothermia was maintained using a cooling blanket. Continuous EEG monitoring was commenced and he was loaded with phenytoin as per protocol. Maintenance fluids were commenced at 70% of his calculated daily requirements and non-nutritive feeds administered for gut protection.

The following day his paralysis was stopped and his sedation reduced to allow assessment of his neurological status. As his sedation lightened he had another period of intracranial hypertension, which responded to another dose of mannitol and re-sedation. A repeat CT scan was arranged which revealed a slight increase in the size of the subdural haematoma. The neurosurgeons were contacted and he was taken back to the operating room for a craniotomy and drainage of his haematoma. Again he was transferred back to PICU where he was sedated and paralysed for a further 24 hours.

The following day his sedation was again reduced and his paralysis stopped. As he awoke his ICP remained stable and the neurosurgeons were able to clinically evaluate him and exclude a neck injury. Later that day he was successfully extubated to facemask oxygen.

Over the following 48 hours he continued to improve and appeared to be neurologically intact. His ICP monitor was removed on day 5 following no further incidents of raised ICP. On day 6 he was transferred from PICU to the ward.

Discussion

In the United Kingdom head injury is the most common cause of death in children aged 1–15 years and accounts for 15% of deaths in this age group. Head injuries are commonly caused by road traffic accidents, falls or child abuse (in infancy) and there may be associated injuries. Indeed, between 10% and 40% of head-injured children will have associated injuries such as intra-abdominal trauma and long bone fractures. The possibility of spinal injuries must never be overlooked in head-injured children.

Initial assessment and management

A history of the accident will provide useful information about the mechanism of injury. Factors indicating a potentially serious head injury include involvement in a road traffic accident or a fall from a height, loss of consciousness, children who are not fully conscious and responsive, neurological deficit such as convulsions or limb weakness. In this scenario a fall from the roof and a depressed conscious level indicated a severe injury.[2]

When assessing an injured child with a potential head injury it is essential to adopt a structured approach.[3]

Initially a **primary survey** should be conducted during which any life-threatening conditions should be identified. These must be dealt with prior to assessing the head injury or associated injuries. Assessment follows the ABC pattern:

A Airway with cervical spine control and 100% oxygen
B Breathing
C Circulation.

In the case discussed, the child's airway was well maintained and there were no obvious breathing difficulties. Cervical spine stabilization was secured by the paramedics with a hard collar and sandbags. Intravenous access was successful. Blood was taken at this time for baseline tests and a fluid bolus, $20\,ml.kg^{-1}$, was given to correct the circulatory compromise. The effect of the fluid bolus should be assessed and further fluid given if clinically indicated. A brief neurological assessment can then be made to assess conscious level. The AVPU score is used initially and comprises four categories:

A Alert
V Responds to voice
P Responds to pain
U Unresponsive.

This child's initial evaluation would have been 'P' (responds to pain). A more detailed neurological examination can then be performed at a later stage, using the Glasgow coma score if the child is 4 years or older or the Children's coma score for those under 4 years.

X-rays taken at this stage should include a lateral cervical spine, chest and pelvis.

Analgesia is important even in the presence of a head injury and should be given after initial neurological assessment because pain may result in raised ICP. This child's pain was controlled with morphine and a femoral nerve block.

With an AVPU score of P it is imperative that the patient's airway and breathing are carefully re-assessed and elective intubation considered. Clearly in this instance intubation would require a rapid sequence induction with cricoid pressure and additional skilled assistance to maintain neck stability with manual in-line traction.

Once the primary survey has been completed and the patient is stable and adequately resuscitated, the **secondary survey** may be commenced. This involves a head to toe examination, including a log-roll to examine the back of the patient. A fractured femur was the only associated injury identified in the case scenario.[4] It is important to note that a fractured femur is an extremely painful and distracting injury and the patient may not complain of abdominal pain even in the presence of intra-abdominal pathology. If there is any concern about the abdominal examination, there should be a low threshold for performing additional investigations such as an abdominal ultrasound or CT scan.

In any head-injured patient one should look carefully for any signs of base of skull fracture, in particular nasal bleeding or clear fluid draining from the nose. Nasogastric tubes and intubation via the nasal route are best avoided until a base of skull fracture has been excluded.

Finally a urinary catheter should be inserted so that urine output can be monitored and accurate fluid balance evaluated.

Assessment and management of head injury

Brain damage is caused by the effects of the injury itself, but further damage may occur from hypoxia, hypercapnia, systemic hypotension and raised ICP.[5] The aim is to avoid secondary damage by maintaining ventilation and circulation and avoiding raised ICP.

This child's clinical condition (depressed conscious level with GCS of 10) was indicative of a severe injury. The CT scan revealed a subdural haematoma that did not require immediate neurosurgical intervention.

ICP monitoring is a useful adjunct while the patient is anaesthetized because neurological assessment of the anaesthetized patient is extremely difficult. In this instance a Codman intraparenchymal ICP monitor was inserted. This monitor consists of a microsensor transducer, which is inserted via a small burr hole into the brain parenchyma. It is easy to insert and provides a reasonably accurate measure of ICP. In contrast the 'Gold standard' ICP monitor is the intraventricular drain (IVD), which gives a very accurate measurement of ICP and also allows for drainage of cerebrospinal fluid, which can be used as a treatment modality to reduce ICP. Insertion of an IVD is technically more challenging however and carries a significantly higher risk of morbidity.

Having an ICP monitor in situ allows the anaesthetist to identify any rises in ICP and to maintain cerebral perfusion pressure (CPP) (cerebral perfusion pressure = mean arterial blood pressure – intracranial pressure) at the required level, dependent on the child's age.

Noradrenaline (norepinephrine) may be used to increase mean arterial blood pressure in order to achieve an adequate CPP. In this case a single episode of raised ICP occurred in the operating room. This responded to hyperventilation and mannitol. A repeat CT scan was performed to ensure that the subdural haematoma had not increased in size and that there was no significant mass effect. If deterioration had occurred then neurosurgical review and possible intervention would have been appropriate (as occurred later during the child's stay on PICU).

The general clinical measures to prevent intracranial hypertension are outlined in Appendix 1. They include maintenance of adequate ventilation and arterial oxygenation, maintenance of adequate CPP, sedation and paralysis, control of body temperature, seizure prophylaxis, fluid restriction and serial neurological evaluation.

Learning points

- Traumatic brain injury in children is relatively common.
- Cervical spine immobilization is mandatory until the cervical spine has been cleared clinically and radiologically.
- A structured approach must be adopted when assessing a child who has sustained a traumatic head injury – a primary survey, appropriate resuscitation followed by a secondary survey.
- The severity of the head injury should be assessed both clinically and with further investigations such as CT scans.
- Neurosurgical advice should be sought.
- Other injuries are common and include abdominal injures and long bone fractures.
- The aim of initial management of a head-injured child is to avoid secondary brain injury.
- Secondary brain injury can be prevented by a structured approach to the management of raised ICP and maintenance of CPP, adequate seizure control, avoidance of pyrexia[6] and regular re-assessment.[7]

Appendix 1

General measures to prevent intracranial hypertension

This protocol consists of a series of general measures designed to prevent raised intracranial pressure and then a critical care pathway for the treatment of inadequate cerebral perfusion.

1. Elevation of head of bed to 30°
2. Midline positioning of head to avoid jugular venous outflow obstruction
3. Maintenance of adequate ventilation/arterial oxygenation
   - Aim to maintain $PaO_2 > 100$ mmHg if possible, and ventilate to normocapnia $PaCO_2$ 35–40 mmHg. Maintain Hb > 10 g.dl^{-1}.
   - Avoid positive end-expiratory pressure (PEEP) >10 cmH_2O as this may impair cerebral venous return and increase ICP. However, the overriding priority is to improve oxygenation, and if this necessitates a high level of PEEP, then such a compromise may have to be accepted.
4. Maintenance of adequate CPP
   - Prior to insertion of ICP monitor one should aim to maintain an adequate mean arterial blood pressure:
     55 mmHg for infants 0–12 months
     65 mmHg for children 1–5 years
     75 mmHg for children 5–10 years
     90 mmHg for children > 10 years
   - Once ICP monitoring is established CPP should guide management. Aims for CPP are as follows:
     40 mmHg for infants 0–12 months
     50 mmHg for children 1–5 years
     60 mmHg for children 5–10 years
     70 mmHg for infants > 10 years
5. Sedation and paralysis
   - Patients should be sedated using morphine and midazolam infusions.
   - Neuromuscular blockade with vecuronium infusion should be considered in order to aid control of minute ventilation and raised ICP, and to prevent shivering in patients who are actively cooled.
6. Control of body temperature
   - Maintain normothermia. This may require active cooling and paralysis.
7. Seizure prophylaxis
   - Administer phenytoin 15 mg.kg^{-1} loading dose and then regular maintenance regimen for 14 days. Beware of phenytoin side-effect profile. Consider measuring phenytoin levels.
   - If the patient is receiving neuromuscular blocking drugs continuous EEG monitoring may be beneficial. Consider routine EEG in all patients to exclude non-convulsive status.
8. Maintenance fluids/feeding
   - Initial maintenance fluids should be isotonic saline restricted to 70% daily requirements.
   - Enteral feeding should be commenced within 72 hours where possible. Aim to replace 140% resting metabolism expenditure in non-paralysed patients and 100% in paralysed patients. Hyperglycaemia should be avoided in the first 24 hours following injury.
   - Ensure that plasma sodium levels are maintained at the high end of the normal range (> 140 mmol.l^{-1}). If necessary administer 3% saline 5 ml.kg^{-1} by slow infusion and recheck plasma sodium.
9. Ensure correct endotracheal suctioning practice to avoid ICP spikes
   - preoxygenation
   - mild hyperventilation
   - fentanyl bolus 1–2 µg.kg^{-1}
10. Serial neurological examination

Appendix 2

Care pathway for treatment of inadequate cerebral perfusion pressure

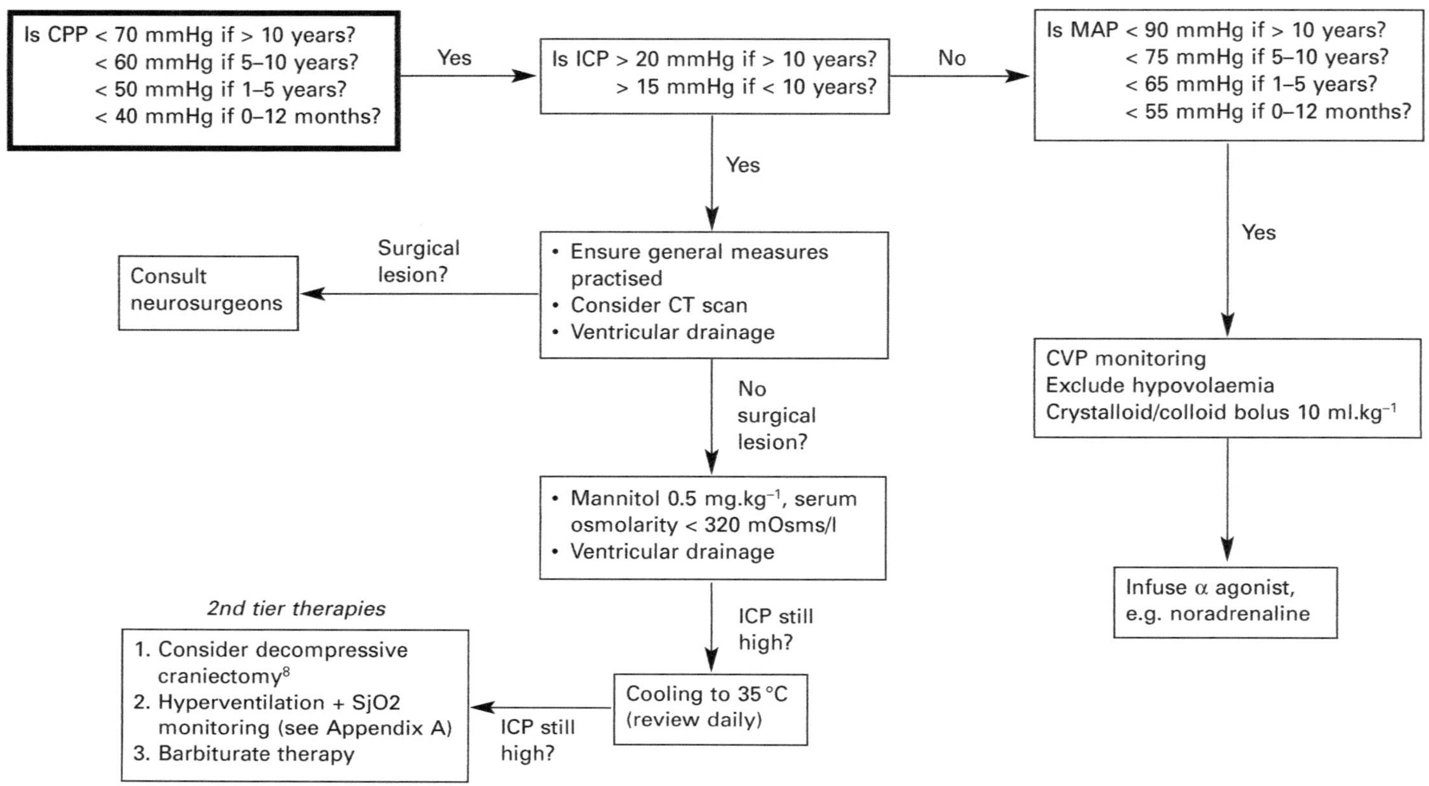

References

1. Holly LT, Kelly DF, Counelis GJ et al. Cervical spine trauma associated with moderate and severe head injury: incidence, risk factors, and injury characteristics. *J Neurosurg* 2002; 96(Suppl 3): 285–291.
2. Wang, MY, Kim KA, Griffith PM et al. Injuries from falls in the pediatric population: an analysis of 729 cases. *J Pediatr Surg* 2001; 36: 1528–1534.
3. APLS. The Practical Approach, 3rd edn. BMJ Publishing Group, 2001.
4. Mendelson SA, Dominick TS, Tyler-Kabara E et al. Early versus late femoral fracture stabilization in multiply injured pediatric patients with closed head injury. *J Pediatr Orthop* 2001; 21: 594–599.
5. Reckate HL. Head injuries: management of primary injuries and prevention of secondary damage. A consensus conference on Pediatric Neurosurgery. *Childs Nerv Syst* 2001; 17: 632–634.
6. Natale JE, Joseph JG, Helfaer MA, Shaffner DH. Early hyperthermia after traumatic brain injury in children: risk factors, influence on length of stay, and effect on short-term neurological status. *Crit Care Med* 2000; 28: 2608–2615.
7. Givner A, Gurney J, O'Connor D et al. Reimaging in pediatric neurotrauma: factors associated with progression of intracranial injury. *J Pediatr Surg* 2002; 37: 381–385.
8. Taylor A, Butt W, Rosenfeld J et al. A randomized trial of very early decompressive craniectomy in children with traumatic brain injury and sustained intracranial hypertension. *Childs Nerv Syst* 2001; 17:154–162.

Further reading

Katz J, Steward D (eds). *Anaesthesia and Uncommon Paediatric Diseases*, 2nd edn. WB Saunder Company, 1993.

Morgan G, Mikhail M (eds). *Clinical Anesthesiology*, 2nd edn. Aplleton and Lange, 1996.

Anaesthesia and Intensive Care for the Neurosurgical Patient. Walters Ingram and Jenkinson. Blackwell, 1994.

35

Paediatric transport medicine: retrieval of a 2-year-old girl with meningococcal septicaemia

Stephen C Marriage

Introduction

The last decade has witnessed fundamental changes in the provision of paediatric intensive care (PIC) in the UK. The adoption of a series of national reports and guidelines has resulted in the development of a regional network of lead centres for PIC and paediatric retrieval services.[1–3] From the moment it is determined that a child needs transfer for definitive treatment, successful management of the most seriously ill children requires an ongoing dialogue to be established between a referring hospital and the lead centre for PIC. An interchange of clinical information and advice will enable a child's care to proceed smoothly through resuscitation, stabilization, transfer and on to intensive care.

Meningococcal septicaemia remains a devastating illness in children, despite the successful introduction of a conjugate vaccine against the C strain of the disease.[4] Progression is rapid, with a high mortality among those children who develop multiorgan failure.[5–8] Successful management requires a thorough, co-ordinated approach, with attention to detail, anticipation of cardiovascular, haematological and metabolic disturbances and the early institution of aggressive supportive therapy.

The following case highlights both the management of meningococcal septicaemia and the particular issues involved in the management of a critically ill child who is to be retrieved by a paediatric transport team.

Case history

A 2-year-old girl presented to the emergency department of her local hospital, having been found collapsed at home. She had previously been well, with no history of recurrent infections and had been fully immunized, including immunizations for *Haemophilus influenzae* and Type C meningococcus. The evening prior to admission she had developed a fever, aching legs and had vomited once. She had been given paracetamol suspension at 6 pm. Her parents had checked on her throughout the evening and had given her a second dose of paracetamol at midnight before going to bed. On waking they entered her bedroom to find her grey and unresponsive, with a widespread non-blanching rash. They immediately called for an ambulance and were brought directly to the emergency department.

On admission she was taken straight to the resuscitation area where a presumptive diagnosis of meningococcal septicaemia was made. Both the on-call paediatric and anaesthetic specialist registrars (SpR) were called to the department. She was given high-flow oxygen via a facemask and monitoring was commenced. Neither pulse oximetry nor cuff blood pressures were recordable. ECG monitoring revealed a tachycardia of 180 bpm. Her capillary refill time was greater than 8 seconds. For the purposes of resuscitation her weight was estimated at 12 kg using the formula:

$$\text{Weight (kg)} = [\text{Age (years)} + 4] \times 2$$

It proved impossible to establish venous access and an intraosseous (IO) needle was inserted into her right tibia. A blood glucose estimation on the small amount of aspirate obtained was 2.1 mmol.l^{-1}. She was immediately treated with 20 ml.kg^{-1} (240 ml) of 0.9% saline followed by 5 ml.kg^{-1} (60 ml) of 10% dextrose. A dose of cefotaxime 100 mg.kg^{-1} (1.2 g) was administered via the IO needle. At this point a peripheral venous cannula was successfully inserted and a small amount of blood obtained. A venous blood gas analysis was performed, with the remainder of the sample being sent for a full blood count and biochemical profile.

The initial blood gas estimation revealed:

Parameter	Result
pH	7.115
pCO_2 (kPa)	5.78
pO_2 (kPa)	4.1
Bicarbonate ($mmol.l^{-1}$)	6.18
Base deficit	–14.0

At this point a second bolus of 0.9% saline was administered and contact made with the local lead centre for PIC, located some 80 miles away.

As soon as the referral call was received, the most senior available clinician (in this case a consultant) was called to take the referral, in order to minimize the need for repetition of clinical details. Apart from the details given above, the PIC consultant asked for details of the respiratory rate and work of breathing; evidence of urine output, as a marker of organ perfusion, and for the pupillary responses to be checked. Her respiratory rate was raised at 45 breaths min^{-1}; she had a dry nappy that had been in place all night, and her pupils were 3 mm in diameter but responded sluggishly to light.

At this point the PIC consultant made some suggestions regarding her acute management. The circumstances suggested that it was likely the child would require further volume resuscitation. A third bolus of fluid was advised in order to prime the circulation in preparation for moving on to rapid sequence induction (RSI). Senior anaesthetic and paediatric staff had already been called to attend and she was in an environment – the emergency department resuscitation area – suitable for progression to intubation if required. It was suggested that an infusion of dobutamine be set up, to run at $10\,\mu g.kg^{-1}.min^{-1}$ via the peripheral cannula; a standard formula for making the infusion was also made available in order that there would be no change in concentration during and following transfer. Having optimized the cardiovascular situation as much as possible, recommendations for proceeding to intubation were made. A selection of drugs were chosen to limit a drop in the systemic vascular resistance. In this case fentanyl 25 µg, midazolam 1 mg and vecuronium 1.5 mg were suggested.

The child was orally intubated with a 4.5-mm endotracheal tube. Non-invasive blood pressure measurements remained unobtainable but her heart rate and perfusion remained unchanged during the procedure. She was sedated with a continuous infusion of midazolam at $120\,\mu g.kg^{-1}.hr^{-1}$ and intermittent boluses of fentanyl and vecuronium. No portable ventilator was available; the anaesthetic SpR continued hand ventilation, while her consultant obtained central venous access with a femoral, single-lumen 20g cannula. The condition of the child meant that obtaining central venous access proved a difficult procedure. By the time both intubation and central venous cannulation had been achieved, the retrieval team had arrived.

Having provided telephone support and advice to the SpRs at the referring hospital, preparation was made at the lead centre for rapid mobilization of a transfer team. The team consisted of an experienced nurse and appropriate medical staff to manage a sick child with meningococcal septicaemia: a consultant in addition to a trainee. Transport for the team was requested from the ambulance authority and while awaiting its arrival, sedation and inotrope infusions were prepared. An appropriate transport ventilator was selected and checked before setting out.

Having arrived at the bedside, the retrieval team immediately introduced themselves and took a handover from the nursing and medical teams. While the nurse transferred monitoring onto the portable retrieval monitor, one doctor met the family and explained the retrieval process, while the other examined the child. Saturations were 92% in 100% oxygen. She was transferred directly onto the paediatric transport ventilator, with a positive end-expiratory pressure set at $6\,cmH_2O$. Capillary refill remained prolonged, despite $80\,ml.kg^{-1}$ of fluid in resuscitation. The heart rate was 172 bpm. The central venous cannula was wired and a 4.5 French Gauge triple-lumen cannula inserted. Monitoring revealed a central venous pressure (CVP) of 8 mmHg.

Blood analyses revealed the following:

Arterial blood gases

Parameter	Result
pH	7.236
pCO_2 (kPa)	4.66
pO_2 (kPa)	6.7
Bicarbonate ($mmol.l^{-1}$)	8.54
Base deficit	–11.3

Laboratory results

Parameter	Result
FBC	Hb $7.4\,g.dl^{-1}$; WCC 2.3 (Neuts $1.1 \times 10^9 l^{-1}$); platelets $34 \times 10^9 l^{-1}$
U&Es	Na^+ 133; K^+ 2.7; creat 103; urea 8.9; Ca^{2+} 2.04
Clotting screen	PT 30/14 secs; INR 2.1; APTR 2.5

The tachycardia, low systolic blood pressure, relatively low CVP and persistent base deficit all suggested that despite substantial volume resuscitation the vascular compartment remained underfilled. Blood, fresh frozen plasma (FFP) and platelets were obtained to provide further volume support and to correct the low haemoglobin and coagulopathy. Potassium and calcium corrections of 0.2 $mmol.kg^{-1}$ were administered via the central venous line, each over 20 minutes, in addition to bicarbonate 1 $mmol.kg^{-1}$. Having performed a round of therapeutic correction, the child's condition was reassessed.

A chest X-ray was obtained and the position of the endotracheal tube noted to be satisfactory. Her cuff blood pressure was now recordable at 73/51 mmHg and her heart rate had fallen to 156 bpm. The dobutamine infusion was converted to a central infusion of dopamine, and epinephrine (adrenaline) added in order to maintain a satisfactory blood pressure. Further volume was given, up to a total of 120 $ml.kg^{-1}$ and consisting of crystalloid, albumin 4.5%, FFP, blood and platelets. A urinary catheter was inserted but only a small amount of urine obtained. Infusions of morphine, midazolam and vecuronium were started. The process of reassessment was repeated until a sufficient degree of stability for transportation was obtained.

Having achieved stability, the child was carefully moved to the ambulance trolley. A final check of vital signs was made, the ventilator moved from wall to bottled oxygen supply and the child transported to the ambulance. A set of observations was taken, the ventilator plugged into the ambulance oxygen supply and a smooth, steady journey back to the PIC unit (PICU) requested. The team was present in the referring hospital for 2 hours and 35 minutes and took a further 80 minutes to return to base. The trip back was uneventful; the child required intensive care support, including mechanical ventilation, inotropic support and peritoneal dialysis for 5 days. She made a full recovery with no neurological deficit.

Discussion

Assessment

Meningococcal disease remains a devastating disease of childhood, characterized by rapid progression and a high mortality in the most severe cases. The incidence of the disease varies greatly from country to country. In Europe, for example, the highest rates are found in Ireland, Scotland and Iceland where the annual incidence approaches 10 : 100,000 of the population, whereas in central Europe the incidence may be an order of magnitude lower. Although the diagnosis is usually apparent in the face of a purpuric rash, it is important to think about the diagnosis when seeing any unwell child. Although 80% of children with proven septicaemia will present with a non-blanching rash, 13% will have an atypical rash and 7% no rash at all.[9] On suspicion, and having made an initial assessment of the child's condition, vascular access should be obtained and either cefotaxime or ceftriaxone administered. Further management should then proceed in accordance with standard paediatric resuscitation guidelines such as those taught on the Advanced Paediatric Life Support course and with specialist guidance such as that provided to all emergency departments in the UK by the Meningitis Research Foundation (MRF).[10]

Over the years a variety of severity scores have been developed for children with meningococcal disease, varying in complexity and ease of use.[7] Most recently, the product of the neutrophil and platelet counts has been shown to be a simple score that can identify the most severe cases of acute meningococcal disease.[11] Nevertheless, none of these scores provide any guide to acute management, which will always rely on appropriate but aggressive resuscitation, assiduous attention to detail and the early involvement of teams with specialist experience.

Definitive management

In any acute situation, it is easy to overlook elements of the clinical examination unless they are requested systematically. Each PICU has a referral form onto which clinical parameters are recorded; those not immediately offered are requested to gain a more complete picture of the child's condition. In order that advice given by the lead centres is consistent, protocols regarding the management of the more common paediatric emergencies are available in many units, providing a suggested ongoing management strategy. An example of such a guideline is shown in Figures 35.1 and 35.2. The management steps reflect those of the more complex MRF guidance, but prioritize interventions in terms of airway management, assessment and support of breathing and cardiovascular interventions. Public health issues, including disease notification and prophylaxis of intimate contacts are also highlighted.

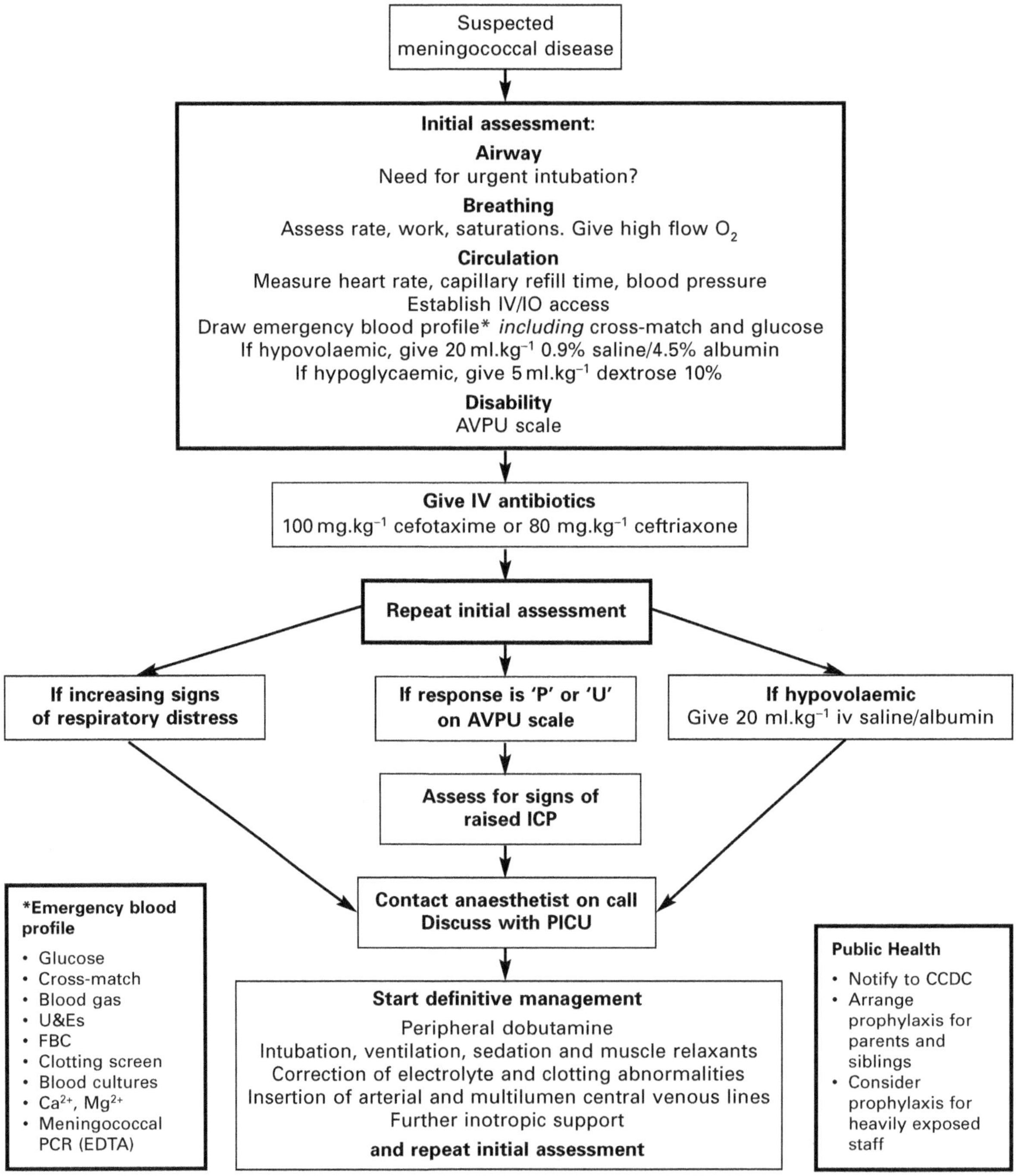

AVPU, alert, responds to voice, responds to pain, unresponsive; ICP, intracranial pressure; PCR, polymerase chain reaction; CCDC, Consultant in Communicable Disease Control

Figure 35.1
Initial assessment and management.

Airway

Indications for intubation: uncompensated shock; ↓ LOC; pulmonary oedema; impending transfer
Considerations: need for rapid sequence induction; potential exacerbation of hypotension
Suggested technique: **Give volume resuscitation before and during induction**
If time, commence iv dobutamine infusion before induction (see below)

Suggested agents:	**fentanyl**	**2–5 μg.kg^{-1}**
	midazolam	**50–100 μg.kg^{-1}**
	suxamethonium	**2 mg.kg^{-1}**

Breathing

Ventilate to normocapnia
Set PEEP to 5–6 cmH_2O (possible pulmonary oedema)
Optimize oxygenation
Site arterial line and monitor ABGs: reassess hourly, with simultaneous blood glucose estimations

Circulation

Commence peripheral iv dobutamine @ 10 μg.kg^{-1}.min^{-1}
(15 mg.kg^{-1} dobutamine made up to 50 ml with 0.9% saline: 2 ml.hr^{-1} ≡ (10 μg.kg^{-1}.min^{-1})

Place multilumen central venous catheter: monitor CVP

Maintain CVP with volume infusions at ≈ 12 cmH_2O
(give 4.5% albumin, FFP and blood as indicated, using 10–20 ml.kg^{-1} boluses)

Consider epinephrine (adrenaline) as second inotrope @ 0.2 μg.kg^{-1}.min^{-1}
(0.3 mg.kg^{-1} adrenaline made up to 50 ml with 0.9% saline: 2 ml.hr^{-1} ≡ 0.2 μg.kg^{-1}.min^{-1})

Expect and correct electrolyte abnormalities
(Hypokalaemia, hypocalcaemia and hypomagnesaemia all occur commonly
Treat each with 0.2 mmol.kg^{-1} of the relevant cation, diluted to 20 ml with normal saline and infused centrally over 20 mins)

Treat coagulopathy
(FFP for prolonged APTR; Vitamin K (0.25 mg.kg^{-1}) for prolonged INR; cryoprecipitate (5 ml.kg^{-1}) if fibrinogen < 1 g.l^{-1})

Disability

Assess GCS prior to intubation, including pupillary responses

Titrate infusions of sedation and muscle relaxant to effect
(Suggested infusions

morphine	1 mg.kg^{-1} made up to 50 ml with 0.9% saline:	1 ml.hr^{-1} ≡ 20 μg.kg^{-1}.hr	(Give 20–40 μg.kg^{-1}.hr^{-1})
midazolam	5 mg.kg^{-1} made up to 50 ml with 0.9% saline:	1 ml.hr^{-1} ≡ 100 μg.kg^{-1}.hr	(Give 100–150 μg.kg^{-1}.hr^{-1})
vecuronium	3 mg.kg^{-1} made up to 50 ml with 0.9% saline:	1 ml.hr^{-1} ≡ 60 μg.kg^{-1}.hr	(Give 60–180 μg.kg^{-1}.hr^{-1})

If meningococcal meningitis is clinically apparent, monitor for signs of ↑ ICP
(Dilated/asymmetric pupils, ↑ BP and bradycardia. Treat with 2.5 ml.kg^{-1} 20% mannitol, then urgent cranial CT scan if stable)

LOC, level of consciousness; PEEP, positive end-expiratory pressure; ABGs, aterial blood gases; CVP, central venous pressure; FFP, fresh frozen plasma; APTR, activated partial thromboplastin time ratio; GCS, Glasgow coma scale; ICP, intracranial pressure; BP, blood pressure; CT, computed tomography

Figure 35.2
Ongoing management.

In this case the circumstances suggested it was likely that the child would require further volume resuscitation, but would be at risk of developing pulmonary oedema as part of the disease process.[12] Both increased vascular permeability and myocardial dysfunction contribute to the development of pulmonary oedema but this should not deflect clinicians from aggressive fluid therapy, which is associated with increased survival.[13] A third bolus of fluid was suggested in order to prime the circulation in preparation for moving on to RSI. It was suggested that an infusion of dobutamine be set up via the peripheral cannula; as an inotrope with vasodilating properties, dobutamine may be infused safely through a peripheral vein in children, although extravasation injuries may still occur. Standard formulae for making all infusions are made available in order that there is no change in concentration during the process of moving to the retrieval team's infusions and pumps.

Having optimized the cardiovascular situation as far as possible, recommendations for proceeding to intubation were made. In these circumstances the need for intubation is not dictated by the development of frank respiratory failure, pulmonary oedema or the inability to protect an airway, but is an elective procedure enabling definitive management to proceed: establishment of central venous and arterial access, urinary catheterization; reduction in the work of breathing and of oxygen consumption,[14] and as a prelude to transportation. Even if a child is able to protect their airway and is maintaining saturations well, intubation and ventilation will allow other vital aspects of care to proceed. In a situation such as this, where the development of hypotension during RSI is a concern, the selection of drugs should be such as to avoid lowering the systemic vascular resistance as far as is possible. Here, fentanyl, midazolam and vecuronium were suggested. The MRF guidelines recommend the use of thiopentone and suxamethonium which have the benefit of being short-acting but may lead to an exacerbation of hypotension.[10] If a short-acting agent is preferred, ketamine has the advantage of providing an increase in systemic vascular resistance, even in the presence of endotoxaemia.[15]

Finally, some recommendations were made as to ongoing care. Once intubated, the priority should be to establish central venous access. Inotropic support may then be moved to a central route, venous blood gases checked, and a complete set of bloods sent to the laboratory, to include a repeat full blood count, clotting screen and biochemical profile; blood grouping and the preparation of blood products; blood cultures and meningococcal polymerase chain reaction (PCR) (EDTA sample). Arterial access, urinary catheterization, placement of a nasogastric tube and chest X-ray may then be undertaken.

Preparation for retrieval

Having provided telephone support and advice to the SpRs at the referring hospital, preparation was made at the lead centre for rapid mobilization of a transfer team. Transport for the team was requested from the ambulance authority and while awaiting its arrival, sedation and inotrope infusions were prepared. A transport ventilator appropriate to the age and weight of the child was selected and its functioning tested before setting out. Before leaving, final contact was made with the admitting team for a progress report on the child who had just been successfully intubated by the consultant anaesthetist. A mobile phone number was given so that the team could be updated with any significant developments while en route.

The retrieval team were able to use the time during the journey to the referring centre to plan their management strategy and to allocate tasks between the members of the team. Working in the unaccustomed environment of another hospital, with a critically ill child, distressed relatives and unfamiliar equipment and staff presents particular challenges in terms of organization, tact and diplomacy. Preparation can help minimize these challenges and ensure that less pressing tasks are not overlooked.

Stabilization and transportation

The cardiovascular parameters and persistent base deficit both suggested that despite substantial volume resuscitation the vascular compartment remained underfilled. Children with meningococcal septicaemia may require enormous volumes of resuscitation fluid – equivalent to two or three times their circulating blood volume – during the first 24 hours following presentation.[16] Blood and FFP were obtained to provide further volume support and to correct the low haemoglobin and coagulopathy. Both hypokalaemia and hypocalcaemia have long been recognized as common features of children presenting with septic shock, despite the acidosis and renal dysfunction that would normally promote hyperkalaemia.[17,18] Bicarbonate, although its use remains controversial, was administered in order to improve pH and hence myocardial contractility.

Although nasal intubation is often preferred in terms of stability in children undergoing transportation, in view of the marked coagulopathy this was deemed unsafe and not undertaken. A chest X-ray was obtained to confirm a satisfactory position of the endotracheal tube. It is also essential to ensure that the tube is adequately fixed. The physical movement of a critically ill child is the time at which acute deterioration due to physiological or equipment-related events is most likely to occur. Close attention must be paid to ensuring that the endotracheal tube, vascular access, monitoring leads and other equipment are not pulled or disconnected in the process of moving.

During the return journey the retrieval team perform regular observations of ventilatory and haemodynamic status. On longer journeys, blood gas analyses may be performed using a portable blood gas analyser. Interventions are only undertaken if absolutely necessary. To this end, a pack of intubation equipment, bolus sedation and resuscitation drugs and syringes of colloid are drawn up to be used if required. The aim is for the return journey to be uneventful, minimizing the amount of work that has to be performed in the difficult working environment of an ambulance. This also helps to minimize the anxiety of the parents, who often find the separation from their child during their transfer to intensive care extremely distressing.[19]

Outcome

The development of PICUs, together with centralized retrieval services, has greatly altered the pattern of provision of care for critically ill children in the UK.[20] To what extent this has translated into a measurable reduction in mortality remains contested, although many units across the UK have reported a fall in mortality rates to as low as 2% in recent years.[21–23] This impressively low mortality is due not only to the institution of improved intensive care provision but also to a concerted community campaign and the efforts of parents and carers, general practitioners and district general hospital staff.

For survivors, the outcome from meningococcal disease is generally good. Of all forms of bacterial meningitis, meningococcal meningitis has the fewest sequelae. A small proportion of children with meningococcal septicaemia may develop purpura fulminans, a condition characterized by widespread ecchymoses and vascular insufficiency of the extremities. Often treated with fasciotomies, a minority of these children go on to need amputation of digits or limbs.[24,25] In general, however, the rash heals without scarring and children go on to make a full physical recovery.

Learning points

- Treatment of children with meningococcal septicaemia requires the early involvement of PIC teams, with specialist expertise.
- Early, aggressive fluid therapy is associated with an improved outcome.
- As soon as intravenous access is gained a glucose stix should be measured and appropriate antibiotics administered.
- Early intubation should be considered in all children who still show signs of shock after initial fluid resuscitation.
- Care must be taken with the choice of agents used to perform rapid sequence induction to prevent a drop in cardiac output.
- Transfer to the regional PICU should be undertaken in all children who require both ventilatory and inotropic support.
- In the best centres the mortality is as low as 2%, with the majority of children making a full recovery.

References

1. Paediatric Intensive Care: Report from Alan Langlands, Chief Executive of the NHS Executive, to the Secretary of State for Health; NHS Executive, May 1996.
2. Standards for Paediatric Intensive Care; Paediatric Intensive Care Society, 1996.
3. Paediatric Intensive Care, A Framework for the Future: Report from the National Co-ordinating Group on Paediatric Intensive Care to the Chief Executive of the NHS Executive; NHS Executive, 1997.
4. Balmer P, Borrow R, Miller EJ. Impact of meningococcal C conjugate vaccine in the UK. *Med Microbiol* 2002; 51: 717–722.
5. Duncan A. New therapies for severe meningococcal disease but better outcomes? *Lancet* 1997; 350: 1564–1565.
6. Kirsch EA, Barton RP, Kitchen L, Giroir BP. Pathophysiology, treatment and outcome of meningococcemia: a review and recent experience. *Pediatr Infect Dis J* 1996; 15: 967–979.
7. Derkx HHF, van den Hoek J, Redekop WK et al. Meningococcal disease: a comparison of eight severity scores in 125 children. *Intensive Care Med* 1996; 22: 1433–1441.

8. Castellanos-Ortega A, Delgado-Rodriguez M, Llorca J et al. A new prognostic scoring system for meningococcal septic shock in children. Comparison with three other scoring systems. *Intensive Care Med* 2002; 28: 341–351.
9. Marzouk O, Thomson AP, Sills JA et al. Features and outcome in meningococcal disease presenting with maculopapular rash. *Arch Dis Child* 1991; 66: 485–487.
10. Available online at: http://www.meningitis.org/uploads/Paed%20Early%20manage%20poster%20for%20website%204th%20edition.pdf
11. Peters MJ, Ross-Russell RI, White D *et al.* Early severe neutropenia and thrombocytopenia identifies the highest risk cases of acute meningococcal disease. *Ped Crit Care Med* 2001; 2: 225–231.
12. Pollard AJ, Britto J, Nadel S et al. Emergency management of meningococcal disease. *Arch Dis Child* 1999; 80: 290–296.
13. Carcillo JA, Davis AL, Zaritsky L. Role of early fluid resuscitation in pediatric septic shock. *JAMA* 1991; 266: 1242–1245.
14. Hussain SN, Roussos C. Distribution of respiratory muscle and organ blood flow during endotoxic shock in dogs. *J Appl Physiol* 1985; 59: 1802–1808.
15. Koga K, Ogata M, Takenaka I et al. Ketamine suppresses tumor necrosis factor-alpha activity and mortality in carrageenan-sensitized endotoxin shock model. *Circ Shock* 1994; 44: 160–168.
16. Nadel S, De Munter C, Britto J et al. Albumin: saint or sinner? *Arch Dis Child* 1998; 79: 384–385.
17. Mauger DC. Hypokalaemia as a consistent feature of fulminant meningococcal septicaemia. *Aust Paediatr J* 1971; 7: 84–86.
18. Gauthier B, Trachtman H, Di Carmine F *et al.* Hypocalcemia and hypercalcitoninemia in critically ill children. *Crit Care Med* 1990; 18: 1215–1219.
19. Colville G, Orr F, Gracey D. 'The worst journey of our lives': parents' experiences of a specialised paediatric retrieval service. *Intensive Crit Care Nurs* 2003; 19: 103–108.
20. Pearson G, Barry P, Timmins C et al. Changes in the profile of paediatric intensive care associated with centralisation. *Intensive Care Med* 2001; 27: 1670–1673.
21. Thorburn K, Baines P, Thomson A et al. Mortality in severe meningococcal disease. *Arch Dis Child* 2001; 85: 382–385.
22. Booy R, Habibi P, Nadel S et al. Reduction in case fatality rate from meningococcal disease associated with improved healthcare delivery. *Arch Dis Child* 2001; 85: 386–390.
23. Tibby SM, Murdoch IA, Durward A. Mortality in meningococcal disease: please report the figures accurately. (Letter) *Arch Dis Child* 2002; 87: 559.
24. Davies MS, Nadel S, Habibi P et al. The orthopaedic management of peripheral ischaemia in meningococcal septicaemia in children. *J Bone Joint Surg Br* 2000; 82: 383–386.
25. Wheeler JS, Anderson BJ, De Chalain TM. Surgical interventions in children with meningococcal purpura fulminans – a review of 117 procedures in 21 children. *J Pediatr Surg* 2003; 38: 597–603.

Index

Page numbers in *italics* indicate figures or tables.

For Product Safety Concerns and Information please contact our EU representative GPSR@taylorandfrancis.com Taylor & Francis Verlag GmbH, Kaufingerstraße 24, 80331 München, Germany

Batch number: 10732714

Printed by Printforce, the Netherlands